Palliative Care

Editor

ERIC WIDERA

MEDICAL CLINICS
OF NORTH AMERICA

www.medical.theclinics.com

Consulting Editor
JACK ENDE

May 2020 • Volume 104 • Number 3

ELSEVIER

1600 John F. Kennedy Boulevard • Suite 1800 • Philadelphia, Pennsylvania, 19103-2899

http://www.theclinics.com

MEDICAL CLINICS OF NORTH AMERICA Volume 104, Number 3
May 2020 ISSN 0025-7125, ISBN-13: 978-0-323-73366-3

Editor: Katerina Heidhausen
Developmental Editor: Kristen Helm

Medical Clinics of North America (ISSN 0025-7125) is published bimonthly by Elsevier Inc., 360 Park Avenue South, New York, NY 10010-1710. Months of publication are January, March, May, July, September, and November. Business and editorial offices: 1600 John F. Kennedy Boulevard, Suite 1800, Philadelphia, PA 19103-2899. Periodicals postage paid at New York, NY, and additional mailing offices. Subscription prices are USD $295.00 per year (US individuals), $654.00 per year (US institutions), $100.00 per year (US Students), $353.00 per year (Canadian individuals), $850.00 per year (Canadian institutions), $200.00 per year for (foreign students), $100.00 per year for (Canadian students), $422.00 per year (foreign individuals), and $850.00 per year (foreign institutions). To receive student/resident rate, orders must be accompanied by name of affiliated institution, date of term, and the signature of program/residency coordinator on institution letterhead. Orders will be billed at individual rate until proof of status is received. Foreign air speed delivery is included in all Clinics' subscription prices. All prices are subject to change without notice. **POSTMASTER:** Send address changes to *Medical Clinics of North America*, Elsevier Health Sciences Division, Subscription Customer Service, 3251 Riverport Lane, Maryland Heights, MO 63043. **Customer Service: Telephone: 1-800-654-2452** (U.S. and Canada); **1-314-447-8871** (outside U.S. and Canada). **Fax: 314-447-8029. E-mail: journalscustomerserviceusa@ elsevier.com** (for print support); **journalsonlinesupport-usa@elsevier.com** (for online support).

Reprints. For copies of 100 or more of articles in this publication, please contact the Commercial Reprints Department, Elsevier Inc., 360 Park Avenue South, New York, NY 10010-1710. Tel.: 212-633-3874; Fax: 212-633-3820; E-mail: reprints@elsevier.com.

Medical Clinics of North America is also published in Spanish by McGraw-Hill Interamericana Editores S. A., P.O. Box 5-237, 06500 Mexico, D.F., Mexico.

Medical Clinics of North America is covered in *MEDLINE/PubMed (Index Medicus), Current Contents, ASCA, Excerpta Medica, Science Citation Index,* and *ISI/BIOMED.*

PROGRAM OBJECTIVE

The goal of the *Medical Clinics of North America* is to keep practicing physicians up to date with current clinical practice by providing timely articles reviewing the state of the art in patient care.

TARGET AUDIENCE

All practicing physicians and other healthcare professionals.

LEARNING OBJECTIVES

Upon completion of this activity, participants will be able to:
1. Review essential primary palliative care topics to enhance or improve competence when caring for patients living with serious illness.
2. Explain various approaches to managing pain and non-pain symptoms for patients living with serious illness.
3. Discuss application of accurate prognostication by combining clinical judgement and evidence- based methods and tools.

ACCREDITATION

The Elsevier Office of Continuing Medical Education (EOCME) is accredited by the Accreditation Council for Continuing Medical Education (ACCME) to provide continuing medical education for physicians.

The EOCME designates this journal-based CME activity for a maximum of 13 *AMA PRA Category 1 Credit*(s)™. Physicians should claim only the credit commensurate with the extent of their participation in the activity.

All other healthcare professionals requesting continuing education credit for this enduring material will be issued a certificate of participation.

DISCLOSURE OF CONFLICTS OF INTEREST

The EOCME assesses conflict of interest with its instructors, faculty, planners, and other individuals who are in a position to control the content of CME activities. All relevant conflicts of interest that are identified are thoroughly vetted by EOCME for fair balance, scientific objectivity, and patient care recommendations. EOCME is committed to providing its learners with CME activities that promote improvements or quality in healthcare and not a specific proprietary business or a commercial interest.

The planning committee, staff, authors and editors listed below have identified no financial relationships or relationships to products or devices they or their spouse/life partner have with commercial interest related to the content of this CME activity:
Meera Agar, MBBS, MPC, FRACP, FAChPM, PhD; Bimal H. Ashar, MD, MBA, FACP; Rachelle E. Bernacki, MD, MS; Shirley H. Bush, MBBS, DRCOG, DCH, MRCGP, PgDip Pall Med, FAChPM; Kimberly Angelia Curseen, MD; Emily Galenbeck, BA; Quintesia Grant, MD, PhD; David A. Gruenewald, MD; David J. Horn, MD; Nelia Jain, MD, MA; C. Bree Johnston, MD, MPH; Anne Kelly, LCSW; Marilu Kelly, MSN, RN, CNE, CHCP; Wing Fun Leo-To, PharmD, MA, MDE, BCPS; Cari Levy, MD, PhD; Kate Magid, MPH; Monica Malec, MD; Emily J. Martin, MD; Kanako Y. McKee, MD; Mary Lynn McPherson, PharmD, MA, MDE, BCPS; Sarah S. Mills, MD, MPH; Brigit C. Palathra, MD; Cynthia X. Pan, MD, FACP; Joseph W. Shega, MD; Christian T. Sinclair, MD; Benjamin M. Skoch, DO, MBA; Jeyanthi Surendrakumar; Jabeen Taj, MD; Shaida Talebreza, MD; Paul E. Tatum, MD, MSPH, CMD, AGSF, FAAHPM; Gregg Vandekieft, MD, MA; Eric Widera, MD

UNAPPROVED/OFF-LABEL USE DISCLOSURE

The EOCME requires CME faculty to disclose to the participants;
1. When products or procedures being discussed are off-label, unlabelled, experimental, and/or investigational (not US Food and Drug Administration [FDA] approved); and
2. Any limitations on the information presented, such as data that are preliminary or that represent ongoing research, interim analyses, and/or unsupported opinions. Faculty may discuss information about pharmaceutical agents that is outside of FDA-approved labelling. This information is intended solely for CME and is not intended to promote off-label use of these medications. If you have any questions, contact the medical affairs department of the manufacturer for the most recent prescribing information.

TO ENROLL

To enroll in the *Medical Clinics of North America* Continuing Medical Education program, call customer service at 1-800-654-2452 or sign up online at http://www.theclinics.com/home/cme. The CME program is available to subscribers for an additional annual fee of USD 300.00.

METHOD OF PARTICIPATION

In order to claim credit, participants must complete the following;
1. Complete enrolment as indicated above.
2. Read the activity.
3. Complete the CME Test and Evaluation. Participants must achieve a score of 70% on the test. All CME Tests and Evaluations must be completed online.

CME INQUIRIES/SPECIAL NEEDS

For all CME inquiries or special needs, please contact elsevierCME@elsevier.com.

MEDICAL CLINICS OF NORTH AMERICA

SERIES OF RELATED INTEREST

Clinics in Geriatric Medicine
https://www.geriatric.theclinics.com/
Primary Care: Clinics in Office Practice
https://www.primarycare.theclinics.com/

Contributors

CONSULTING EDITOR

JACK ENDE, MD, MACP
The Schaeffer Professor of Medicine, Perelman School of Medicine, University of Pennsylvania, Hospital of the University of Pennsylvania, Philadelphia, Pennsylvania, USA

EDITOR

ERIC WIDERA, MD
Professor of Medicine, Division of Geriatrics, Department of Medicine, Program Director, Geriatric Medicine Fellowship, University of California, San Francisco (UCSF), Director, Hospice and Palliative Care, San Francisco VA Health Care System, San Francisco, California, USA

AUTHORS

MEERA AGAR, MBBS, MPC, FRACP, FAChPM, PhD
Professor of Palliative Medicine, IMPACCT (Improving Palliative, Aged and Chronic Care Through Clinical Research and Translation) Faculty of Health, University of Technology Sydney, Ultimo, New South Wales, Australia

RACHELLE E. BERNACKI, MD, MS
Director of Quality Initiatives, Senior Physician, Adult Palliative Care, Department of Psychosocial Oncology and Palliative Care, Dana-Farber Cancer Institute, Serious Illness Care Program, Ariadne Labs, Assistant Professor, Harvard Medical School, Boston, Massachusetts, USA

SHIRLEY H. BUSH, MBBS, DRCOG, DCH, MRCGP, PgDip Pall Med, FAChPM
Associate Professor, Department of Medicine, Division of Palliative Care, University of Ottawa, Clinical Scientist, Bruyère Research Institute, Clinician Investigator, Ottawa Hospital Research Institute, Physician, Palliative Care, Bruyère Continuing Care, The Ottawa Hospital, Ottawa, Ontario, Canada

KIMBERLY ANGELIA CURSEEN, MD, FAAHPM
Director of Outpatient Supportive Care, Emory Palliative Care Center, Associate Professor, Division of Palliative Medicine, Department of Family and Preventive Medicine, Emory University School of Medicine, Atlanta, Georgia, USA

EMILY GALENBECK, BA
Professional Research Assistant, Research, Rocky Mountain Regional Veterans Affairs Medical Center, Denver-Seattle Center of Innovation, Aurora, Colorado, USA

QUINTESIA GRANT, MD, PhD
Attending, Palliative and Supportive Care, Grady Memorial Hospital, Associate Hospice Medical Director, Harbor Grace Hospice, Director of Palliative Medicine Education, Grady

Memorial Hospital, Assistant Professor, Division of Palliative Medicine, Department of Family and Preventive Medicine, Atlanta, Georgia, USA

DAVID A. GRUENEWALD, MD
Medical Director, Palliative Care and Hospice Service, Geriatrics and Extended Care Service, VA Puget Sound Healthcare System, Associate Professor of Medicine, Division of Gerontology and Geriatric Medicine, Department of Medicine, University of Washington School of Medicine, Seattle, Washington, USA

DAVID J. HORN, MD
Assistant Professor, Department of Emergency Medicine, Division of Geriatrics, General Internal Medicine and Palliative Medicine, University of Arizona, University of Arizona College of Medicine, Tucson, Arizona, USA

NELIA JAIN, MD, MA
Physician, Adult Palliative Care, Department of Psychosocial Oncology and Palliative Care, Dana-Farber Cancer Institute, Instructor in Medicine, Harvard Medical School, Boston, Massachusetts, USA

CATHERINE BREE JOHNSTON, MD, MPH
Division of Geriatrics, General Internal Medicine and Palliative Medicine, Professor, Department of Medicine, University of Arizona College of Medicine, University of Arizona, Tucson, Arizona, USA

ANNE KELLY, LCSW
San Francisco VA Health Care System, San Francisco, California, USA

WING FUN LEO-TO, PharmD, BCPS
Clinical Pharmacy Coordinator, NewYork-Presbyterian Queens, Flushing, New York, USA; Affiliate Clinical Faculty, College of Pharmacy and Health Science, St John's University, Jamaica, New York, USA

CARI LEVY, MD, PhD
Principal Investigator, Research, Rocky Mountain Regional Veterans Affairs Medical Center, Denver-Seattle Center of Innovation, Professor, Division of Health Care Policy and Research, School of Medicine, University of Colorado, Aurora, Colorado, USA

KATE MAGID, MPH
Health Science Specialist, Research, Rocky Mountain Regional Veterans Affairs Medical Center, Denver-Seattle Center of Innovation, Aurora, Colorado, USA

MONICA MALEC, MD
Associate Professor of Medicine, Section of Geriatrics and Palliative Medicine, Department of Medicine, University of Chicago, Chicago, Illinois, USA

EMILY J. MARTIN, MD
Assistant Clinical Professor, Division of General Internal Medicine and Health Services Research, Department of Medicine, University of California, Los Angeles, Los Angeles, California, USA

KANAKO Y. McKEE, MD
Associate Clinical Professor, Division of Geriatrics, Department of Medicine, University of California, San Francisco, San Francisco VA Health Care System, San Francisco, California, USA

MARY LYNN McPHERSON, PharmD, MA, MD, BCPS
Professor and Executive Director, Advanced Post-Graduate Education in Palliative Care, Executive Program Director, Online Master of Science in Palliative Care, Department of Pharmacy Practice and Science, University of Maryland School of Pharmacy, Baltimore, Maryland, USA

SARAH S. MILLS, MD, MPH
Dell Medical School, The University of Texas at Austin, Austin, Texas, USA

BRIGIT C. PALATHRA, MD
Assistant Professor of Clinical Medicine, Weill Cornell Medical College, New York, New York, USA; Associate Program Director, Hospice and Palliative Medicine Fellowship, Division of Palliative Medicine and Geriatrics, NewYork-Presbyterian Queens, Flushing, New York, USA

CYNTHIA X. PAN, MD, FACP, AGSF
Chief, Division of Palliative Medicine and Geriatrics, Designated Institution Official of Graduate Medical Education, NewYork-Presbyterian Queens, Flushing, New York, USA; Associate Professor of Clinical Medicine, Weill Cornell Medical College, New York, New York, USA

JOSEPH W. SHEGA, MD
Associate Professor of Medicine, Vitas Healthcare, Miami, Florida, USA; University of Central Florida, Orlando, Florida, USA

CHRISTIAN T. SINCLAIR, MD, FAAHPM
Associate Professor, Division of Palliative Medicine, University of Kansas Medical Center, Kansas City, Kansas, USA

BENJAMIN M. SKOCH, DO, MBA
Assistant Professor, Division of Palliative Medicine, University of Kansas Medical Center, Kansas City, Kansas, USA

JABEEN TAJ, MD
Site Director, Hospice and Palliative Medicine, Emory University Hospital, Medical Director, Cardiac Palliative Care, Emory Palliative Care Center, Assistant Professor, Medicine, Emory University School of Medicine, Atlanta, Georgia, USA

SHAIDA TALEBREZA, MD, AGSF, FAAHPM
Section Chief, Geriatric and Palliative Medicine, George E. Wahlen Salt Lake City Veterans Affairs Medical Center, Associate Professor, Division of Geriatrics, University of Utah School of Medicine, Salt Lake City, Utah, USA

PAUL E. TATUM, MD, MSPH, CMD, AGSF, FAAHPM
Dell Medical School, The University of Texas at Austin, Austin, Texas, USA

GREGG VANDEKIEFT, MD, MA
Palliative Care Program, Providence St. Joseph Health Southwest Washington Region, Olympia, Washington, USA; Associate Medical Director, Palliative Practice Group, Institute for Human Caring at Providence St. Joseph Health, Gardena, California, USA; Clinical Associate Professor of Family Medicine, Department of Family Medicine, University of Washington School of Medicine, Seattle, Washington, USA

ERIC WIDERA, MD
Professor of Medicine, Division of Geriatrics, Department of Medicine, Program Director, Geriatric Medicine Fellowship, University of California, San Francisco (UCSF), Director, Hospice and Palliative Care, San Francisco VA Health Care System, San Francisco, California, USA

Contents

Palliative medicine is specialized medical care for people with serious illness. Serious illness is one with high risk of mortality that negatively affects quality of life or function or is burdensome in symptoms, treatments, or caregiver stress. Palliative care improves symptom management and addresses the needs of patients and families, resulting in improved patient and caregiver quality of life and reduced symptom burden and health care utilization. Hospice is palliative care for patients with a prognosis of 6 months or less and is appropriate when goals are to avoid hospitalization and maximize time at home for patients who are dying.

Clinicians working with seriously ill patients need the skills to effectively communicate with patients and their families throughout the trajectory of illness. Common communication tasks that arise in the care of seriously ill patients include advance care planning, delivering serious news, discussing prognosis, eliciting values, and medical decision making. Clinicians often use goals of care conversations to facilitate these tasks. Similar to other procedures, goals of care conversations require a systematic, evidence-based approach to ensure quality and value. This article provides a framework that clinicians can follow to effectively communicate with seriously ill patients and families and promote patient-centered care.

Prognostication is a vital aspect of decision making because it provides patients and families with information to establish realistic and achievable goals of care, is used in determining eligibility for certain benefits, and helps in targeting interventions to those likely to benefit. Prognostication consists of 3 components: clinicians use their clinical judgment or other tools to estimate the probability of an individual developing a particular outcome over a specific period of time; this prognostic estimate is communicated in accordance with the patient's information preferences; the prognostic estimate is interpreted by the patient or surrogate and used in clinical decision making.

Older adults, particularly those late in life, are at higher risk for medication misadventure, yet bear the burden of increasing polypharmacy. It is incumbent on practitioners who care for this vulnerable population to use one or more approaches to deprescribe medications that impose a greater burden than benefit, including medically futile medications. It is essential that health care providers use compassionate communication skills when explaining these interventions with patients and families, pointing out that this is a positive, patient-centric intervention.

Managing pain in patients with serious illness can be complex. However, pain is often a prominent symptom in patients with malignant and nonmalignant serious illness and providers have to be adept at balancing effective pain management and safety. Clinicians should start with a standard pain assessment that lays important groundwork for developing a tailored multimodal approach to pain management. It is important to identify physical causes of pain and also existential causes. Opioids are not always appropriate but are still an important tool for managing pain. Basic opioid management and safe practices are essential when managing this population.

Anorexia and cachexia, nausea and vomiting, and constipation are gastrointestinal symptoms that commonly accompany serious illness. Basic science and clinical research continue to improve the understanding of their pathophysiology. Thorough assessment necessitates history, physical examination, and laboratory and diagnostic testing. Pharmacologic management attempts to counteract or reverse the underlying pathophysiologic mechanisms that accompany each symptom, which may benefit from a multimodal approach to achieve adequate control. Future improvements in management require investments in clinical research to determine the efficacy of novel agents along with comparator studies to better understand which treatments should be used in what sequence or combination.

Respiratory symptoms are common in patients living with serious illness, both in cancer and nonmalignant conditions. Common symptoms include dyspnea (breathlessness), cough, malignant pleural effusions, airway secretions, and hemoptysis. Basic management of respiratory symptoms is within the scope of primary palliative care. There are pharmacologic and nonpharmacologic approaches to treating respiratory symptoms. This article provides clinicians with treatment approaches to these burdensome symptoms.

> The purpose of this article is to present evidence on the efficacy and safety of medical cannabis as a therapy for symptom management in palliative care. This article provides an overview of the evidence on the risks and benefits of using medical cannabis for the indications of chronic pain, cancer-related pain, cancer cachexia, dementia, and Alzheimer's disease. Currently, there is insufficient evidence to determine the effectiveness and safety of cannabinoids for most reviewed indications, with the exception of chronic pain. Future research is required before palliative care clinicians can make evidence-based decisions on the integration of medical cannabis as adjunct therapies.

> Delirium is a prevalent acute neurocognitive condition in patients with progressive life-limiting illness. Delirium remains underdetected; a systematic approach to screening is essential. Delirium at the end of life requires a comprehensive assessment. Consider the potential for reversibility, illness trajectory, patient preference, and goals of care before proceeding with investigations and interventions. Management should be interdisciplinary, and nonpharmacologic therapy is fundamental. For patients with refractory and severe agitation or perceptual disturbance, judicious use of medication may also be required. Carers and family should be seen as partners in care and be involved in shared decision making about care.

> The varied physical, social, and psychological stressors that accompany advanced disease can be burdensome and cause intense emotional suffering, hindering the ability of patients and families to cope in day-to-day life and negatively affecting quality of life. This article addresses key concepts for the assessment and management of commonly encountered types of psychological distress in serious illness including grief, prolonged grief, major depressive disorder, death contemplation, and suicidal ideation.

> Medical emergencies at the end of life require recognition of patients at risk, so that a comprehensive assessment and plan of care can be put in place. Frequently, the interventions depend on the patient's underlying prognosis, location of care, and goals of care. The mere presence of a medical emergency often rapidly changes an estimated prognosis. Education of the patient and family may help empower them to adequately handle many situations when clinicians are not available.

Some patients with terminal and degenerative illnesses request assistance to hasten death when suffering is refractory to palliative care, or they strongly desire to maximize their autonomy and dignity and minimize suffering. Palliative sedation (PS), voluntarily stopping eating and drinking (VSED), and physician-assisted death (PAD) are possible options of last resort. A decision to choose PS can be made by an informed surrogate decision maker, whereas intact decision-making capacity is required to choose VSED or PAD. For all palliative treatments of last resort, the risk of harm is minimized by the use of checklists, and establishment of policies and procedures.

Burnout is common in physicians who care for patients with serious illness, with rates greater than 60% in some studies. Risk factors for burnout include working on small teams and/or in small organizations, working longer hours and weekends, being younger than 50 years, burdensome documentation requirements, and regulatory issues. Personal factors that can protect against burnout include mindfulness, exercise, healthy sleep patterns, avoiding substance abuse, and having adequate leisure time. Institutional and work factors that can buffer against burnout include working on adequately staffed teams, having a manageable workload, and minimally burdensome electronic health record documentation.

Foreword

Completing the Circle of Care

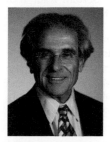

Jack Ende, MD, MACP
Consulting Editor

Palliative care completes the circle of medical care. It makes medical care whole. Palliative care exists because the manifestations of illness are not delimited by diagnosis, nor are symptoms necessarily eradicated by disease-specific treatment. When patients are left on their own to deal with difficult and long-lasting, even life-altering, symptoms like pain, dyspnea, anorexia, and debilitating grief, care becomes fractional. Likewise, care becomes fragmented when patients turn to their principal providers, be they primary care providers or specialists, for help with these life-altering symptoms, and those principal providers are not as skilled in symptom management as they may be in diagnosis and treatment.

The field of palliative care exists to provide patients with more comprehensive care, addressing symptom management and complementing diagnosis and disease treatment. Whether that care is provided by a palliative care specialist and team, brought in for the purpose of managing debilitating symptoms, or provided by the patient's principal provider, is likely to be determined by local resources, and patient and provider preferences. Who delivers the high-level palliative care is not a key issue. What is critical, however, is that the patient receives the best possible palliative care. Our commitment as health care professionals demands nothing less.

This issue of *Medical Clinics of North America* titled, *Palliative Care*, is as important as it is timely. Much of palliative care is, and likely will be, delivered by patients' principal providers. They, myself included, need to know about the latest advances in palliative care and be armed with the most up-to-date, evidence-based information the discipline has to offer.

That is how the field of palliative care completes the circle of medical care. It allows medical care to be more holistic and humanistic: holistic, not in the sense of melding traditional with complementary approaches, although it may do that to some extent, but to bring to patients for the entirety of their journeys, the same level of expertise that characterizes diagnosis and treatment. Palliative care also enables providers to

Med Clin N Am 104 (2020) xv–xvi
https://doi.org/10.1016/j.mcna.2020.02.002
0025-7125/20/© 2020 Published by Elsevier Inc.

practice medicine more humanistically. Palliative care embodies our concerns for the patient as a person. Francis Peabody's essay,[1] "The Care of the Patient," cannot be read often enough. It ends as follows: "One of the essential qualities of the clinician is interest in humanity, for the secret of the care of the patient is in caring for the patient."

Editor Eric Widera and his team of authors have produced an important volume of great value to physicians, and therefore, to their patients as well. I hope you find it enriching and educational.

Jack Ende, MD, MACP
The Schaeffer Professor of Medicine
Perelman School of Medicine of the University of Pennsylvania
Hospital of the University of Pennsylvania
5033 West Gates Pavilion 3400 Spruce Street
Philadelphia, PA 19104, USA

E-mail address:
jack.ende@uphs.upenn.edu

REFERENCE

1. Peabody FW. The care of the patient. JAMA 1927;88:877–82.

Preface
Primary Palliative Care

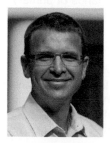

Eric Widera, MD
Editor

Palliative care focuses on improving quality of life for patients with serious illness and their families. This type of care includes providing relief from pain and/or other distressing symptoms, integrating psychosocial and spiritual aspects of care, assisting with difficult decision making, and supporting patients, families, and other medical teams. Palliative care can be provided concurrently with life-prolonging or curative therapies as needed from time of diagnosis, and it is appropriate at any age or stage of serious illness.

Specialty palliative care consists of care by an interprofessional team of doctors, nurses, social workers, chaplains, and other individuals with expertise in palliative medicine, who work with patients' other doctors to provide care that matches patients' goals. The vast majority of palliative care delivered in the United States is delivered not by these specialists in hospice and palliative care but by clinicians ranging from internists, family medicine doctors, oncologists, and others who care for seriously ill patients. This type of palliative care provided by clinicians who are not palliative care specialists is called "primary" palliative care, and it is the focus of this issue of *Medical Clinics of North America*.

All clinicians who care for seriously ill patients should be able to deliver competent primary palliative care. This issue is directed at primary palliative care clinicians who are aiming to improve their own abilities to care for those living with serious illness. This issue contains many of the most important primary palliative care topics, beginning with a comprehensive overview of the field of hospice and palliative care. The issue continues with articles that bring expert perspective on having goals-of-care discussions with patients and family members, prognostication, and recognizing and managing polypharmacy in advanced illness.

In addition, this issue covers an approach to managing pain and nonpain symptoms in those with serious illness, including respiratory and gastrointestinal symptoms, delirium, and the role that cannabis plays in symptom management. Further articles

Med Clin N Am 104 (2020) xvii–xviii
https://doi.org/10.1016/j.mcna.2020.02.001
0025-7125/20/© 2020 Published by Elsevier Inc.

medical.theclinics.com

go over how best to manage grief and depression in those with serious illness, urgent medical conditions at the end of life, an overview of options of last resort (palliative sedation, physician aid in dying, and voluntary cessation of eating and drinking), and how to care for oneself while delivering primary palliative care.

I am grateful to the authors for their outstanding contributions to this issue and to the publisher for allowing us this opportunity to highlight the importance of primary palliative care and to enhance the skills of all clinicians providing care for those with serious illness.

Eric Widera, MD
Division of Geriatrics
Department of Medicine
University of California–San Francisco
4150 Clement St, Box 181G
San Francisco, CA 94121, USA

E-mail address:
Eric.widera@ucsf.edu

Hospice and Palliative Care

An Overview

Paul E. Tatum, MD, MSPH, CMD*, Sarah S. Mills, MD, MPH

KEYWORDS

- Hospice • Palliative care • Serious illness • Interdisciplinary team • End of life

KEY POINTS

- Palliative medicine is for anyone with serious illness, not just those who are dying. In other words, palliative care is for anyone with a condition that carries a high risk of mortality, has a negative impact on quality of life and daily function, and/or is burdensome in symptoms, treatments, or caregiver stress.
- Although palliative care can be delivered by specialists for more complicated cases, palliative care is really the work of all physicians caring for patients with serious illness.
- Hospice is a subtype of palliative medicine that specifically focuses on end-of-life care for patients with a prognosis of 6 months or less.
- There is a substantial evidence base that palliative care improves patient outcomes, including better symptom management and clearer communication, resulting in improved patient satisfaction. Palliative care and hospice also improve caregivers' experiences.

INTRODUCTION

Of the advances in medicine in the past half century, the development of hospice and the integration of palliative medicine into health systems have been among the most impactful. Although advances in cardiology, transplantation medicine, and cancer care capture the public imagination, hospice and palliative medicine's development has been just as transformational. Hospice was once a countercultural program primarily for patients dying with cancer to get care away from the traditional medical system. In short time, from the creation of the hospice benefit in 1982 to the current day, hospice has become the standard for delivering quality end-of-life care. As of 2017, 48.2% of Medicare decedents received hospice care.[1] Over the past 30 years, end-of-life care has changed from being primarily based in the hospital to approximately a quarter of deaths occurring at home.[2] Likewise, hospital-based palliative care has become a norm. By 2015, more than 85% of hospitals had palliative care programs in place.[3] In short, incorporating palliative medicine into routine care of patients with serious illness and involvement of hospice before death are now considered best

Dell Medical School, University of Texas in Austin, 1501 Red River Street, Austin, TX 78701, USA
* Corresponding author.
E-mail address: Paul.Tatum@austin.utexas.edu

Med Clin N Am 104 (2020) 359–373
https://doi.org/10.1016/j.mcna.2020.01.001
0025-7125/20/© 2020 Elsevier Inc. All rights reserved.

practice. It is the job of all providers who care for patients with serious illness to provide basic palliative care and refer to specialty palliative care when appropriate.

This issue of the *Medical Clinics of North America* reviews the core palliative skills, including communication, prognostication, and symptom management. This article presents a historical look at the development of hospice and palliative care and provides an overview of the key issues in hospice and palliative care.

HOW DID MODERN HOSPICE AND PALLIATIVE CARE DEVELOP?

The founder of the modern hospice movement was Dame Cicely Saunders. Saunders founded St Christopher's Hospice in London in 1967. Observing the unrelieved suffering of patients while working as a social worker led Saunders to first attend nursing school and then medical school. She developed the concept of total pain, officially defined in 1964 as "including not only physical symptoms but also mental distress and social or spiritual problems."[4] In addition to developing clinical programs, Dr Saunders emphasized research into quality end-of-life care. Her observations established that regularly scheduled opioid doses could provide pain relief, while allowing patients to remain alert and responsive.[5]

In the United States, Florence Wald of the Yale School of Nursing went on sabbatical to work at St Christopher's Hospice and learn their model. She then established the United States' first hospice in Bradford, Connecticut.[6] Dr Josefina Magno also studied at St Christopher's Hospice and established a pilot hospice program, which led to the modern payment model used today, resulting in formalization of hospice as a Medicare benefit that occurred in 1982.[7]

Palliative care owes its name to Dr Balfour Mount, a surgical oncologist at the Royal Victoria Hospital of McGill University in Montreal, Canada. Due to the negative connotations of the word hospice in French-speaking Quebec, he coined the term, *palliative care*.[8] The first hospital-based palliative care programs in the United States were the Wayne State University School of Medicine program dating to 1985 and the Cleveland Clinic program developed by Dr Declan Walsh in 1987.[9,10]

WHAT IS PALLIATIVE CARE?

The question, What is palliative care?, is surprisingly difficult to answer succinctly and many formal definitions of palliative care exist. Likely, the complex definition is one reason talking to patients about palliative care is challenging. Although the definition of cardiology according to the American Heart Association is "the branch of medicine that studies diseases of the heart" or, at the most complex, cardiology's definition might expand to include the words "and blood vessels," cardiology's definition is 10 words total and is clearer to most people than pages written about palliative medicine.[11]

The National Consensus Project for Quality Palliative Care defines palliative care: "Beneficial at any stage of a serious illness, palliative care is an interdisciplinary care delivery system designed to anticipate, prevent, and manage physical, psychological, social, and spiritual suffering to optimize quality of life for patients, their families and caregivers. Palliative care can be delivered in any care setting through the collaboration of many types of care providers. Through early integration into the care plan of seriously ill people, palliative care improves quality of life for both the patient and the family."[12]

The 2015 Institute of Medicine report *Dying in America* defines palliative care as "care that provides relief from pain and other symptoms, supports quality of life, and is focused on patients with serious advanced illness and their families. Palliative care may begin early in the course of treatment for a serious illness and may be delivered in a number of ways across the continuum of health care settings, including in the home, nursing homes, long-term acute care facilities, acute care hospitals, and outpatient clinics"[13] (**Box 1**).

Both the Center to Advance Palliative Care and the American Cancer Society define palliative care as "specialized medical care for people with serious illness. It focuses on providing relief from the symptoms and stress of a serious illness. The goal is to improve the quality of life for both the patient and the family."[14,15]

Many common threads emerge that shape an understanding of the question, What is palliative care? Some important themes to note are that palliative care is for patients with serious disease and that palliative treatment can start at any time of the disease trajectory. In addition, the focus of care is on both patients and families or caregivers as opposed to just on the patient. A common barrier to palliative care is the providers' false impression that a patient "is not ready for palliative care." Palliative care happens at the same time, however, as curative or life-prolonging therapy. There is no dichotomy of needing to choose 1 path or the other, unlike in hospice, where the regulations require a prognosis of 6 months or less (**Fig. 1**).

WHICH PATIENT SHOULD RECEIVE PALLIATIVE CARE?

Anyone with a serious illness is appropriate for palliative care. Serious illness has been defined as "a condition that carries a high risk of mortality, negatively impacts quality of life and daily function, and/or is burdensome in symptoms, treatments, or caregiver stress."[16,17]

Palliative care often is offered late in the course of disease, after curative treatments have been exhausted. Delay in palliative care referral may lead to suboptimal symptom management, increased suffering, less advance care planning, more hospitalizations, and unplanned hospital deaths.[18,19]

Box 1
National Academy of Medicine core components of quality palliative care

Frequent assessment of the patient's physical, emotional, social, and spiritual well-being

Management of emotional distress

Offer referral to expert-level palliative care

Offer referral to hospice if the patient has a prognosis of 6 months or less

Management of care and direct contact with patient and family for complex situations by a specialist-level palliative care physician

Round-the-clock access to coordinated care and services

Management of pain and other symptoms

Counseling of patient and family

Family caregiver support

Attention to the patient's social context and social needs

Attention to the patient's spiritual and religious needs

Regular personalized revision of the care

Adapted from Institute of Medicine. 2015. Dying in America: Improving Quality and Honoring Individual Preferences Near the End of Life. Washington, DC: The National Academies Press; with permission.

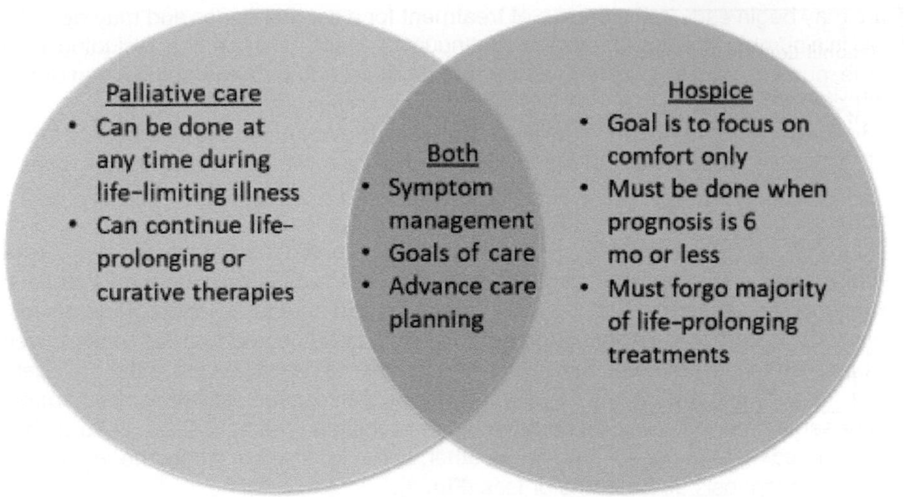

Palliative care
- Can be done at any time during life-limiting illness
- Can continue life-prolonging or curative therapies

Both
- Symptom management
- Goals of care
- Advance care planning

Hospice
- Goal is to focus on comfort only
- Must be done when prognosis is 6 mo or less
- Must forgo majority of life-prolonging treatments

Fig. 1. Similarities and differences of hospice and palliative care.

Many specialty societies support the early use of palliative care. The American Society of Clinical Oncology recommends early integration of palliative care alongside oncology care and states that any patient with a high symptom burden or any patient with advanced disease is appropriate.[20] The American College of Chest Physicians strongly supports the position that palliative care for patients with "an acute devastating or chronically progressive pulmonary or cardiac disease and his/her family should be an integral part of cardiopulmonary medicine."[21] The American Heart Association and the American Stroke Association state, "palliative care should be integrated into the care of all patients with advanced cardiovascular disease and stroke early in the disease trajectory."[22]

Still, despite these and other strong position statements promoting early referral to palliative care, wide adoption of this practice is slow.[13] To attempt to help providers identify appropriate patients, several tools have been created that can help target patients and families in need.

WHAT DOES PALLIATIVE CARE DO?

Palliative care works through the interdisciplinary process to meet the needs of patients, although the structure of the team may vary and palliative care delivery models differ greatly by geographic location and principal care focus (inpatient vs outpatient, cancer focus vs multimorbidity, and so forth). The National Consensus Project for Quality Palliative Care has defined 8 domains of palliative care delivery that represent the ideal interdisciplinary team structure and are listed in **Table 1**.[23] Physical, psychological, social, and spiritual components of patient care are addressed within the patient's unique cultural context to meet the whole needs of the patient.

Comprehensive assessments by palliative care teams have been shown to identify unmet needs. For heart failure patients for example, the median number of symptoms identified by comprehensive assessment is 9.[24] Even assessing symptoms that clinicians are ill equipped to improve, such as body dysmorphia or financial distress, is important because it provides a greater understanding of a patient's situation. Comprehensive symptom assessment builds provider trust, provides insight into

Table 1
National Consensus Project for Quality Palliative Care 8 domains of palliative care delivery

Structure and processes of care	IDT that includes physicians, nurses, chaplains, social workers, and pharmacists. Defined elements of assessment and care planning
Physical	Assessment and treatment of symptoms, and care planning, emphasizing patient-directed and family-directed holistic care
Psychological and psychiatric	Psychological and psychiatric care needs in context of serious illness
Social	Assessing and addressing patient and family social support needs
Spiritual	Spiritual, religious, and existential needs, including the importance of screening for unmet needs
Cultural	Cultural context that influences both the way in which care is delivered and the experience of care by patient and family from time of diagnosis, through death and bereavement
End of life	Symptoms and situations that focus on the final days and weeks of life
Ethical and legal	Advance care planning, surrogate decision making, and regulatory and legal considerations, focusing on ethical imperatives and processes to support patient autonomy

Adapted from National Consensus Project for Quality Palliative Care. Clinical Practice Guidelines for Quality Palliative Care, 4th edition. Richmond, VA: National Coalition for Hospice and Palliative Care; 2018; with permission.

patient struggles, and helps clinicians monitor those patients at greater risk for clinical depression or anxiety.[23,25]

In addition, palliative care informs patients and families about their illness trajectories and prognosis after a careful assessment of patient preferences regarding medical disclosure. Patients diagnosed with serious illness may ask, "How long have I got?" What they often are asking along with that question is, "What is going to happen?" Palliative care teams talk about serious illness, the likely trajectory of the disease, and the various needs the patients may have along the way.[26] For example, many patients need to move from independent living to an assisted-living or other care facility along the course of their illness. By anticipating future challenges, frantic, last minute, and potentially traumatic moves can be avoided.

In order to negotiate these complex conversations with families, it is important to assess how the patients and the families prefer to make decisions. Decision-making preferences are a spectrum: one end is paternalistic model, where physicians decide for the patient; the other end is an informed decision-making model, where patients and families gather the information from the clinicians and decide independently; and the middle is a shared decision-making model, as demonstrated in **Fig. 2**.[27]

Paternalistic Decision Making	Shared Decision Making	Informed Decision Making

Fig. 2. Spectrum of decision-making preference. (*Data from* White DB, Malvar G, Karr J, et al. Expanding the paradigm of the physician's role in surrogate decision-making: an empirically derived framework. Crit Care Med 2010;38(3):743–750.)

The expert communicator assesses how families prefer to make decisions and then adjust the delivery of information accordingly. Shy of expert level, all physicians should be aware that this spectrum does exist and seek to broaden communication strategies.

WHO PROVIDES PALLIATIVE CARE?

Primary palliative care is being delivered every day by physicians of all specialties caring for patients with serious illness. When physicians are addressing basic symptom management, evaluating social and emotional impacts and contexts for disease, discussing patient prognosis, or introducing hospice, physicians are practicing primary palliative care.[28] In addition to primary palliative care, which is also known as generalist palliative care, specialist palliative care can be conceptualized as secondary or tertiary palliative care. The primary, secondary, and tertiary palliative care models are represented in **Fig. 3**. Secondary palliative care models include a board-certified specialist leading an interdisciplinary palliative care team, whereas tertiary models are practiced at academic medical centers, where the most complex cases are practiced, researched, and taught.[29]

All physicians who care for patients who have serious illness should develop primary palliative care skills, including basic pain and symptom management as well as conversations skills around prognosis, end of life, and the introduction of hospice as a treatment option for patients and families. These are important skills necessary to meet the needs of patients with serious illness. Just as primary care physicians, for example, are not cardiologists, they still need to manage their patient's atrial fibrillation and coronary artery disease to a point, and refer when appropriate. Similarly, all physicians need these basic conversation skills and, again, may refer when appropriate to specialty palliative care for more complex cases.

HOW WELL DOES PALLIATIVE CARE WORK?

Palliative care has been well studied, and studies consistently show that palliative care improves patients' quality of life, leads to greater advance care planning, and

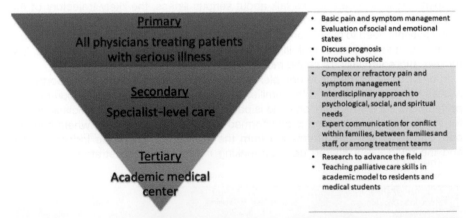

Fig. 3. Primary, secondary, and tertiary palliative care. (*Data from* Quill TE, Abernethy AP. Generalist plus specialist palliative care—creating a more sustainable model. N Engl J Med 2013;368(13):1173-1175; and von Gunten CF. Secondary and Tertiary Palliative Care in US Hospitals. JAMA 2002;287(7):875-881.)

improves caregiver satisfaction, while resulting in lower health care utilization and therefore expenses.[30,31] Palliative care leads to significant improvement in pain and symptom burden ratings after palliative care involvement in part due to a dedicated focus on comprehensively identifying all of patients' symptoms.[30,32] Patients also report improved communication between physicians and patients with palliative consultation as well as improved emotional support and higher patient satisfaction.[33] Also, patients are more likely to use hospice earlier rather than in the last few days before death and less likely to receive intensive care at the end of life, which may be burdensome.[34] In addition, patients have shorter length of stays with a reduction potentially in both in intensive care unit days and total days in hospital.[35,36] Palliative care can have greater impact if consulted in the emergency department (ED) prior to hospital admission.[37] There is even some evidence that suggests that palliative care can be associated with improved survival in cancer patients, especially if the palliative consultation occurs within the first 3 months of diagnosis.[38,39] In addition to palliative care models for cancer, palliative care has been demonstrated to improve care in chronic illness, such as congestive heart failure and chronic lung disease.[34,40] Patients have a better experience. They have better health. Mortality is not worsened and is possibly improved, and utilization of futile care goes down. The cost savings is estimated at thousands of dollars per patient with the greatest savings seen in cancer patients and those with high illness burden.[41]

WHAT IS HOSPICE?

Hospice is a system of care delivery for patients at the end of life. Hospice eligibility is based on a set of rules developed as part of the Medicare hospice benefit first established by act of Congress in 1982. By Congressional statute, hospice is specifically limited to patients with a prognosis of 6 months or less. Hospice care is covered under Medicare, Medicaid, and most private insurance plans and managed care organizations. Hospice in 2017 cared for approximately 1.5 million Medicare beneficiaries.[27] Although the average (mean) length of stay from admission to death was 89 days, the median length of stay was only 18 days because approximately a third of beneficiaries were on hospice for less than a week.[42]

Hospice is a philosophy of care and a system of care delivery, not a place. Not infrequently, however, hospitalized patients decline hospice services under the mistaken belief that hospice is a place and hospice discharge in their minds would not allow them to go home.

WHERE DOES HOSPICE PROVIDE CARE?

Hospice has 4 levels of care: routine hospice care, general inpatient care (GIP), continuous home care, and inpatient respite care. Routine hospice care is the most common type of care level, and it occurs at whatever place the patient resides routinely, which can be home, assisted living, long-term care, or adult board and care home. GIP is for acute symptom management that cannot be managed in another setting. GIP care may be provided in a Medicare-certified hospital, a dedicated hospice inpatient facility, or a nursing facility with around-the-clock registered nurse availability. Continuous care is for crisis management, such as a severe pain exacerbation, terminal agitation, or status epilepticus, where skilled care is provided but within the home setting rather than relocating. The continuous care services must be predominantly nursing care for at least 8 hours but may be supplemented with caregiver and hospice aide services to maintain the patient at home during the crisis. Respite care is intended to provide temporary relief to the patient's caregiver. Although respite care can be provided in hospital or hospice facility, it usually is provided in a long-term care facility for a few days to enable the caregiver to rest and be able to return the patient to home.

WHO SHOULD BE REFERRED TO HOSPICE?

Ideally, referrals to hospice would be based on patient need for increased care support over the course of care of a terminal illness. The formal criteria from Medicare, however, are based on prognosis and require a prognosis of 6 months or less. Unfortunately, physicians are notoriously inaccurate when it comes to prognostication, and patients often are reluctant to ask about prognosis.[43] Further complicating matters, hospice patients often have multiple, chronic illnesses, making prognostication far more complex than when the hospice benefit originally was designed when most patients had cancer. Perhaps the complexities of prognosis explain why 28% of hospice patients die within 7 days or less and the median length of stay for hospice is a mere 24 days despite the potential benefit duration of 6 months.[1]

Strategies to guide hospice referrals are listed in **Box 2**. A first step is to recognize that a patient may have a terminal illness. The surprise question helps clinicians think about prognosis is a way that accommodates clinical uncertainty and performs reasonably well. Rather than asking, Will this patient die in 6 months? the surprise question merely asks, Would you be surprised if the patient were to die? Although the surprise question was not designed as a formal prognostic tool but rather as a screening tool for hospice or palliative care eligibility, 16 studies have looked at the surprise question utilizing prognostication metrics. Although it performs only

---

Box 2
When to refer to hospice for a hospice eligibility evaluation

Screening questions

For the clinician
  Would you be surprised if the patient dies in the next 6 mo/y?
    If answer is no, prognosis may support hospice use. Follow-up with patient about hospice options and care preferences. HMD confirms prognostic estimates.

For the terminally ill patient
  Have you thought about where you want to be at the time of your death? Is location important?
    If preferred site of death is home, recommend hospice as hospice allows patients to remain in their preferred site of death (home, assisted living, etc.)

Clinical clues

Functional decline and can no longer do activities of daily living

Repeat hospitalizations, and patient does not want to be hospitalized

Ongoing weight loss with no reversible cause (>10% in 6 months)

Cancer progression and no longer chemotherapy eligible due to functional status

Multiple chronic illnesses with general deterioration

Required elements

Two physicians (referring physician and HMD) conclude that prognosis is <6 months

+

Patient elects for comfort-focused care and forgoes life-prolonging treatments modestly, the surprise question can help predict mortality, but it performs better for cancer opposed to noncancer diagnoses as.[44] Combining the surprise question with other clinical predictors may improve prognostic accuracy.[45] Formal prognostic calculators, such as those found at eprognosis.ucsf.edu, also may help with recognition of patients eligible for hospice.

In addition to prognosis, patient or family preferences and care needs may be a key guiding factor that it is time for hospice referral. Identifying the need for increased care support at home or declining performance status may trigger hospice referral, assuming the prognostic criteria can be met. Patient inability to care for activities of daily living is associated with higher mortality.[46]

Clinical encounters after repeat hospitalizations are another ideal time to revisit patient goals and preferences. When a patient with chronic progressive disease with multiple hospitalizations describes suffering related to hospital stays and wishes to avoid rehospitalization, hospice reduces rehospitalization episodes.[47] Although having a conversation about a patient's preferred site of death is a challenge to both patients and clinicians, it is important because patients whose preferred place of death is unknown are more likely to be admitted to the hospital for end-of-life care.[48] Simply asking the question, Have you thought about where you want to be at the time of your death? can be a powerful way to make a hospice referral more effective. If a patient's preferred site of death is home, recommending hospice can be a key way to match patient goals because hospice allows patients to remain in their preferred site of care at the time of death.

HOW IS A PATIENT DETERMINED TO BE ELIGIBLE FOR HOSPICE?

For patients to be eligible for hospice, 3 components are required to be met:

1. Two physicians certify the patient is terminally ill.
2. The patient accepts palliative care for comfort instead of care with intent to cure the underlying terminal illness.
3. The patient or surrogate formally signs a statement of hospice benefit election.

Terminal illness is defined as having a life expectancy of 6 months or less. Given the great prognostic uncertainty associated with some conditions, however, the terminal illness time frame of 6 months is specifically described by federal statute as "if the disease runs its normal course."[49] Terminal illness may be certified by a primary care physician or the main outpatient treating specialist, such as an oncologist or cardiologist, but also may be made by a hospitalist or post–acute care physician in the setting of an acute event. In addition to the referring physician's certification, the hospice medical director (HMD) serves as the second physician to confirm a prognosis of 6 months or less.

The Centers for Medicare and Medicaid Services (CMS) has published guidelines for the determining terminal status that rely heavily on decline in clinical status.[50] Clinicians referring patients to hospice can help the admission team by painting a clear picture of decline and noting the irreversibility of the decline where appropriate. CMS recommends documenting progression of disease in 4 key areas, including clinical status, symptoms, signs, and laboratory results. Clinical status supporting eligibility may include recurrent infections (pneumonia/pyelonephritis/sepsis) or progressive inanition, defined as weight loss of at least 10% body weight in the past 6 months or decreasing midarm circumference, observations of signs of weight loss, decreasing serum albumin or cholesterol, or dysphagia with recurrent aspiration or inadequate oral intake.

CMS also cites other key areas consistent with hospice eligibility, including decline in functional status due to progression of disease, progressive decline in cognition in the setting of dementia, and progression to assistance with activities of daily living. In addition, progressive stages 3 to 4 pressure ulcers despite optimal care may be cited as evidence of poor prognosis. Finally, an increase in ED visits, hospitalizations, and physician visits also may justify decline and a terminal prognosis.

CMS also has published disease-specific prognosis determination guidelines. For the referring physician, making the general referral is adequate and it is the hospice admission team's job to help apply the disease-specific guidelines. Because prognosis often is difficult to determine, there sometimes are complexities in the patient story that are not apparent to chart abstraction alone. If a patient is determined to be ineligible by the hospice admission team, consider asking for a direct discussion with the HMD. Direct conversation between the HMD and referring physician can help refine the prognostic evaluation guided by patient characteristics and CMS' non–disease-specific and disease-focused guidelines.

WHAT SHOULD A PATIENT EXPECT FROM HOSPICE?

Hospice care is provided by the interdisciplinary group (IDG), previously referred to as the interdisciplinary team [IDT], which coordinates care and attends to both the patient and the patient's caregivers. **Fig. 4** graphically presents the members of the IDG. Each IDG is led by an HMD or a hospice associate physician (previously referred to as associate medical director), who directs the IDG in anticipating patient symptoms and care needs. The hospice IDG then creates and continuously updates the hospice plan of care.

In addition to the role of HMD, each patient has an attending physician of record. The patient may designate as the attending physician the primary care physician or a specialist treating the underlying terminal illness. If the patient cannot identify a physician to fulfill this role or if the physician declines to participate, the HMD also

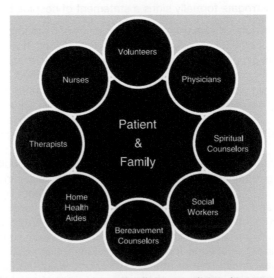

Fig. 4. Interdisciplinary team in hospice and palliative medicine. (*From* NHPCO Facts and Figures: Hospice Care in America. Alexandria, VA: National Hospice and Palliative Care Organization, Rev. ed. April 2018; with permission.)

may serve in the attending physician role. The attending physician manages the care and symptom management of the patient. Although the attending physician may make home visits, often the direct home visits are made by the hospice nurse who coordinates care with the attending physician. Attending physicians are responsible for prescribing necessary medications and updating the care plan as needed.

The hospice IDG can vary its services as needed to meet the needs of the patient. Nursing visits may occur weekly or biweekly, depending on the intensity of need, and can be increased to daily if symptom management requires. Social workers and pastoral care likewise make a visit within 5 days of admission as part of the comprehensive assessment and attend to the patient's emotional, social, and spiritual needs on a regular basis (often 1 visit every 2 weeks with increasing visits, as needed). Nurse home health aides can be added as a patient's ability to attend to activities of daily living decline, but such visits are limited to a few times a week. The entire IDG works to help the patient's family and caregivers gain skills to provide care, but hospice does not provide around-the-clock care. A patient who is unable to care for activities of daily living may require relocation to a higher level of care (assisted living or long-term care) if caregivers are not available or capable of meeting care needs as a patient declines. The expenses associated with long-term care are not covered as part of the hospice benefit.

As the patient approaches death, the intensity of service needed to keep the patient at home may increase. Medicare has revised payments to adjust for the more intensive hospice service needed in the initial hospice weeks and again in the last 2 weeks of life. Finally, hospice provides bereavement resources for the patient's family for the year after death.

WHAT IS THE HOSPICE RECERTIFICATION PROCESS, AND WHY IS A PATIENT SOMETIMES DISCHARGED FROM HOSPICE?

When a patient is admitted to hospice, the certification period is limited to only 3 months. The hospice IDG must recertify that the patient still meets the eligibility criteria for hospice by the 90th day. The second hospice benefit period is also a 90-day certification, whereas subsequent benefit periods need to be recertified every 60 days. Although the hospice benefit is designed for a prognosis of 6 months, there is no maximum time that one can receive hospice under Medicare. In 2017%, 86% of hospice patients who died did so in less than 6 months.[1]

Recertification of the terminal illness after the first benefit period is the responsibility of the HMD, not the referring physician. The hospice IDG gathers data that support the terminal prognosis and data that document further decline. The HMD must complete a narrative that presents the evidence for ongoing certification and formally sign the recertification document. After the first two 90-day hospice benefit periods, subsequent recertifications require a face-to-face encounter to evaluate the life expectancy of 6 months or less. The face-to-face encounter may be performed by the HMD or a nurse practitioner.

If a patient's prognosis appears to have improved over the course of hospice care and no longer is consistent with a prognosis of 6 months or less, the patient is discharged. In 2017, of the patients cared for by hospice, 6.7% had hospice-initiated live discharges because the patients were no longer considered terminally ill.[1]

HOW CAN IT BE ENSURED THAT A PATIENT RECEIVES HIGH-QUALITY HOSPICE CARE?

CMS has been collecting standardized hospice quality data via the Hospice Item Set, which is endorsed by the National Quality Forum, since 2014, and, although most hospices perform moderately well, only 4% receive a perfect score, with the greatest substantial variation occurring in the domain of pain score assessment, where only 78% of hospices perform well.[51] A recent Office of Inspector General report highlights the need for care in referring to high-quality hospices. According to the report, 18% of hospices were considered poor performers, meaning the hospice had at least 1 serious deficiency or at least 1 substantiated severe complaint during state survey or survey by accrediting organizations.[52] Hospice quality data are publicly reported on the Web site Hospice Compare (https://www.medicare.gov/hospicecompare/), which allows comparison of hospice agencies' quality data.

For professional improvement in hospice care for providers, additional hospice training can be found through the resources of the National Hospice and Palliative Care Organization or the American Academy of Hospice and Palliative Medicine. For the practicing physician who plans to practice as an HMD but is unable to do hospice and palliative fellowship training, there is a formal credentialing through the Hospice Medical Director Certification Board, which addresses the core roles and administrative, regulatory, legal, and ethical responsibilities of the hospice physician.

ACKNOWLEDGMENTS

The authors wish to thank Imelda Vetter, MLIS, for assistance with the preparation of this article.

DISCLOSURE

Dr P.E. Tatum is a director at large of the board of the American Academy of Hospice and Palliative Medicine, and he is a member of the Geriatrics and Palliative Care Standing Committee of the National Quality Forum.

REFERENCES

1. NHPCO facts and figures: hospice care in America. Rev edition. Alexandria (VA): National Hospice and Palliative Care Organization; 2019. Available at: https://www.nhpco.org/wp-content/uploads/2019/07/2018_NHPCO_Facts_Figures.pdf.
2. Teno JM, Gozalo P, Trivedi AN, et al. Site of death, place of care, and health care transitions among US medicare beneficiaries, 2000-2015. JAMA 2018;320:264–71.
3. Dumanovsky T, Rogers M. Trends in hospital palliative care from the National Palliative Care Registry™. J Pain Symptom Manag 2017;53:422.
4. Saunders C. The symptomatic treatment of incurable malignant disease. Prescr J 1964;4(4):68–73.
5. Saunders C. The evolution of palliative care. J R Soc Med 2001;94(9):430–2.
6. Wall PD. 25 volumes of pain. Pain 1986;25(1):1–4.
7. Josephina Bautista Magno. BMJ 2003;327(27):753. Available at: www.hospicecare.org.
8. Loscalzo MJ. Palliative care: an historical perspective. Hematology 2008;1:465.
9. Carlson RW, Devich L, Frank RR. Development of a comprehensive supportive care team for the hopelessly ill on a university hospital medical service. JAMA 1988;259(3):378–83. Available at: http://www.ncbi.nlm.nih.gov/pubmed/3336162. Accessed August 22, 2019.
10. Walsh D. The Harry R. Horvitz Center for Palliative Medicine (1987-1999): development of a novel comprehensive integrated program. Am J Hosp Palliat Med 2001;18(4):239–50.

11. American Heart Association Definition of Cardiology. Available at: http://www.heart. org/HEARTORG/Encyclopedia/Heart-Encyclopedia_UCM_445084_ContentIndex. jsp?levelSelected=3. Accessed August 26, 2019.

12. Ferrell BR, Twaddle ML, Melnick A, et al. National consensus project clinical practice guidelines for quality palliative care guidelines, 4th Edition. J Palliat Med 2018;21(12):1684-9.

13. Dying in America: improving quality and honoring individual preferences near the end of life. National Academies Press; 2015. https://doi.org/10.17226/18748.

14. No Title. Center to advance palliative care. Available at: https://www.capc.org/ about/palliative-care/. Accessed August 22, 2019.

15. No title. Available at: https://www.cancer.org/treatment/treatments-and-side-effects/palliative-care.html. Accessed August 22, 2019.

16. Kelley AS. Defining "serious illness". J Palliat Med 2014;17(9):985.

17. Kelley AS, Bollens-Lund E. Identifying the population with serious illness: the "denominator" challenge. J Palliat Med 2018;21(S2):S7-16.

18. Fischer SM, Gozansky WS, Sauaia A, et al. A practical tool to identify patients who may benefit from a palliative approach: the CARING criteria. J Pain Symptom Manage 2006;31(4):285-92.

19. Teno JM, Gozalo PL, Bynum JPW, et al. Change in end-of-life care for medicare beneficiaries: Site of death, place of care, and health care transitions in 2000, 2005, and 2009. JAMA 2013;309(5):470-7.

20. Ferrell BR, Temel JS, Temin S, et al. Integration of palliative care into standard oncology care: American society of clinical oncology clinical practice guideline update. J Clin Oncol 2017;35(1):96-112.

21. Selecky PA, Eliasson AH, Hall RI, et al. Palliative and end-of-life care for patients with cardiopulmonary diseases: American College of Chest Physicians position statement. Chest 2005;128(5):3599-610.

22. Braun LT, Grady KL, Kutner JS, et al. Palliative care and cardiovascular disease and stroke: a policy statement from the American Heart Association/American Stroke Association. Circulation 2016;134(11):e198-225.

23. Clinical practice guidelines for quality palliative care. 4th edition. National Coalition for Hospice and Palliative Care Clinical Practice Guidelines for Quality Palliative Care; 2018. Available at: https://www.

24. Blinderman CD, Homel P, Billings JA, et al. Symptom distress and quality of life in patients with advanced congestive heart failure. J Pain Symptom Manage 2008; 35(6):594-603.

25. Jagosh J, Donald Boudreau J, Steinert Y, et al. The importance of physician listening from the patients' perspective: enhancing diagnosis, healing, and the doctor-patient relationship. Patient Educ Couns 2011;85(3):369-74.

26. Delgado-Guay M, Ferrer J, Rieber AG, et al. Financial distress and its associations with physical and emotional symptoms and quality of life among advanced cancer patients. Oncologist 2015;20(9):1092-8.

27. White DB, Malvar G, Karr J, et al. Expanding the paradigm of the physician's role in surrogate decision-making: an empirically derived framework. Crit Care Med 2010;38(3):743-50.

28. Quill TE, Abernethy AP. Generalist plus specialist palliative care - creating a more sustainable model. N Engl J Med 2013;368(13):1173-5.

29. Von Gunten CF. Perspectives on care at the close of life secondary and tertiary palliative care in US hospitals. vol. 287. 2002. Available at: www.jama.com.

30. Kavalieratos D, Corbelli J, Zhang D, et al. Association between palliative care and patient and caregiver outcomes: a systematic review and meta-analysis. JAMA 2016;316(20):2104–14.
31. Lustbader D, Mudra M, Romano C, et al. The impact of a home-based palliative care program in an accountable care organization. J Palliat Med 2017;20(1). https://doi.org/10.1089/jpm.2016.0265.
32. Armstrong B, Jenigiri B, Hutson SP, et al. The impact of a palliative care program in a rural appalachian community hospital: a quality improvement process. Am J Hosp Palliat Med 2013;30(4):380–7.
33. Bernacki RE, Block SD. Communication about serious illness care goals: a review and synthesis of best practices. JAMA Intern Med 2014;174(12):1994–2003.
34. Sidebottom AC, Jorgenson A, Richards H, et al. Inpatient palliative care for patients with acute heart failure: Outcomes from a randomized trial. J Palliat Med 2015;18(2):134–42.
35. Khandelwal N, Kross EK, Engelberg RA, et al. Estimating the effect of palliative care interventions and advance care planning on ICU utilization: a systematic review. Crit Care Med 2015;43(5):1102–11.
36. Chen CY, Thorsteinsdottir B, Cha SS, et al. Health care outcomes and advance care planning in older adults who receive home-based palliative care: a pilot cohort study. J Palliat Med 2015;18(1):38–44.
37. Wu FM, Newman JM, Lasher A, et al. Effects of initiating palliative care consultation in the emergency department on inpatient length of stay. J Palliat Med 2013; 16(11):1362–7.
38. Temel JS, Greer JA, Muzikansky A, et al. Early palliative care for patients with metastatic non-small-cell lung cancer. N Engl J Med 2010;363(8):733–42.
39. Bakitas M, Tosteson T, Li Z, et al. The ENABLE III randomized controlled trial of concurrent palliative oncology care. J Clin Oncol 2014;32(15_suppl):9512.
40. Higginson IJ, Bausewein C, Reilly CC, et al. An integrated palliative and respiratory care service for patients with advanced disease and refractory breathlessness: a randomised controlled trial. Lancet Respir Med 2014;2(12):979–87.
41. May P, Normand C, Cassel JB, et al. Economics of palliative care for hospitalized adults with serious illness: A meta-analysis. JAMA Intern Med 2018;178(6):820–9.
42. Medicare Payment Advisory Commission. Report to congress: medicare payment policy. March 2019.
43. Glare P, Virik K, Jones M, et al. Predictions in terminally ill cancer patients terminally ill cancer patients. Current 2003;327(February 2005):1–6.
44. Downar J, Goldman R, Pinto R, et al. The "surprise question" for predicting death in seriously ill patients: a systematic review and meta-analysis. CMAJ 2017; 189(13):E484–93.
45. Cohen LM, Ruthazer R, Moss AH, et al. Predicting six-month mortality for patients who are on maintenance hemodialysis. Clin J Am Soc Nephrol 2010;5(1):72–9.
46. Stineman MG, Xie D, Pan Q, et al. All-cause 1-, 5-, and 10-year mortality in elderly people according to activities of daily living stage. J Am Geriatr Soc 2012;60(3): 485–92.
47. Tangeman JC, Rudra CB, Kerr CW, et al. A hospice-hospital partnership: Reducing hospitalization costs and 30-day readmissions among seriously ill adults. J Palliat Med 2014;17(9):1005–10.
48. Ali M, Capel M, Jones G, et al. The importance of identifying preferred place of death. BMJ Support Palliat Care 2019;9(1):84–91.
49. Certification of terminal illness. Fed Regist 2011;76(150):47331. Codified at 42 CFR §418.22.

50. Local Coverage Determination (LCD) for hospice determining terminal status (L33393). Available at: https://www.cms.gov/medicare-coverage-database/details/lcd-details.aspx?LCDId=33393&ContrId=272&ver=2&ContrVer=1&CntrctrSelected=272*1&Cntrctr=272&name=National+Government+Services%2C+Inc.+(06004%2C+HHH+MAC)&DocType=All&s=56&bc=AggAAAIAAAAAAA%3D%3D&. Accessed August 21, 2019.
51. Zheng NT, Li Q, Hanson LC, et al. Nationwide quality of hospice care: findings from the centers for medicare & medicaid services hospice quality reporting program. J Pain Symptom Manage 2018;55(2):427–32.e1.
52. Chiedi JM. Hospice deficiencies pose risks to medicare beneficiaries hospice deficiencies pose risks to medicare beneficiaries what OIG found 2019.

Goals of Care Conversations in Serious Illness

A Practical Guide

Nelia Jain, MD, MA[a,b,*], Rachelle E. Bernacki, MD, MS[b,c,d]

KEYWORDS

- Communication • Serious illness care • Goals of care • Values and preferences
- Prognosis

KEY POINTS

- Excellent communication is needed to promote patient-centered care.
- Goals of care conversations are an opportunity to engage patients in shared decision making regarding serious illness care.
- Quality communication ensures that medical treatments or interventions offered align with patients' values and preferences.
- Communication skill acquisition requires training, practice, and feedback to develop proficiency and expertise.

INTRODUCTION

As a clinician involved in caring for patients with serious illness, one frequently is tasked with helping patients and their families navigate various points of the patient's illness trajectory. Excellent communication is required to ensure that the care provided is patient centered and aligns with the patient's values and preferences. Clinicians working with seriously ill patients engage in various communication tasks, including advance care planning, delivering serious news, discussing prognosis, and engaging in goals of care conversations. Although in practice these communication tasks are often conflated, important distinctions exist among these types of discussions, all of which encompass a unique skill set. Advance care planning is "a process that supports adults at any

[a] Adult Palliative Care, Department of Psychosocial Oncology and Palliative Care, Dana-Farber Cancer Institute, 450 Brookline Avenue, JF 805D, Boston, MA 02215, USA; [b] Harvard Medical School, 25 Shattuck Street, Boston, MA 02215, USA; [c] Adult Palliative Care, Department of Psychosocial Oncology and Palliative Care, Dana-Farber Cancer Institute, Harvard Medical School, 450 Brookline Avenue, JF 821, Boston, MA 02215, USA; [d] Serious Illness Care Program, Ariadne Labs, 401 Park Drive, 3rd floor, Boston, MA 02215, USA
* Corresponding author.
E-mail address: Nelia_Jain@dfci.harvard.edu
Twitter: @njanej (N.J.); @rbernack (R.E.B.)

Med Clin N Am 104 (2020) 375–389
https://doi.org/10.1016/j.mcna.2019.12.001
0025-7125/20/© 2019 Elsevier Inc. All rights reserved.

age or stage of health in understanding and sharing their personal values, life goals, and preferences regarding future medical care."[1] After a patient is diagnosed with a serious illness and experiences a change in health state, additional exploration of the patient's values and preferences to help guide medical decision making may be warranted and occurs in the context of goals of care conversations. As patients navigate transition points throughout their illness trajectory, clinicians are often called on to deliver serious news or updated prognostic assessments, which lead to further goals of care conversations. For the purpose of this article, the authors focus on the communication strategies used to conduct successful goals of care conversations.

Frequently, clinicians' understanding of goals of care conversations is limited to urgent conversations that occur after recognition of an acute change in a patient's condition. As a result, many clinicians equate goals of care conversations with conversations that occur in an acute, inpatient setting, reserved specifically to address patients' preferences regarding life-sustaining interventions or to perform a code status discussion. When patients and families are faced with urgent decision making in acute, "crisis" situations, they are often emotionally overwhelmed and have difficulty comprehending complex medical information.[2] Ideally, goals of care conversations should occur earlier in the illness, beginning at the time of diagnosis, and be revisited throughout the illness trajectory; these discussions are often termed "serious illness conversations."[3] These discussions are an iterative process, designed to periodically check in with the patient and family to convey medical updates or revisit the risks, benefits, and alternatives of treatment options throughout the patient's disease course. Earlier conversations allow patients and families to engage in thoughtful discussions that shift the focus away from specific medical treatments to a broader exploration of the patients' values and preferences. This foundation guides patients, families, and clinicians toward an effective shared decision-making framework that ensures treatment choices and medical recommendations align with patients' goals.

APPROACH TO GOALS OF CARE CONVERSATIONS

Goals of care conversations are an essential aspect of providing quality care for patients with serious illness. Patients rely on a variety of values, experiences, and sources to aid in medical decision making. Patients view discussions regarding goals of care, treatment options, and prognosis as important sources of medical information and expect their physicians to bring them up.[4,5] Although many clinicians agree on the importance of conducting such conversations, fewer than 1 in 5 physicians who routinely care for patients aged 65 and older report engaging their patients in conversations about serious illness care.[6] Without these conversations, physicians are unaware of the factors that influence patients' decisions regarding serious illness care or the values and preferences that contribute to these decisions.[7] A lack of exploration of goals in serious illness care moves the focus away from the patient, often resulting in care that is inconsistent with patient wishes.

For the majority of clinicians, goals of care discussions are challenging and often avoided owing to a variety of factors. Frequently cited barriers include lack of training, insufficient time, failure to recognize the need for the conversation, discomfort with discussing prognosis or end-of-life issues, uneasiness responding to strong emotion, concerns about patients losing hope, and a desire to avoid conflict.[8-11] Clinicians also hesitate owing to their perception that patients and families often struggle to accept poor prognoses and have difficulty understanding the limitations of life-sustaining treatments; further, clinicians lack agreement among themselves regarding treatment decisions.[9,12] These barriers lead to clinicians being reluctant to have these conversations and initiating discussions about patients' goals and values infrequently and in later stages of illness.[8] Those clinicians who do initiate such conversations often lack a systematic approach and variably document the results of these discussions.[10,13]

By embracing a broader understanding of the value of goals of care communication, clinicians may begin to view these discussions as a forum for patients and clinicians to exchange information and formulate a mutually agreed upon care plan. These conversations are important opportunities for clinicians to assess a patient's illness understanding, deliver clinical updates, elicit a patient's values and treatment preferences, share prognostic information, and review treatment options. Patients, similarly, can benefit from these conversations by receiving important updates about their clinical condition, processing emotional responses to a declining health status, asking questions relevant to their condition or treatment options, providing insight into their unique values and beliefs that inform their approach to making medical decisions, and actively participating in formulating an individualized treatment plan. Patients who have an opportunity to speak to their physicians about the nature of their illness and serious illness care preferences have been shown to experience less psychological distress, report better quality of life, and receive care at the end of life that is more consistent with their preferences.[3,14–16]

Physicians with formal training or working in systems with formal mechanisms to assess patients' wishes and goals are more likely to value the importance of these conversations.[6] Physicians with the knowledge and access to a systematic approach to serious illness conversations also feel more comfortable with the content of these conversations and find the experience more rewarding.[6,17] Clinicians should view goals of care conversations as they would any other procedure and, likewise, expect that developing proficiency in communicating about serious illness goals requires training and practice to ensure quality and effectiveness. Numerous communication frameworks, conversation guides, and training programs are available to clinicians and patients to promote quality goals of care conversations (**Table 1**).[11,18–24] Additionally, clinician reimbursement for time spent conducting advance care planning conversations began in 2016 and helps to address clinicians' concerns regarding time constraints.[25] Patients are accepting of goals of care discussions being initiated by multiple team members, including nurses, social workers, and care coordinators.[12,26] Investing in interprofessional training in facilitating goals of care discussions can distribute the responsibility and offload any one member of the health care team.

This article provides a systematic framework that all clinicians may use to approach goals of care conversations with their patients. Not all discussions will require that clinicians cover all conversation elements in one sitting. However, by familiarizing oneself with the themes that commonly arise in goals of care discussions, the clinician can work toward building a skill set to successfully navigate these discussions and improve the quality and value of such conversations. Increased clinician confidence and investment in conducting conversations about serious illness care goals can aid to move conversations earlier in trajectory, allow clinicians to take ownership of these conversations, and ensure the dissemination of relevant outcomes with the remainder of health care team.

PREPARE FOR THE DISCUSSION

Before conducting a goals of care conversation, clinicians should engage in adequate preparation. In the planning phase, a thorough review of relevant medical facts pertaining to the patient's care is valuable. Information gathering should include

Table 1
Select communication resources

Communication Resource	Description	Audience	Tools
Serious Illness Care Program https://www.ariadnelabs.org/areas-of-work/serious-illness-care/	Intervention to facilitate more, better, and earlier conversations between clinicians and seriously ill patients	Clinicians Health Systems	Serious Illness Conversation Guide (available in multiple languages) Training, coaching, implementation, and reference materials for clinicians System for documenting conversation in the health record
VitalTalk https://www.vitaltalk.org/	Resources and courses to strengthen clinicians' communication skills	Clinicians	In-person workshops Online courses Conversation guides and videos VitalTalk App
Respecting Choices https://respectingchoices.org/	Model for advance care planning geared toward creating a health care culture of patient-centered care	Clinicians Health Systems	Online communication curricula Design and implementation packages In-person certification courses
PREPARE https://prepareforyourcare.org	Website that assists patients and families to have conversations with clinicians and make medical decisions regarding advance care planning	Patients and families	Question guides, videos and pamphlets to facilitate conversations Advance directives Toolkit for groups Resources in Spanish and English
The Conversation Project https://theconversationproject.org/	Public engagement initiative to help individuals speak to loved ones about their wishes regarding end-of-life care	Patients and families	Conversation starter and health care proxy kits Guide for beginning conversation with health care team Resources available in multiple languages

Data from Refs.[11],[18–24]

discussion with a patient's longitudinal providers such as his or her primary care provider or oncologist and relevant specialists. By reviewing available documentation pertaining to a patient's advance directives and summaries of prior goals of care discussions, clinicians gain insight into a patient's previously delineated values and preferences. In addition, critical information regarding psychosocial aspects of a patient's care or pertinent family dynamics can be obtained by discussion with additional members of the health care team, such as social workers, care managers, and nurses.

There are numerous benefits to multidisciplinary communication in advance of a goals of care discussion. Such communication creates an opportunity for clinicians to familiarize themselves with all team members involved in a patient's care and learn from each other's contributions. Based on each team members' unique interactions with the patient and family, clinicians can often anticipate questions or concerns that may arise and strategize the best method to address them. Clinicians also have the opportunity to compare relevant data and ensure consensus with respect to treatment options, prognostic estimates, and medical recommendations. If consensus is not present, further discussion may be needed to reconcile differences in medical opinions or reach agreement on multiple appropriate courses of action. In doing so, clinicians can construct a unified agenda and intended outcomes for the meeting.[27] Additionally, advanced preparation allows clinicians to identify key health care participants who should be present for the goals of care discussion.

The acuity of a patient's condition and the practice setting in which the goals of care discussion take place often inform the extent to which advanced preparation and multidisciplinary communication may occur. By holding conversations earlier in the disease trajectory, the clinician has enough opportunity to solicit input from relevant health care team members along the way, as well as include team members in ongoing goals of care discussions when appropriate. However, in caring for patients who experience an acute change in their clinical condition, clinicians may not always have sufficient time to prepare for a goals of care discussion in advance. In these situations, timely identification of relevant health care team members and arranging for a discussion in the form of a brief care team meeting before meeting with the patient and/or family is useful to review key aspects of the patient's care and formulate a recommended treatment plan. These care team meetings, also referred to as "premeetings," are an opportunity to ascertain which team member is most appropriate to lead the meeting, as well as anticipate the roles and contributions of other team members present.

Finally, by planning for goals of care conversations in advance, clinicians can provide sufficient notice to patients and families. Clinicians should identify an appropriate meeting space and arrange for an interpreter if needed. Ideally, the patient should be in attendance and participate in the discussion. If the patient's condition prohibits his or her participation, clinicians should ensure that the patient's health care proxy is present for the meeting. If there are numerous family members involved in a patient's care or a health care proxy has not been designated, the health care team can request the family identify a representative to be present at the meeting as well as assume the responsibility to disseminate key updates and outcomes of the meeting to other family members.

INTRODUCE THE PURPOSE OF THE DISCUSSION AND SET AN AGENDA

Once adequate preparation has occurred and all of the key participants have gathered, the clinician selected to lead the meeting may begin. The discussion should start with introductions of all individuals present and their relationship to the patient or role in his or her care. The lead clinician may then convey the purpose for the meeting. Importantly, this introduction should be followed by inviting the patient and family to share their understanding of the reason for the discussion as well as any questions or concerns they are hoping to have addressed. Negotiating the agenda is helpful in setting reasonable expectations for what is able to be addressed, reviewing ground rules for the discussion, and minimizing unexpected questions or concerns being raised later in the discussion.[28] The patient and family's responses also provide insight for the clinicians into their readiness for the discussion, allowing clinicians to tailor the quantity of information and manner of delivery accordingly.[29]

ASSESS ILLNESS UNDERSTANDING, COPING STYLE, AND PROGNOSTIC AWARENESS

After establishing a mutually agreed upon agenda, clinicians may then proceed with assessing the patient and family's understanding of the patient's medical condition. This information can be elicited by asking, "What have you heard from your health care team about your illness?" Although clinicians may be tempted to interrupt when discussing medical details, they should continue to listen and explore the patient's and family's illness understanding to best guide further discussion. The clinician can glean information about the illness experience by asking questions such as, "What changes have you noticed throughout the illness?" The clinician should attend to the information that is shared by the patient and family as well as topics that seem to be avoided. In addition, clinicians can collect valuable data from observing family dynamics as well as the emotional state of the patient and family.

By actively listening to the patient and family, the clinician becomes aware of their illness understanding, level of prognostic awareness, and preparedness to hear additional medical updates. The information shared may also provide insight regarding the patient and family's coping styles. Clinicians may be surprised if patients share an overly optimistic or unrealistic sense of the illness trajectory or prognosis; however, this is commonly encountered. Among patients with recent diagnoses of incurable cancer, for example, high rates of inaccurate prognostic understanding exist.[30] Furthermore, a patient may maintain hope for an unrealistic treatment outcome even while acknowledging that this outcome is different from the treatment goal of their physician.[30]

Clinicians can experience discomfort when addressing patients with low prognostic awareness or those who seem to be reluctant to hear news that would counteract their hoped-for outcomes. Clinicians should pause to examine the root of their discomfort. Some may worry they will face a challenging conversation ahead. Others may jump to the assumption that the patient and family are unrealistic and any attempts to relay medical updates or need for reevaluation of treatment options will be futile. In responding to such patients, clinicians should begin with broad, open-ended questions, such as, "When you look to the future, what are you most hopeful for?" In posing such a question, clinicians are acknowledging that, although the delivery of serious news or prognosis may impact a particular hope of a patient such as a hope for a cure or a longer life expectancy, seriously ill patients often possess multiple hopes that may still be achieved.[31] Similarly, the clinician can use this time to obtain information about any concerns that might inform the patient's decision making by asking, "What worries you the most about the future when you think about your illness?" Patients' responses to such questions can help to guide the clinician in how best to deliver medical updates and prognostic information. Although clinicians may mistakenly believe a patient's expression of unrealistic hopes represents poor prognostic understanding, an exploration of his or her worries may reveal an acknowledgment of the severity of the illness.

Clinicians should exercise caution in replying cognitively and attempting to correct a patient or family's inaccurate illness or prognostic understanding. They should also be careful not to assume denial prematurely, because a the patient's and family's statements may be more reflective of their hopes and expressions of anticipatory grief rather than a true lack of understanding of the seriousness of the underlying illness.[29,30] Patients facing serious illness experience a pendulum swing in the level of realistic awareness they possess with respect to their prognosis and illness trajectory.[32] A patient's ability to cope and integrate serious news throughout the course of their illness is impacted by their coping style and their family's level of prognostic awareness. A patient's illness understanding and prognostic awareness can be enhanced when he or she possesses adaptive coping behaviors. Furthermore, patients with caregivers who possess a greater prognostic awareness are more easily able to integrate a realistic understanding of their illness compared with those with caregivers with lower prognostic awareness.[32] Regardless of the patient's and family's level of illness understanding, prognostic awareness, and coping style, each patient and family system will be unique in their willingness and ability to integrate new information, adapt to changes in their medical condition, and preferences for receiving information. Promoting accurate illness understanding is often an ongoing process, likely requiring multiple conversations over time.

DELIVER MEDICAL UPDATES AND PROGNOSTIC INFORMATION

Patients and families are more likely to feel listened to and respected if the clinician summarizes what he or she heard about their illness understanding before moving the conversation forward.[27] This summary also allows the clinician to address any gaps in illness understanding. Once these gaps have been reconciled, clinicians can proceed with delivering medical updates. In delivering serious news or prognostic information, clinicians may struggle with the best timing and method to approach these discussions. Although most patients and families wish to receive such information directly from their health care team, they are often more receptive when given the option to defer receiving information until they are ready.[33] Clinicians may assess readiness by asking permission from the patient and family before proceeding further in the discussion. This readiness may be elicited by posing the question, "How much information would you like about what lies ahead with your illness?"[11] Additional questions such as, "If I have information about specific time frames, would that be information you are interested in hearing?" can further help the clinician to titrate the information presented based on individual preferences.[34]

In some situations, patients and families may remain reluctant to hear such information when asked. In these situations, the clinician should acknowledge the difficulty of these discussions, explore underlying reasons that may be explain their hesitation, and recognize ambivalence. Simultaneously, clinicians should gauge how important this information is to the discussion. If there is a clear need based on the clinical situation, such as evidence of rapid clinical deterioration or concern that a patient is engaging in poor decision making owing to an incomplete illness understanding, clinicians should negotiate methods to proceed with the discussion.[35] In such instances, clinicians may gently pursue this conversation by "naming the dilemma."[32,33] For example, clinicians may explain their inability to discuss the risks and benefits of future treatment options without first relaying information about prognosis. Other strategies to consider include offering to discuss the information with a proxy rather than the patient directly or relaying prognostic information in terms of function rather than specific timeframes. Clinicians often discover that, by providing context for the necessity of the discussion while maintaining an empathetic and flexible approach, patients and families may be more receptive and able to integrate information in a manner that allows them to make the best decisions for themselves.

After asking permission and negotiating patient and family preferences for information, clinicians may proceed with delivering serious news and prognostic information. This approach is often referred to as ask–tell–ask (**Table 2**).[28] The information should be presented succinctly and avoid medical jargon. Information is best received when given directly. Often, both positive and negative framing is used through hope/worry statements, which are effective ways to convey prognostic information. For example, a clinician may state, "I hope you continue to feel well for as long as possible, and I worry that, based on the condition, this is as strong as you will feel."[20,32,36] Normalizing the inherent uncertainty in conveying information about future projections for a seriously ill patient helps to set realistic expectations while maintaining a sense of hope.[37] Approaching updates on serious illness in this manner will help to continue the discussion in a patient-centered manner and promote a therapeutic alliance between the clinician and the patient.

EXPECT AND RESPOND TO EMOTION

In all serious illness discussions, clinicians should anticipate and be prepared to respond to emotions from patients and families. Hearing news about changes in one's condition or worries about a limited life expectancy may provoke a strong emotional response from a patient or family member. Although a patient's response may sound like a request for more information, the clinician should attend to clues, such as a patient's body language, that might suggest he or she is still emotionally processing the news and is not ready to hear more information. Clinicians may experience discomfort in the presence of strong emotions and worry that their actions directly caused a patient or family member to become upset. More often, a strong emotional reaction is a positive sign that the information that needed to be conveyed was appropriately received and internalized.

Clinicians should be cautious not to respond from a place of discomfort by offering false reassurance or backtracking on the information delivered, because this tactic may lessen the credibility of the information conveyed or the patient and family's confidence in the clinician. Instead, the clinician should use empathic actions or statements to respond to emotions. Examples include the use of therapeutic silence or offering a "NURSE" statement (**Table 3**).[28] Statements such as "I wish things were different" help the clinician align with patients' hopes while acknowledging the reality of a poor prognosis.[38] Patients who feel supported by their clinician may be more willing to

Table 2 Ask-tell-ask	
Ask	Ask the patient about his or her illness understanding. Ask the patient what questions he or she has about the illness. Ask the patient about information preferences
Tell	Communicate serious news, medical updates, prognostic information and/or treatment options.
Ask	Ask the patient to summarize the information you conveyed. Ask the patient for permission to move forward in the conversation.

Data from Back AL, Arnold RM, Baile WF, et al. Approaching Difficult Communication Tasks in Oncology. CA Cancer J Clin 2005;55(3):164-177.

Table 3	
NURSE statements	
Naming	"I can see that hearing this information was upsetting."
Understanding	"I can't imagine how difficult it is to hear this news."
Respecting	"I can see how committed you are to doing everything you can to feel as well as possible."
Supporting	"I will remain an active part of your care team as we navigate the next steps."
Exploring	"Tell me more about how you are feeling right now."

Data from Back AL, Arnold RM, Baile WF, et al. Approaching Difficult Communication Tasks in Oncology. CA Cancer J Clin 2005;55(3):164-177.

expand upon their concerns. Clinicians should carefully listen to patients' responses because they often provide valuable insight into distressing aspects of the illness experience, anticipated losses, and worries about the future that the patient may not have previously expressed. Clinicians should continue to explore patient's emotions using statements, such as, "Tell me more about how you are feeling," until they feel the patient is ready to move on in the conversation. Clinicians may then proceed by requesting the patient and family to summarize the new information they heard to check for understanding, followed by asking permission to continue the discussion.

EXPLORE PATIENTS' VALUES AND PREFERENCES

Some patients and families may remain emotionally overwhelmed such that additional discussion should be deferred until a later time. Clinicians should be prepared that addressing goals of care may require multiple discussions over the course of a patient's illness, particularly if permitted by the clinical circumstances. For those patients who are willing to continue or for whom additional discussion is warranted based on the clinical situation, the clinician can gradually shift the focus of the discussion to an exploration of the patient's values and preferences, which will further inform downstream recommendations regarding next steps in the treatment plan. Clinicians should intentionally refrain from asking about patients' preferences regarding specific treatments when opening these discussions to keep the focus of the discussion on understanding who the patient is as a person and what hopes and goals are most important to him or her. Engaging patients in discussion regarding their values and preferences may help patients to move past the discomfort of dealing with an uncertain future and refocus the discussion to how best to care for the patient in the present.[37]

Interviews with patients facing serious illness have demonstrated that patient preferences are impacted by the burden of treatment, type of outcome anticipated, and the likelihood of the outcome occurring.[4] Therefore, an exploration of a patient's preferences and values should include an understanding of an acceptable quality of life to the patient in terms of function and level of dependency, as well as tradeoffs the patient is willing to accept to achieve important goals. Clinicians may inquire about patients' general views about cognitive and functional states or ask after specific situations patients have experienced or observed. Questions such as, "Have you experienced anything throughout the course of your illness or observed something a family member with serious illness has gone through that you considered unacceptable?" may help the clinician to guide the patient through the discussion. Additionally, a clinician may ask, "If you become sicker, how much are you willing to go through in order to gain more time?" as a means to understand tradeoffs that a patient is willing to accept.[11] The patient's responses can help the clinician to consider treatment options that would have the highest likelihood of helping a patient to realize particular hopes and goals while avoiding those that may pose unacceptable burdens or outcomes.

In discussing patients' values and preferences, clinicians should be prepared that patients may describe conflicting preferences or outcomes that diverge from expressed values.[39] In these situations, clinicians should ask patients to prioritize their values to help guide decision making. However, clinicians are likely to encounter a subset of patients who are unable to clearly prioritize their values or may require additional time and ongoing discussion to do so.[40] Revisiting patients' values and preferences is useful as patients may demonstrate evolving treatment preferences throughout the course of their illness, particularly after viewing these decisions in the context of changes in their health state. Clinicians should also note that patients' preferences may vary based on cultural beliefs. These beliefs may impact the type of information they desire, who they would like to be present for goals of care discussions, the extent to which family members are expected to participate in decision making, and which treatments they are willing to pursue or forgo.[41,42] Clinicians should maintain a curiosity and openness to learning about patients' values and preferences and how these may be informed by their beliefs, community, and other aspects of their life such as cultural, religious, or spiritual traditions.[43] In doing so, the clinician can continue to foster a patient-centered approach that respects the unique values and beliefs of varying cultures while also recognizing that individuals will vary in their adoption and application of these values and beliefs within their unique illness experience.

DISCUSS TREATMENT OPTIONS AND MAKE A RECOMMENDATION

After the clinician has taken the opportunity to understand a patient's values and preferences regarding important goals, acceptable tradeoffs, and standards for quality of life, the clinician can address specific treatment options. Clinicians should engage patients in a shared decision-making process, in which they provide information to the patients while also support the patient's decision-making process.[44] Information about treatment options should be framed in the context of burdens or benefits posed by the various options and the likelihood of achieving particular outcomes. Importantly, a patient's values, beliefs, and preferences may also provide sufficient guidance that particular treatments would not meet a patient's goals or would pose unacceptable burdens. The clinician should not feel obligated to present every treatment option available and instead should tailor the treatments offered based on information gained from the preceding discussion.

After a discussion of available treatment options, the clinician should check in with the patient and family to ensure accurate understanding of each option. Rather than passively allowing the patients and families to navigate these treatment options independently, the clinician should remain actively engaged in the deliberation process. In doing so, the clinician demonstrates nonabandonment and an ongoing investment in the patient's well-being. The extent of the clinician's involvement should depend on preferences of the patient and family and cannot be assumed based on the type of decision at hand.[45] Part of the clinician's responsibility in the decision-making process is to emphasize the importance of individual preference in selecting the best treatment option while also acknowledging the extent of uncertainty that inherently exists regarding projected treatment outcomes.[44] The clinician can also assist patients and families by incorporating relevant decision support tools such as videos, print and web-based media, or formal decision aids, which have been shown to improve communication and patient knowledge and preparation for treatment choices in the care of seriously ill patients.[46,47] One such decision support tool relies on scenario planning using best case and worst case scenarios to assist patients and families in managing the uncertainty that often surrounds treatment options. By combining the clinician's interpretation of medical facts with a personalization of scenarios to address the patient's values and concerns, this decision aid reaffirms a patient-centered approach while providing greater access to patients and families of the causal relationship between treatment choices and likely outcomes (**Fig. 1**).[48,49]

Finally, clinicians play a critical role in the medical decision-making process by offering the patient and family a recommendation. Patients vary in where they lie on the shared decision-making continuum and desire for physician input. Clinicians may assess the patient and family's willingness to hear a recommendation by asking, "Would it be helpful if I shared my recommendation regarding the treatment options?"[28,50] For patients and families who are receptive, the clinician should outline a recommendation with accompanying rationale. Clinicians should be careful to avoid personal values and preferences from informing their recommendation. Instead, clinicians should rely on the information obtained about the patient's values and preferences to offer a recommendation that best aligns with the patient's priorities.[50]

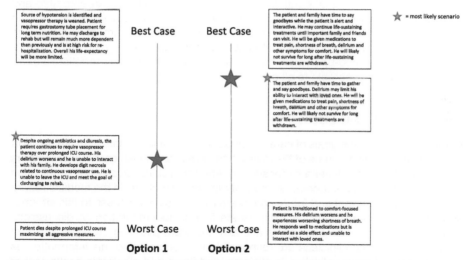

Fig. 1. Example of best case and worst case scenario. Case scenario: A 64-year-old man with coronary artery disease status post coronary artery bypass graft surgery, systolic heart failure with estimated ejection fraction of 25%, and remote bladder cancer is admitted to the intensive care unit with presumed septic shock from a urinary source. He has experienced hypoxic respiratory failure due to volume overload with prolonged intubation and is now status post tracheostomy. He is delirious but intermittently awake and interactive with loved ones. Despite receiving aggressive interventions for the past three weeks, he remains dependent on vasopressor therapy. You conduct a goals of care discussion with the patient's wife to determine best next steps. She shares that her husband has overcome multiple illnesses in the past and would want to continue the current level of interventions if there is a chance that he could discharge to a rehab and begin efforts toward walking and regaining independence. You present two options. Option 1: Continue present management. Option 2: Transition to comfort-focused measures. (*Adapted from* Schwarze ML. Best Case/Worst Case Training Program. UW - Madison Department of Surgery; 2016. Available at: https://www.hipxchange.org/BCWC. Accessed Dec 18 2019; with permission.)

FINALIZE THE TREATMENT PLAN

The final step in completing a goals of care conversation is to finalize a treatment plan. As noted, patients and families may feel too overwhelmed to finalize a decision at the conclusion of the discussion. In nonurgent clinical situations, the clinician can validate their emotions and suggest further discussion at a later time. In more urgent circumstances, the clinician may need to continue to explore patient hesitation or ambivalence related to decision making. Patients and families may not always agree with a clinician's recommendation or they may hesitate to forgo potentially beneficial treatments even if they are associated with significant risk or burden. In these situations, consideration of a time-limited trial may be beneficial, in which medical treatments are trialed over a prespecified period of time with close monitoring for prespecified outcomes.[51] Patients, families, and clinicians should leave the discussion with a clear understanding of which treatments are being pursued, the timeframe in which the patient's clinical condition will be reevaluated, and any downstream treatment options that may be considered in future discussions. Reviewing the finalized treatment plan with all involved parties also creates an opportunity to address any areas of conflict or disagreement. An inability to reach consensus is typically a reflection of underlying emotion and anticipatory grief in an understandably distressing situation. Addressing conflict requires recognition of the presence of disagreement as well as identification of the type of conflict.[52] Clinicians should maintain an empathic and nonjudgmental position, with incorporation of interdisciplinary colleagues as needed for additional support to all parties in navigating areas of disagreement. By reframing the discussion toward the patient's interests and reinforcing a commitment to formulating a mutually agreed-upon plan, clinicians can often successfully negotiate a treatment plan that is acceptable to all parties.[52,53]

FOLLOW-UP AFTER THE DISCUSSION

At the conclusion of the goals of care conversation, the clinician should make an effort to communicate the outcome of the meeting to all relevant health care team members as well as establish the timeframe for subsequent discussions. Quality communication includes documenting outcomes of goals of care conversations in the medical record to ensure that all current and future care team members have access to this information. At present, significant variability exists in the documentation of discussions regarding patient's goals and values and advance care planning owing to a lack of consensus on which clinicians are responsible for documenting this information as well as a lack of standardization in clinician workflows and electronic health record design.[13] Barriers to documentation about serious illness care preferences may be overcome by focusing efforts on patient-centered, clinician-centered, and systems-centered interventions, such as creating patient-friendly advance directives, encouraging a clinician quarterback to take ownership of documentation, and designating a specific site in the electronic health record to serve as the single source of truth. These measures will facilitate access to summaries of previous goals of care discussions and advance care planning documents pertaining to health care proxy, life-sustaining treatment, and code status preferences.[11,54] Last, as with any other process of clinical skill acquisition, the development of optimal goals of care communication requires practice and feedback. Therefore, the clinician may benefit from debriefing with other colleagues present during the discussion to review what went well during the conversation, opportunities for improvement, and strategies to implement in subsequent discussions.

SUMMARY

Clinicians caring for seriously ill patients are often tasked with engaging patients and families in goals of care conversations to convey medical updates or make medical decisions in the context of changes in disease status. Serious illness communication is an iterative process that requires ongoing discussion and reevaluation. Conversations that are held earlier in the disease course afford clinicians better opportunities to elicit patients' values and preferences and help patients plan in advance of changes in their underlying condition. Clinicians who invest in systematic approaches to such communication tasks are more likely to have empathic, high-quality conversations with patients and families. Such conversations enable clinicians and patients to engage in shared-decision making that promotes patient-centered care and aligns medical treatments and interventions with patients' values, preferences, and treatment goals.

DISCLOSURE

The authors have nothing to disclose.

REFERENCES

1. Sudore RL, Lum HD, You JJ, et al. Defining advance care planning for adults: a consensus definition from a multidisciplinary Delphi Panel. J Pain Symptom Manag 2017;53(5):821–32.e1.
2. Block SD. Psychological considerations, growth, and transcendence at the end of life: the art of the possible. JAMA 2001;285(22):2898–905.
3. Bernacki R, Paladino J, Neville BA, et al. Effect of the serious illness care program in outpatient oncology. JAMA Intern Med 2019;179(6):751–9.
4. Fried TR, Bradley EH, Towle VR, et al. Understanding the treatment preferences of seriously ill patients. N Engl J Med 2002;346(14):1061–6.
5. Petrillo LA, McMahan RD, Tang V, et al. Older adult and surrogate perspectives on serious, difficult, and important medical decisions. J Am Geriatr Soc 2018; 66(8):1515–23.
6. Fulmer T, Escobedo M, Berman A, et al. Physicians' views on advance care planning and end-of-life care conversations. J Am Geriatr Soc 2018;66(6):1201–5.
7. Desharnais S, Carter RE, Hennessy W, et al. Lack of concordance between physician and patient reports on end-of-life care discussions. J Palliat Med 2007;10(3):728–40.
8. Dunlay S, Foxen JL, Cole T, et al. A survey of clinician attitudes and self-reported practices regarding end-of-life care in heart failure. Palliat Med 2015;29(3):260–7.
9. Ethier J-L, Paramsothy T, You JJ, et al. Perceived barriers to goals of care discussions with patients with advanced cancer and their families in the ambulatory setting. J Palliat Care 2018;33(3):125–42.
10. Keating NL, Landrum M, Rogers SO, et al. Physician factors associated with discussions about end-of-life care. Cancer 2010;116(4):998–1006.
11. Bernacki RE, Block SD. Communication about serious illness care goals: a review and synthesis of best practices. JAMA Intern Med 2014;174(12):1994–2003.
12. You JJ, Downar J, Fowler RA, et al. Barriers to goals of care discussions with seriously ill hospitalized patients and their families: a multicenter survey of clinicians. JAMA Intern Med 2015;175(4):549–56.
13. Dillon E, Chuang J, Gupta A, et al. Provider perspectives on advance care planning documentation in the electronic health record: the experience of primary

care providers and specialists using advance health-care directives and physician orders for life-sustaining treatment. Am J Hosp Palliat Med 2017;34(10): 918–24.

14. Mack JW, Weeks JC, Wright AA, et al. End-of-life discussions, goal attainment, and distress at the end of life: predictors and outcomes of receipt of care consistent with preferences. J Clin Oncol 2010;28(7):1203–8.

15. Wright AA, Zhang B, Ray A, et al. Associations between end-of-life discussions, patient mental health, medical care near death, and caregiver bereavement adjustment. JAMA 2008;300(14):1665–73.

16. Detering K, Hancock AD, Reade MC, et al. The impact of advance care planning on end of life care in elderly patients: randomised controlled trial. BMJ 2010;340: c1345.

17. Lakin JR, Koritsanszky LA, Cunningham R, et al. A systematic intervention to improve serious illness communication in primary care. Health Aff 2017;36(7): 1258–64.

18. Baile WF, Buckman R, Lenzi R, et al. SPIKES—a six-step protocol for delivering bad news: application to the patient with cancer. Oncologist 2000;5(4):302–11.

19. Childers JW, Back AL, Tulsky JA, et al. REMAP: a framework for goals of care conversations. J Oncol Pract 2017;13(10). https://doi.org/10.1200/jop.2016. 018796.

20. Ariadne Labs. Serious illness care resources. Available at: https://www. ariadnelabs.org/areas-of-work/serious-illness-care/resources/#Downloads&% 20Tools. Accessed July 31, 2019.

21. Vital talk. Available at: https://www.vitaltalk.org/. Accessed August 12, 2019.

22. Respecting choices. Available at: https://respectingchoices.org/. Accessed August 12, 2019.

23. PREPARE for your care. Available at: https://prepareforyourcare.org/welcome/. Accessed August 12, 2019.

24. The Conversation Project. Available at: https://theconversationproject.org/. Accessed August 12, 2019.

25. Jones CA, Acevedo J, Bull J, et al. Top 10 tips for using advance care planning codes in palliative medicine and beyond. J Palliat Med 2016;19(12):1249–53.

26. Izumi S. Advance care planning. Am J Nurs 2017;117(6):56–61.

27. Billings AJ, Block SD. Part III: a guide for structured discussions. J Palliat Med 2011;14(9):1058–64.

28. Back AL, Arnold RM, Baile WF, et al. Approaching difficult communication tasks in oncology1. CA Cancer J Clin 2005;55(3):164–77.

29. Weiner JS, Roth J. Avoiding Iatrogenic harm to patient and family while discussing goals of care near the end of life. J Palliat Med 2006;9(2):451–63.

30. Nipp RD, Greer JA, El-Jawahri A, et al. Coping and prognostic awareness in patients with advanced cancer. J Clin Oncol 2017;35(22). https://doi.org/10.1200/ jco.2016.71.3404.

31. Feudtner C. The breadth of hopes. N Engl J Med 2009;361(24):2306–7.

32. Jackson VA, Jacobsen J, Greer JA, et al. The cultivation of prognostic awareness through the provision of early palliative care in the ambulatory setting: a communication guide. J Palliat Med 2013;16(8):894–900.

33. Clayton JM, Butow PN, Tattersall M. When and how to initiate discussion about prognosis and end-of-life issues with terminally ill patients. J Pain Symptom Manag 2005;30(2):132–44.

34. Back AL, Arnold RM. Discussing prognosis: "How much do you want to know?" Talking to patients who are prepared for explicit information. J Clin Oncol 2006; 24(25):4209–13.

35. Back AL, Arnold RM. Discussing prognosis: "How much do you want to know?" Talking to patients who do not want information or who are ambivalent. J Clin Oncol 2006;24(25):4214–7.

36. Lakin JR, Jacobsen J. Softening our approach to discussing prognosis. JAMA Intern Med 2019;179(1):5.

37. Smith AK, White DB, Arnold RM. Uncertainty — the other side of prognosis. N Engl J Med 2013;368(26):2448–50.

38. Quill TE, Arnold RM, Platt F. "I Wish Things Were Different": expressing wishes in response to loss, futility, and unrealistic hopes. Ann Intern Med 2001;135(7):551.

39. Howard M, Bansback N, Tan A, et al. Recognizing difficult trade-offs: values and treatment preferences for end-of-life care in a multi-site survey of adult patients in family practices. BMC Med Inform Decis Mak 2017;17(1):164.

40. Modes ME, Engelberg RA, Downey L, et al. Toward understanding the relationship between prioritized values and preferences for cardiopulmonary resuscitation among seriously ill adults. J Pain Symptom Manag 2019. https://doi.org/10.1016/j.jpainsymman.2019.06.011.

41. Sharma RK, Hughes MT, Nolan MT, et al. Family understanding of seriously-ill patient preferences for family involvement in healthcare decision making. J Gen Intern Med 2011;26(8):881–6.

42. Barclay JS, Blackhall LJ, Tulsky JA. Communication strategies and cultural issues in the delivery of bad news. J Palliat Med 2007;10(4):958–77.

43. Crawley LM, Marshall PA, Lo B, et al. Strategies for culturally effective end-of-life care. Ann Intern Med 2002;136(9):673.

44. Elwyn G, Frosch D, Thomson R, et al. Shared decision making: a model for clinical practice. J Gen Intern Med 2012;27(10):1361–7.

45. Kon AA. The shared decision-making continuum. JAMA 2010;304(8):903–4.

46. El-Jawahri A, Mitchell SL, Paasche-Orlow MK, et al. A randomized controlled trial of a CPR and intubation video decision support tool for hospitalized patients. J Gen Intern Med 2015;30(8):1071–80.

47. Austin AC, Mohottige D, Sudore RL, et al. Tools to promote shared decision making in serious illness: a systematic review. JAMA Intern Med 2015;175(7):1213–21.

48. Schwarze ML, Taylor LJ. Managing uncertainty — harnessing the power of scenario planning. N Engl J Med 2017;377(3):206–8.

49. Schwarze ML. Best case/worst case training program. Madison (WI): UW - Madison Department of Surgery; 2016. Available at: https://www.hipxchange.org/BCWC. Accessed August 12, 2019.

50. Jacobsen J, Blinderman C, Alexander C, et al. "I'd recommend ..." How to incorporate your recommendation into shared decision making for patients with serious illness. J Pain Symptom Manag 2018;55:1224–30.

51. Quill TE, Holloway R. Time-limited trials near the end of life. JAMA 2011;306(13):1483–4.

52. Back AL, Arnold RM. Dealing with conflict in caring for the seriously ill: "It Was Just Out of the Question. JAMA 2005;293(11):1374–81.

53. Bloche GM. Managing conflict at the end of life. N Engl J Med 2005;352(23):2371–3.

54. Sudore RL, Boscardin J, Feuz MA, et al. Effect of the PREPARE website vs an easy-to-read advance directive on advance care planning documentation and engagement among veterans: a randomized clinical trial. JAMA Intern Med 2017;177(8):1102.

Prognostication in Serious Illness

Emily J. Martin, MD[a],*, Eric Widera, MD[b,c]

KEYWORDS

- Prognosis • Decision making • Goals of care • Communication • Palliative care
- Patient-centered care • Palliative medicine • End-of-life care

KEY POINTS

- Prognosis, defined as the likelihood of a patient developing a particular outcome over a specific period of time, is essential to informed, patient-centered, clinical decision making.
- Prognostication involves 3 key components: formulation of the patient's prognosis; communication of the patient's prognosis; and the patient or surrogate's interpretation of the communicated prognosis.
- Prognostic indices are designed to quantify the relative contributions of prognostic variables and to assist clinicians in formulating prognostic estimates.
- A patient-oriented approach is needed when disclosing prognostic information.
- A patient or surrogate's interpretation of the communicated prognosis may be biased by optimism and the perception that the patient's attributes portend a more favorable outcome.

THE ESSENTIAL ROLE OF PROGNOSIS

The path forward would seem obvious if only I knew how many months or years I had left. Tell me three months, I'd just spend time with my family. Tell me one year, I'd have a plan (write that book). Give me ten years, I'd get back to treating diseases.

—*Paul Kalanithi, MD*

Of the 3 pillars of clinical medicine, diagnosis, prognosis, and treatment, one remains largely underprioritized in modern medical practice. Prognosis, the likelihood of a patient developing a particular outcome over a specific period of time, has

[a] Division of General Internal Medicine and Health Services Research, Department of Medicine, University of California, Los Angeles, 757 Westwood Plaza Suite 7501, Los Angeles, CA 90095, USA; [b] Division of Geriatrics, Department of Medicine, University of California, San Francisco, San Francisco, CA, USA; [c] San Francisco Veterans Affairs Health Care System, 4150 Clement Street, Box 181G, San Francisco, CA 94121, USA
* Corresponding author.
E-mail address: ejmartin@mednet.ucla.edu
Twitter: @emilyjeanmartin (E.J.M.); @EWidera (E.W.)

Med Clin N Am 104 (2020) 391–403
https://doi.org/10.1016/j.mcna.2019.12.002
0025-7125/20/© 2019 Elsevier Inc. All rights reserved.

been greatly overshadowed by a pervasive emphasis on diagnosis and treatment.[1] However, prognosis is an essential consideration in the delivery of high-quality, patient-centered care.

Prognostication involves the both the appraisal and the disclosure of a patient's prognosis as well as the interpretation of the disclosed information (**Fig. 1**). In essence, prognostication is the clinician's way of communicating what a patient can reasonably expect of the future with respect to a medical condition or its treatment. A dynamic skill, prognostication involves integrating clinical judgment with evidence-based patient-, disease-, and environment-related factors to make a prediction about the likelihood of a future clinical outcome. Although often equated with a prediction of survival, prognosis can refer to a range of outcomes along a patient's disease trajectory, such as a change in symptom burden, functional ability, or cognition. Given that prognosis frequently shapes a patient's priorities and alters the balance of potential benefits and burdens of a given medical intervention, prognostication is critical to informed shared decision making.[2–8]

BARRIERS TO PROGNOSTICATION

Most patients with serious illness prefer to know what to anticipate as their disease progresses. Yet clinicians are often reluctant to formulate and communicate prognostic estimates,[9–17] especially in the setting of terminal disease or serious illness, when prognostic information is likely to be most relevant. Consequently, patients or their surrogates often lack the information necessary to make informed medical decisions or to establish realistic goals of care.[8,18,19] For example, in a survey of patients with advanced breast cancer, nearly 60% of respondents incorrectly thought that their treatment was curative in intent,[20] and in a study of more than 1000 patients with incurable metastatic lung or colorectal cancer, 74% thought that the intent of chemotherapy was cure.[18] Similarly, in a multicenter study of nearly 600 patients with metastatic cancer, 71% wanted to be told their life expectancy, but only 18% had received this information.[20]

Perhaps the most significant factor limiting clinicians' willingness to engage patients in discussions about expected clinical outcomes is the misconception that prognostic inaccuracy renders such predictions clinically irrelevant.[21–23] It is not uncommon, for example, for a clinician to deflect an opportunity to engage a patient in a discussion about his or her prognosis with the reasoning that one cannot possibly predict the future.

Although it is known that, at least in terms of survival estimates among patients with cancer, clinicians tend to be overly optimistic and are frequently inaccurate, the clinical significance of this inaccuracy is unclear.[23–26] Lam[27] found a strong correlation between predicted and actual survival with an absolute difference in median survival of only 6 days (70 vs 76 days). Similarly, in a metaanalysis including more than 1500

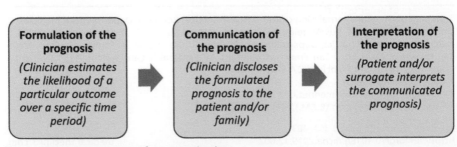

Fig. 1. Three components of prognostication.

patients with cancer, predicted survival of less than 6 months was highly correlated with actual survival, although systematically overestimated.[28] Several reasons for this tendency toward overestimation have been postulated. First, because prognostication is not a routine part of clinical discourse or education, most clinicians are poorly trained in how to formulate prognostic estimates.[16,29,30] Second, most data about patients' actual survival are obtained from clinical trials, which typically select for otherwise healthy patients and are therefore limited in their generalizability.[29] Third, the culture of modern medicine discourages frank discussions of death and dying and has, in turn, fostered professional norms that devalue prognostic estimates and favor optimism over accuracy.[22,29,31]

Unfortunately, even when a clinician has a clear sense of a patient's disease trajectory, prognostic nondisclosure is exceedingly common.[7,18,20,21,31] Clinicians routinely avoid initiating discussions about expected outcomes and often knowingly communicate overly optimistic estimates of survival.[1,32,33] A survey-based study by Lamont and Christakis[23] showed that even when a patient specifically requests prognostic information, approximately two-thirds of surveyed physicians indicated that they would either refuse to disclose this information or intentionally communicate a prognosis that differs from that which they had formulated.

Clinicians cite fear of taking away patients' hope or disrupting the patient-clinician relationship as key barriers to prognostic disclosure.[11,15] There is strong evidence to suggest, however, that these barriers are not well founded. Several studies have shown that prognostic disclosure preserves, and even promotes, hope among patients and their families.[14,34–37] Furthermore, an unfavorable prognosis, when communicated skillfully and with attention to patients' individual needs, does not detract from patients' emotional well-being or weaken the patient-clinician relationship.[20,36–38] Instead, prognostic awareness has been shown to increase emotional and social functioning, reduce anxiety and spiritual distress, and improve the quality of end-of-life care.[39–44] Common barriers to prognostication are summarized in **Box 1**.

FORMULATION OF THE PROGNOSIS

Prognostication, like most aspects of clinical medicine, is both an art and a science, with increased accuracy noted when clinical judgment is combined with evidence-based tools.[45–49] Although many disease-, patient-, and environment-related factors are known to influence the likelihood of a particular clinical outcome, clinicians are often unsure of how to weigh these variables when

---

Box 1
Common barriers to prognostication

Discomfort with the inherent uncertainty of forecasting

Inaccuracy of prognostication tools

Fear of being judged for inaccurate predictions

Discomfort with disclosing serious news

Inadequate communication skills training

Fear of diminishing patients' hope

Fear of causing patients distress or reducing their quality of life

Fear of disrupting the patient-clinician relationship or decreasing patient satisfaction

Guilt associated with not being able to offer curative treatments

formulating a prognostic estimate, especially for patients with noncancer diagnoses, atypical clinical presentations, and multi-comorbidities.

The most common way that clinicians estimate prognosis is through their clinical judgment and experience. Prognostication based on clinical judgment is correlated with actual survival; however, it is subject to various shortcomings that limit prognostic accuracy. In addition to the bias toward overestimation as described above, other studies have shown that clinical predictions tend to be more accurate for short-term prognosis than long-term prognosis and that the length of clinician-patient relationships also appears to increase the odds of making an erroneous prognostic prediction.

Clinician predictions may be improved by integrating within the clinician's judgment some other form of estimating prognosis, such as life tables, published studies, or prognostic indices.[50] Life tables require knowledge of only a few demographic characteristics, most commonly age and gender.[5] However, there tends to be significant variation in life expectancy based on life tables alone (**Table 1**), limiting their clinical applicability. Another method to determine prognosis is to reference published studies in which participants' diseases and demographics closely mirror those of a given patient. Importantly, because studies frequently exclude individuals who have multiple comorbidities or who are frail, prognostic estimates using published studies may often overstate survival.

Lastly, clinicians can use well-validated prognostic indices to help refine their prognostic estimates (**Table 2**). Prognostic indices are tools that use systematically selected characteristics from a particular population, such as age, comorbidities, functional status, and laboratory test results, to calculate a prognostic estimate. Use of any prognostic index requires some understanding of its accuracy, validity, and generalizability. For instance, if a prognostic index was created and tested in a community-based setting, it will likely overestimate prognosis in hospitalized adults.

Considerations of Prognosis in Select Diseases

Cancer

Prognosis for early-stage cancer is primarily based on tumor type, disease burden, and aggressiveness suggested by clinical, imaging, laboratory, pathologic, and molecular characteristics. For more advanced cancers, functional status has consistently demonstrated an association with survival, although length of survival may depend on the underlying cancer. For example, for patients with metastatic cancer with relatively

Table 1
Life table of upper, middle, and lower quartiles of life expectancy for women and men at selected ages

	Women			Men		
Age	Top 75th Percentile	50th Percentile	Lowest 25th Percentile	Top 75th Percentile	50th Percentile	Lowest 25th Percentile
65	26.9	21.2	14.2	24.3	18.3	11.4
70	22.2	16.9	10.7	19.8	14.4	8.5
75	17.8	12.9	7.6	15.6	10.8	6
80	13.6	9.3	5.1	11.8	7.7	4
85	9.9	6.3	3.2	8.5	5.2	2.5
90	6.9	4.1	1.9	5.9	3.4	1.6
95	4.7	2.6	1.2	4.1	2.2	1

Table 2
Examples of commonly used prognostic indices

	Prognostic Index	Patient Population	Web Site
Non-disease-specific examples	Walter 1-y index	Hospitalized adults ≥70 y old	www.ePrognosis.org
	Lee 4- and 10-y index	Community-dwelling adults ≥50 y old	
	Schonberg 5- and 9-y index	Community-dwelling adults ≥65 y old	
Disease-specific examples			
Cancer	Palliative Prognostic Score	Hospice and palliative care patients with advanced solid tumors	www.ePrognosis.org
Dementia	ADEPT	Nursing home residents with advanced dementia	www.ePrognosis.org
Heart failure	Seattle Heart Failure Model	Community-based heart failure patients without significant other comorbidities	http://depts.washington.edu/shfm

good treatment options, such as prostate or breast cancer, prognosis may be considerably longer than someone with pancreatic or biliary cancers, even among patients with poorer functional status. Clinicians can refer to published studies evaluating outcomes associated with specific cancer diagnoses and their treatments. Although this is particularly helpful in cancers whereby treatment modalities are frequently changing, caution is warranted when looking at survival estimates based on published studies because most of these trials do not include patients with poor functional status, multimorbidity, or organ dysfunction.

Advanced dementia
Individuals living with dementia typically have a prolonged period of severe functional disability as the disease progresses to its advanced stages. Unfortunately, estimating short-term prognosis in this patient population is difficult. Individuals with advanced disease may survive for several years with severe functional and cognitive impairments, yet run the risk of developing sudden, life-threatening complications, such as aspiration pneumonias and urinary tract infections. These complications serve as a marker of a very poor short-term survival. In a study of individuals with advanced dementia residing in a nursing home, the 6-month mortality after the development of pneumonia, a febrile episode, or eating difficulties was 47%, 45%, and 39%, respectively.[51] In another study, individuals with advanced dementia who were admitted to the hospital with either pneumonia or a hip fracture had a median survival of approximately 6 months.[52]

Hospice eligibility guidelines for dementia state that individuals need to meet or exceed stage 7a on the Functional Assessment Stage scale (**Table 3**) and must have at least 1 dementia-related complication (aspiration, upper urinary tract infection, sepsis, multiple stage 3–4 pressure injuries, persistent fever, weight loss >10% within 6 months). However, these criteria fail to accurately predict 6-month survival in those with advanced disease. An example of a mortality index that can be used in nursing home residents with advanced dementia is the Advanced Dementia Prognostic Tool (ADEPT), also found on ePrognosis.org. ADEPT can help identify nursing home residents with advanced dementia who are at high risk of death within 6 months, although only marginally better than current hospice eligibility guidelines.[53]

Congestive heart failure

Most deaths from advanced heart failure are preceded by a period of worsening symptoms, functional decline, and repeated hospitalizations as a result of progressive pump failure. Despite significant advances in the treatment of heart failure, the prognosis in patients who have been hospitalized for heart failure remains poor, with a 1-year mortality rate ranging from 20% to 47% after discharge. The prognosis is worse for those with multiple hospitalizations. The median survival in a study of older patients admitted for heart failure declined from 2.4 years in those with 1 hospitalization to 0.6 years for those with 4 hospitalizations.[54] Other indicators of a poor prognosis in heart failure include patient demographic factors, disease severity, comorbid conditions, physical examination findings, and laboratory values. Heart failure–specific prognostic indices often combine many of these factors to help identify patients who have a high short-term mortality.

COMMUNICATION OF THE PROGNOSIS

There are few tasks in clinical medicine that are as challenging, or as important, as skillfully communicating a patient's prognosis. Unfortunately, few clinicians receive formal training in how to effectively communicate prognostic information. To address this need, several communication aids have been developed to guide clinicians through the process of prognostic disclosure and to promote patient-centered communication. Ask-Tell-Ask is a simplified model that highlights the importance of assessing a patient's understanding before and after disclosing important information (**Table 4**). Similarly, the SPIKES (**Box 2**) and NURSE (**Table 5**) frameworks can help lead clinicians through the key considerations when disclosing prognostic information.[55] **Table 6** highlights additional resources related to communicating prognosis.

Table 3	
Summary of functional assessment staging	
Stage 1	No subjective or objective impairments in cognition
Stage 2	Mainly subject complains of forgetting names and misplacing objects
Stage 3	Objective evidence of memory impairment; impairment beginning to affect work performance
Stage 4	Moderate cognitive decline with impairments in instrumental activities of daily living
Stage 5	Difficulty with naming current aspects of their lives with some disorientation
Stage 6 (a-e)	Difficulty dressing, bathing, toileting without assistance. Experiences urinary and fecal incontinence in stage 6d and 6e
Stage 7 (a-f)	Speech declines from <6 intelligible words per day (7a) to one or less (7b). Progressive loss of ability to ambulate (7c), sit up (7d), smile (7e), and hold head up (7f)

Table 4
Ask-tell-ask

		Example Statement
Ask	Clarify what prognostic information the patient wants to know and ask for permission to disclose this information.	"What questions do you have about how your symptoms may change over the next few weeks?"
Tell	Disclose the requested information using simple clear language.	"Your shortness of breath will continue to worsen as your disease progresses."
Ask	Clarify the patient's understanding and interpretation of the disclosed information as well as how this may inform future decisions or goals.	"How does this information impact your preferences about your treatment options?"

Data from Back AL, Arnold RM, Baile WF, et al. Approaching Difficult Communication Tasks in Oncology. CA Cancer J Clin 2005;55(3):164-177.

Setting

Clinicians should prepare for prognostic disclosure. Conversations should ideally be held in a private setting and without disruption. Clinicians should ensure that they are familiar with the case and have reviewed the relevant information ahead of time.

Perception

A key step before prognostic disclosure is evaluating the patient's current understanding of his or her medical condition. Often, a clinician can best assess a patient's understanding through the use of open-ended, exploratory questions; however, for some patients, directed questioning may be required.

Invitation

Clinicians should gauge the patient's desire for prognostic disclosure. Although most patients want to discuss their prognosis with their clinicians, those who prefer not to should have the opportunity to communicate this preference. Clinicians should similarly clarify which outcomes their patients find most relevant and want disclosed. For example, a patient may prefer to not discuss how much time he has left but may want to know what changes in his functional independence he can reasonably expect. Clinicians should also assess patients' preferences regarding how and

Box 2
SPIKES framework for delivering serious news

Setting (eg, ensuring a private location, minimizing interruptions)

Perception (eg, assessing the patient's understanding)

Invitation (eg, clarifying what information the patient wants to know)

Knowledge (eg, stating the information clearly)

Emotion (eg, identifying and responding to patient's emotion with empathy)

Summarize/strategize (eg, determining next steps, closing the encounter)

Adapted from Back AL, Arnold RM, Baile WF, et al. Approaching Difficult Communication Tasks in Oncology. CA Cancer J Clin 2005;55(3):169; with permission.

Table 5
NURSE mnemonic for responding to emotion

	Example Statement
Name the emotion	"This news seems like it's a big surprise for you."
Understand the emotion	"It sounds like you are afraid of what's to come. Is that right?"
Respect/praise the patient/family	"I'm so impressed with the strength you have shown through all of this."
Support	"We're going to make a plan together."
Explore	"What's the most difficult part of this for you?"

Data from Back AL, Arnold RM, Baile WF, et al. Approaching Difficult Communication Tasks in Oncology. CA Cancer J Clin 2005;55(3):164-177.

when they want prognostic information communicated. Attentive listening is key to ensure that the clinician best understands the information needs of each patient.

Knowledge

Prognostic estimates should be communicated clearly and without the use of jargon. Prognostic disclosure is best done through a brief statement that addresses the expected outcome most relevant to the patient while incorporating the patient's communication preferences. For some patients, visual aids may be helpful in conveying information about the likelihood of a particular outcome (**Fig. 2**).

Emotion

Upon disclosing prognostic information, clinicians should anticipate that patients may have an acute emotional response. Although somewhat counterintuitive, a strong emotional reaction often indicates that the information was communicated effectively. Clinicians should allow patients time to process the new information while remaining attentive to their emotional experience. Attending to emotion can be accomplished through therapeutic silence or responding with empathic statements. The mnemonic NURSE highlights ways of responding to patients' emotional cues.[55]

Table 6
Selected resources for communicating prognostic information

Resource	Description	Web Site
VitalTalk	Communication skills training with modules on prognostication	https://www.vitaltalk.org
Serious Illness Care Program	A multifaceted program aimed at improving communication between clinicians and patients with serious illness	https://www.ariadnelabs.org/areas-of-work/serious-illness-care
Palliative Care Fast Facts	Concise, evidence-based, peer-reviewed summaries covering a variety of palliative care topics, including prognostication	http://www.mypcnow.org/fast-facts
Center to Advance Palliative Care	Online courses in prognostication	https://www.capc.org

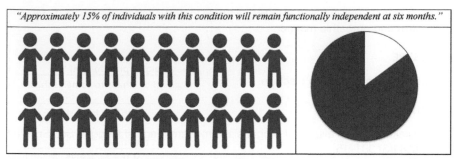

"*Approximately 15% of individuals with this condition will remain functionally independent at six months.*"

Fig. 2. Visual aids can assist in communicating the likelihood of specific clinical outcomes.

Summarize/Strategize

After responding to the patient's emotion, the clinician should assess the patient's understanding of the disclosed information and should address questions that arise. An effort should be made to delineate next steps because this can alleviate uncertainty or trepidation about the immediate plan of care.

INTERPRETATION AND INTEGRATION OF THE PROGNOSIS

The third, yet frequently underacknowledged, component of prognostication is the patient or surrogate's interpretation of the communicated prognosis. Take, for example, a patient with decompensated end-stage liver failure on maximum vasopressor support in the intensive care unit. The patient is not a transplant candidate and is actively dying. The patient's family, however, insists that the patient remains "full code" despite a communicated prognosis of hours to days. A clinician may be tempted to label the family as "in denial" or "unwilling to accept the truth." Alternatively, the clinician may assume that the patient's prognosis was not adequately communicated and therefore may repeatedly attempt to convince the family of the inevitability of the patient's impending death.

However, studies indicate that surrogates rarely base their view of a loved one's prognosis solely on the clinician's prognostic estimate. Instead, these studies suggest that surrogates attempt to balance the clinician's judgment with other factors, including their belief of the patient's intrinsic qualities and will to live; their observations of the patient; their belief in the power of their support and presence; and their optimism, intuition, and faith.[56–58] Furthermore, even in the face of poor prognostic information, patients and surrogates remain optimistic and overestimate survival. Given these findings, it can be helpful to communicate the specific factors influencing the clinician's prognostic estimate because these may also influence the patient or surrogate's interpretation of this information. It is also valuable to ask the patient or surrogate to share how they interpret the communicated prognosis and what other factors influence their beliefs because this can help guide further discussions.

SUMMARY

Prognostication is a key component in clinical decision making and is a fundamental skill for all practicing clinicians. Accurate prognostication allows for clinicians to provide patients and families with realistic options for care given current medical circumstances and aids in determining which interventions offer little chance of benefit because of competing risks of morbidity and mortality. The use of communication aids such as Ask-Tell-Ask and SPIKES can help in delivering prognostic estimates in an effective and empathic manner.

DISCLOSURE

The authors have nothing to disclose.

REFERENCES

1. Christakis NA. The ellipsis of prognosis in modern medical thought. Soc Sci Med 1997;44(3):301–15.
2. Gill TM. The central role of prognosis in clinical decision making. JAMA 2012;307: 199–200.
3. Temel JS, Greer JA, Admane S, et al. Longitudinal perceptions of prognosis and goals of therapy in patients with metastatic non-small-cell lung cancer: results of a randomized study of early palliative care. J Clin Oncol 2011;29(17):2319–26.
4. Murphy DJ, Burrows D, Santilli S, et al. The influence of the probability of survival on patients' preferences regarding cardiopulmonary resuscitation. N Engl J Med 1994;330:545–9.
5. Walter LC, Covinsky KE. Cancer screening in elderly patients: a framework for individualized decision making. JAMA 2001;285(21):2750–6.
6. Wright AA, Zhang B, Ray A, et al. Associations between end-of-life discussions, patient mental health, medical care near death, and caregiver bereavement adjustment. JAMA 2008;300:1665–73.
7. Weeks JC, Cook EF, O'Day SJ, et al. Relationship between cancer patients' predictions of prognosis and their treatment preferences. JAMA 1998;279(21): 1709–14.
8. Smith AK, Williams BA, Lo B. Discussing overall prognosis with the very elderly. N Engl J Med 2011;365(23):2149–51.
9. Fried TR, Bradley EH, O'Leary J. Prognosis communication in serious illness: perceptions of older patients, caregivers, and clinicians. J Am Geriatr Soc 2003; 51(10):1398–403.
10. Ahalt C, Walter LC, Yourman L, et al. "Knowing is better": preferences of diverse older adults for discussing prognosis. J Gen Intern Med 2012;27(5):568–75.
11. Koedoot CG, Oort F, de Haan R, et al. The content and amount of information given by medical oncologists when telling patients with advanced cancer what their treatment options are: palliative chemotherapy and watchful-waiting. Eur J Cancer 2004;40:225–35.
12. Fairchild A, Debenham B, Danielson B, et al. Comparative multidisciplinary prediction of survival in patients with advanced cancer. Support Care Cancer 2014; 22:611–7.
13. Butow PN, Dowsett S, Hagerty RG, et al. Communicating prognosis to patients with metastatic disease: what do they really want to know? Support Care Cancer 2002;10:161–8.
14. Hagerty RG, Butow PN, Ellis PM, et al. Communicating prognosis in cancer care: a systematic review of the literature. Ann Oncol 2005;16:1005–53.
15. Hancock K, Clayton JM, Parker SM, et al. Truth-telling in discussing prognosis in advanced life-limiting illnesses: a systematic review. Palliat Med 2007;21(6): 507–17.
16. Christakis NA. Death foretold: prophecy and prognosis in medical care. Chicago: University of Chicago Press; 1999.

17. Chen AB, Cronin A, Weeks JC, et al. Expectations about the effectiveness of radiation therapy among patients with incurable lung cancer. J Clin Oncol 2013; 31(21):2730–5.

18. Weeks JC, Catalano PJ, Cronin A, et al. Patients' expectations about effects of chemotherapy for advanced cancer. N Engl J Med 2012;367:1616–25.

19. Soylu C, Babacan T, Sever AR, et al. Patients' understanding of treatment goals and disease course and their relationship with optimism, hope, and quality of life: a preliminary study among advanced breast cancer outpatients before receiving palliative treatment. Support Care Cancer 2016;24(8):3481–8.

20. Enzinger AC, Zhang B, Schrag D, et al. Outcomes of prognostic disclosure: associations with prognostic understanding, distress, and relationship with physician among patients with advanced cancer. J Clin Oncol 2015;33(32):3809–16.

21. Daugherty CK, Hlubocky FJ. What are terminally ill cancer patients told about their expected deaths? A study of cancer physicians' self-reports of prognosis disclosure. J Clin Oncol 2008;26:5988–93.

22. Glare PA, Sinclair CT. Palliative medicine review: prognostication. J Palliat Med 2008;11(1):84–103.

23. Lamont EB, Christakis NA. Prognostic disclosure to patients with cancer near the end of life. Ann Intern Med 2001;134:1096–105.

24. Perez-Cruz PE, Dos Santos R, Silva TB, et al. Longitudinal temporal and probabilistic prediction of survival in a cohort of patients with advanced cancer. J Pain Symptom Manage 2014;48:875–82.

25. Stiel S, Bertram L, Neuhaus S, et al. Evaluation and comparison of two prognostic scores and the physicians' estimate of survival in terminally ill patients. Support Care Cancer 2010;18(1):43–9.

26. Christakis NA, Lamont EB. Extent and determinants of error in doctors' prognoses in terminally ill patients: prospective cohort study. BMJ 2000;320(7233):469–72.

27. Lam PT. Accuracy of clinical prediction of survival in a palliative care unit. Prog Palliat Care 2008;16:113–7.

28. Glare P, Virik K, Jones M, et al. A systematic review of physicians' survival predictions in terminally ill cancer patients. BMJ 2003;327:195–200.

29. Hallenbeck JL. Palliative care perspectives. New York: Oxford University Press; 2003.

30. Christakis NA, Iwashyna TJ. Attitude and self-reported practice regarding prognostication in a national sample of internists. Arch Intern Med 1998;158:2389–95.

31. Bradley EH, Hallemeier AG, Fried TR, et al. Documentation of discussions about prognosis with terminally ill patients. Am J Med 2001;111(3):218–23.

32. Field D, Copp G. Communication and awareness about dying in the 1990s. Palliat Med 1999;13(6):459–68.

33. The AM, Hak T, Koëter G, et al. Collusion in doctor-patient communication about imminent death: an ethnographic study. BMJ 2000;321(7273):1376–81.

34. Lin CC, Tsai HF, Chiou JF, et al. Changes in levels of hope after diagnostic disclosure among Taiwanese patients with cancer. Cancer Nurs 2003;26:155–60.

35. Kamihara J, Nyborn JA, Olcese ME, et al. Parental hope for children with advanced cancer. Pediatrics 2015;135(5):868–74.

36. Mack JW, Wolfe J, Cook EF, et al. Hope and prognostic disclosure. J Clin Oncol 2007;25(35):5636–42.

37. Smith TJ, Dow LA, Virago E, et al. Giving honest information to patients with advanced cancer maintains hope. Oncology 2010;24(6):521–5.

38. Zwingmann J, Baile WF, Schmier JW, et al. Effects of patient-centered communication on anxiety, negative affect, and trust in the physician in delivering a cancer diagnosis: a randomized, experimental study. Cancer 2017;123(16):3167.
39. Lee MK, Baek SK, Kim S-Y. Awareness of incurable cancer status and health-related quality of life among advanced cancer patients: a prospective cohort study. Palliat Med 2013;27:144–54.
40. Mack JW, Weeks JC, Wright AA. End-of-life discussions, goal attainment, and distress at the end of life: predictors and outcomes of receipt of care consistent with preferences. J Clin Oncol 2010;28:1203–8.
41. D'Agostino TA, Atkinson TM, Latella LE, et al. Promoting patient participation in healthcare interactions through communication skills training: a systematic review. Patient Educ Couns 2017;10:1247–57.
42. Leung KK, Chiu TY, Chen CY. The influence of awareness of terminal condition on spiritual well-being in terminal cancer patients. J Pain Symptom Manage 2006;31:449–56.
43. Zachariae R, Pedersen CG, Jensen AB, et al. Association of perceived physician communication style with patient satisfaction, distress, cancer-related self-efficacy, and perceived control over the disease. Br J Cancer 2003;88:658–65.
44. Chan WCH. Being aware of the prognosis: how does it relate to palliative care patients' anxiety and communication difficulty with family members in the Hong Kong Chinese context? J Palliat Med 2011;14(9):997–1003.
45. Morita T, Tsunoda J, Inoue S, et al. Improved accuracy of physicians' survival prediction for terminally ill cancer patients using the Palliative Prognostic Index. Palliat Med 2001;15:419–24.
46. Teno JM, Harrell FE Jr, Knaus W, et al. Prediction of survival for older hospitalized patients: the HELP survival model. Hospitalized Elderly Longitudinal Project. J Am Geriatr Soc 2000;48(5 Suppl):S16–24.
47. Knaus WA, Harrell FE Jr, Lynn J, et al. The SUPPORT prognostic model. Objective estimates of survival for seriously ill hospitalized adults. Study to understand prognoses and preferences for outcomes and risks of treatments. Ann Intern Med 1995;122(3):191.
48. Maltoni E, Scarpi E, Pittureri E, et al. Prospective comparison of prognostic scores in palliative care cancer populations. Oncologist 2012;17:446–54.
49. Hamaker ME, Augschoell J, Stauder R. Clinical judgement and geriatric assessment for predicting prognosis and chemotherapy completion in older patients with a hematological malignancy. Leuk Lymphoma 2016;57(11):2560–7.
50. Yourman LC, Lee SJ, Schonberg MA, et al. Prognostic indices for older adults: a systematic review. JAMA 2012;307(2):182–92.
51. Mitchell SL, Teno JM, Kiely DK, et al. The clinical course of advanced dementia. N Engl J Med 2009;361:1529–38.
52. Morrison RS, Siu AL. Survival in end-stage dementia following acute illness. JAMA 2000;298(1):47–52.
53. Mitchell SL, Miller SC, Teno JM, et al. Prediction of 6-month survival of nursing home residents with advanced dementia using ADEPT vs hospice eligibility guidelines. J Am Med Assoc 2010;304(17):1929–35.
54. Setoguchi S, Stevenson LW, Schneeweiss S. Repeated hospitalizations predict mortality in the community population with heart failure. Am Heart J 2007;154:260–6.
55. Back A, Arnold R, Tulsky J. Mastering communication with seriously ill patients: balancing honesty with empathy and hope. New York: Cambridge University Press; 2009.

56. Zier LS, Sottile PD, Hong SY, et al. Surrogate decision makers' interpretation of prognostic information: a mixed-methods study. Ann Intern Med 2012;156(5): 360–6.

57. Char SJL, Evans LR, Malvar GL, et al. A randomized trial of two methods to disclose prognosis to surrogate decision makers in intensive care units. Am J Respir Crit Care Med 2010;182(7):905–9.

58. White DB, Ernecoff N, Buddadhumaruk P, et al. Discordance about prognosis between physicians and surrogate decision makers of critically ill patients. JAMA 2016;315(19):2086–94.

Recognizing and Managing Polypharmacy in Advanced Illness

Shaida Talebreza, MD, AGSF[a],
Mary Lynn McPherson, PharmD, MA, MD, BCPS[b],*

KEYWORDS

- Polypharmacy • Deprescribing • Geriatrics • Advanced illness • Communication

KEY POINTS

- The term "polypharmacy" refers to the regular use of at least 5 medications by an individual.
- Patients with an advanced illness are at heightened risk of adverse effects from polypharmacy, and medication regimens should be pared to the most essential, necessary medications.
- There are several models that may be used in deprescribing in advanced illness, including a systematic mindset that considers the patient's goals of care and medication benefits and burdens, tools that consider the medication list in its totality, and medication-specific guidance.
- Effective communication between health care providers, and with patients and families, is a critically important part of the deprescribing process.

INTRODUCTION: A CALL TO ACTION IN POLYPHARMACY

Although one might be tempted to believe the term "polypharmacy" refers to a patient who frequents several pharmacies, it is typically defined as the regular use of at least 5 medications by an individual.[1] Polypharmacy is growing in prevalence; one study reports that polypharmacy in the United States increased from 8% in 1999 to 2000 to 15% in 2011 to 2012.[2] More than 90% of patients in long-term care facilities receive more than 5 medications.[3] This is particularly concerning in older adults who are more likely to take multiple medications, and are at higher risk for medication-related

[a] Geriatric and Academic Palliative Medicine, Division of Geriatrics, University of Utah School of Medicine, George E. Wahlen Salt Lake City Veterans Affairs Medical Center, 30 North 1900 East SOM AB193, Salt Lake City, UT 84132-0001, USA; [b] Advanced Post-Graduate Education in Palliative Care, Online Master of Science in Palliative Care, Department of Pharmacy Practice and Science, University of Maryland School of Pharmacy Baltimore, 20 North Pine Street, S405, Baltimore, MD 21201, USA
* Corresponding author.
E-mail address: mmcphers@rx.umaryland.edu

Med Clin N Am 104 (2020) 405–413
https://doi.org/10.1016/j.mcna.2019.12.003
medical.theclinics.com

adverse effects.[1] Polypharmacy has been associated with higher symptom burden and lower quality of life for patients with advanced illness.

The solution to polypharmacy is careful assessment of a patient's medication regimen and discontinuing medications that are harmful or medically future. This practice is referred to as "deprescribing," and is defined as "the systematic process of identifying and discontinuing drugs in instances in which existing or potential harms outweigh existing or potential benefits within the context of individual patient's care goals, current level of functioning, life expectancy, values, and preferences."[4] Scott and colleagues[4] recommend a 5-step process for deprescribing:

1. Confirm all medications the patient is taking
2. Evaluate risk of drug-induced harm
3. Determine whether each drug should be discontinued
4. Prioritize medications to discontinue
5. Implement recommendations and monitor the patient

Evidence regarding the effectiveness of deprescribing is limited and outcomes are not definitive, but data suggest this is a safe and feasible practice with some favorable outcomes.[1,5–7]

Anywhere from 40% to 90% of adults surveyed agreed that they take too many medications, and most are willing to discontinue 1 or more of their medications if their prescriber agreed or recommended such.[8–11] Most prescribers, when surveyed, stated they are comfortable deprescribing, but less so if a medication was prescribed by another prescriber, was a guideline-recommended medication, or if the patient or family thought the medication was important to continue.[12]

POLYPHARMACY IN ADVANCED ILLNESS

It would be reasonable to expect that patients living with a serious or advanced illness may have medications added to treat pain and other physical symptoms, but preventive medications and other medically futile medications would be discontinued. But this does not seem to be the case, which is unfortunate because this is a vulnerable population at greater risk for medication-induced adverse effects. Morin and colleagues[13] reported on patients in their last year of life in Sweden from 2007 to 2013. The proportion of patients receiving more than 10 medications increased from 30% to 47%; the investigators concluded that many of these were symptom-relief medications, but also a great number of preventive treatments of nebulous benefit.[13–15] A report of prescribing practices of 179 patients in the last week of life in the Netherlands showed the mean number of medications prescribed was 9 in the 1 week before death, and 6 on the day of death. Almost 30% of this population were receiving a preventive medication on the day of death.[16] It is unclear why this is the case; perhaps prescribers fail to continually reevaluate the appropriateness of each prescribed medication, and medications are added not only for pain and symptom relief, but also to alleviate side effects of other medications (eg, a "prescription cascade").[17]

TOOLS FOR DEPRESCRIBING IN FRAIL OLDER ADULTS AND THOSE WITH ADVANCED ILLNESS

There are many tools available to guide practitioners in deprescribing, but few of them are specific for frail older adults or patients with an advanced illness. Thompson and colleagues[18] conducted an extensive review of the literature and identified 3 main categories of tools that may be appropriate in this situation. A description of each category follows.

Models or Frameworks

This model describes a "way of thinking," an approach to decision making that considers the patient's goals of care, time to benefit of each medication, the patient's life expectancy, clinical status, and whether or not treatment aligns with the patient's goals. Holmes and colleagues[19] provide several examples of using the model they proposed that demonstrates consideration of each of these variables. For example, a 75-year-old highly functional woman with hypertension and osteoarthritis was recently diagnosed with type 2 diabetes mellitus. The patient has an expected life expectancy of 17 years, and her goal is to maximize life span and maintain functionality. It would be appropriate to treat diabetes because benefit will be seen in a time frame less than her expected life span. On the other hand, consider a patient with multiple comorbidities and a prognosis of several months. The patient wishes comfort care and is admitted to hospice. In this case, medications used to treat pain and other symptoms would be appropriate, and medications that are no longer beneficial should be discontinued.[19]

Entire Medication List

This category includes tools that allow for identifying and prioritizing which medications should be discontinued, based on the patient's clinical status.[18] Thompson and colleagues[18,20,21] identified several tools; 2 well-recognized tools into the Geriatric-Palliative algorithm, and the STOPPFrail instrument. The Geriatric-Palliative algorithm poses a series of considerations to the user, such as whether or not an evidence-based consensus exists for the use of the medication in its current context, the indication is valid and relevant for the specific patient, whether or not adverse effects are present and potentially outweigh benefits of therapy, if there is alternate preferred therapy, and if the dosage can be reduced without causing harm.[20] Applying this model to 119 disabled older adults compared with 71 control patients demonstrated a reduction in mortality rates, referrals to acute care facilities, lower costs, and improved quality of life.[20]

STOPPFrail is a list of potentially inappropriate prescribing indicators designed to assist physicians with stopping such medications in older patients (≥65 years) who meet ALL of the criteria listed as follows:

- End-stage irreversible pathology
- Poor 1-year survival prognosis
- Severe functional impairment or severe cognitive impairment or both
- Symptom control is the priority rather than prevention of disease progression[21]

This is a validated instrument containing 27 criteria that indicate potentially inappropriate medications in frail older patients with limited life expectancy.

One would expect the "Beers criteria" (the American Geriatrics Society Beers Criteria for Potentially Inappropriate Medication Use in Older Adults) to be included in this category.[22] However, these criteria, and others, such as the STOPP/START criteria, are not specific for patients who are late in life.[23]

Medication-Specific Guidance

The last set of tools provides detailed guidance of deprescribing specific medications/medication classes. One classic example is the guidance provided on the Web site deprescribing.org, which includes patient and professional educational materials and algorithms.[24] Several examples of approaches to deprescribing specific medications/medication classes are illustrated here.

Statins

Treatment benefits with statin medications include decreased vascular events and mortality, and potential harms include myopathy and fatigue. According to randomized control trial data in older adults, the time to benefit of statins for primary prevention is 2 years for myocardial infarction prevention and 5 years for stroke prevention.[25,26] The time to benefit is shorter for secondary prevention in younger people.[26,27] No specific trials for secondary prevention in patients older than 80 years have been identified.[28] Guides to deprescribing recommend stopping statins (without the need for tapering) in patients with limited prognosis.[28] A review of the benefit of statins in patients with high noncardiovascular mortality risk concluded that statins had little reduction in total mortality in these patients.[28] In patients with life-limiting illness, a randomized control trial suggested that stopping statin medication was not only safe, but also improved quality of life.[29]

Diabetes medications

Treatment benefits for tighter glycemic control include reduction of microvascular complications, such as retinopathy, neuropathy, and nephropathy. Harms include risk of mortality from hypoglycemia. Studies note that older adults with a life expectancy of less than 10 years do not benefit from intensive glycemic control and are at higher risk of hypoglycemia.[30] In addition, the authors of the United Kingdom Diabetes Prevention Study found that patients who received intensive type 2 diabetes control for 10 years and then returned to looser glycemic control had a persistence of benefit of decreased microvascular events for 7 additional years.[31,32] A number of guidelines suggest approximate glycemic targets of 7.0% to 7.5% in healthy older adults with life expectancy of more than 10 years, 7.5% to 8.0% in those with moderate comorbidity and a life expectancy less than 10 years, and 8.0% to 9.0% in those with multiple morbidities and shorter life expectancy.[32,33] A comfort approach to glycemic control is often appropriate for patients with a very limited life expectancy. This approach includes avoidance of hypoglycemia and hyperglycemic symptoms, including thirst and polyuria.

Cholinesterase inhibitors

Benefits of cholinesterase inhibitors (CI) include statistically significant slowing of cognitive decline associated with types of dementia, but the clinical benefits are modest and it is uncertain if these benefits improve patients' daily functioning or reduce their need for supervision.[34] Harms of CIs include diarrhea, urinary incontinence, bradycardia, and appetite disturbance. No studies of CIs have investigated benefits of the mediation beyond 1 year.[34] Before starting a trial of CI medications, the American Geriatrics Society recommends discussing practical treatment goals that can be easily and routinely assessed for efficacy as well as the potential adverse effects, and tapering off of the medication after approximately 12 weeks if the treatment goals are not reached.[33] The University of Sydney provides an algorithm for deprescribing CIs after 1 year of use that includes directions on weaning off the mediation and symptoms to monitor during the tapering off period.[34] Given the lack of established benefit and risk of adverse events, both CIs and memantine generally should be discontinued or avoided in populations with far advanced dementia or short life expectancy.

Bisphosphonates

Benefits of bisphosphonates include reduced fracture risk for patients with low bone mineral density. Harms can include hypocalcemia, renal dysfunction, osteonecrosis of the jaw, and difficulty adhering to medication administration requirements (sitting up for 30 minutes and avoiding food and drink for an hour after taking the medication). The time to benefit of bisphosphonates is 1 to 3 years,[35,36] and therefore may not be beneficial to start in patients with a shorter prognosis than this timeframe. For

Table 1
The goals of care approach to discussing medication changes

Step 1	Introduce the conversation and elicit the patient's overall goals of care. **Why:** • Build trust and rapport. • Determine what matters most to the patient to ensure medication changes will assist them achieve goals meaningful to the patient and avoid unwanted burdens **How:** • I'd like to make sure that we are providing you with the best care possible. What are the things that matter most to you? • What would a great day look like? • What symptoms do we need to manage to help you have more great days? • What symptoms are already well managed?
Step 2	Reflect back the patient's goals and ask permission to proceed with a thorough medication reconciliation. **Why:** • Reflecting back the patient's goals continues to build the therapeutic alliance by letting patients know they have been heard. • Asking permission to proceed with the medication reconciliation demonstrates respect for the patient and allows patients to control the timing of the discussion. Patients with advanced illness can often feel vulnerable and powerless, letting them control the timing of aspects of their care can restore a feeling of autonomy. **How:** • Thanks for sharing that information with me. • *It sounds like it is really important to make sure your [name symptoms] are well managed. It is also really important to us as your health care team to keep you safe as well.* • *For this reason, it is important to look through all your medications together to see if there are any changes that we should make to treat your [symptoms] as effectively and safely as possible.* • *Is now an OK time to go over the medications with you and your family?*
Step 3	Determine the patient's adherence with treatment regimen and perception of medication benefits and risks. **Why:** • Can help clinicians explore if the patient or caregiver has a strong emotional attachment to a potentially harmful medication or is reluctant to start a potentially beneficial medication and assess their readiness to make changes to their medication regimen. **How:** • Are there medications that are prescribed that you aren't taking or that you would like to stop? • How do you feel about taking [medication name]? • What are you hoping [medication name] can do for you? • What worries you about taking [medication name]? • Are you having any [side effects, any trouble with how often you need to take it, problems with the cost of the medication]?
Step 4	Make recommendations about prescribing or deprescribing in alignment with patient goals and with consideration of prognosis. **Why:** • Helping patients understand how medication changes align with their goals is another crucial step in building a therapeutic alliance. • *NOTE:* This alliance may not develop during the first visit with a patient. Clinicians may need to have a series of conversations using effective communication skills to build the trust necessary for patients to be willing to consider the clinician's recommendations.

(continued on next page)

Table 1 (*continued*)	

	How:
	• Can we talk about how your medications fit in with your goals to [name goal] and our goal to keep you safe?
	Prescribe:
	• I recommend we start medication because it will help you reach your goal of…
	Deprescribe:
	• Frequently medications that were once needed are no longer helpful, and in some cases, can even be harmful. From what I know about your goals for your health, I am concerned that [medications] are no longer helpful for you and may be actually harming you.
	• Is it OK if I make a recommendation?
	• *I recommend that we wean you off of [medication]*
	  ○ Because it has already done its job and you'll still benefit from it even when we stop it.
	  ○ Because it is no longer helping you and is actually harming you by [describe adverse effects].

Step 5	Acknowledge the patient's concerns, realign with goals, and provide reassurance.
	Why:
	   Conversations about medication changes may be emotionally difficult for patients with advanced illness, acknowledging this difficulty, aligning with goals, and providing reassurance can build trust.
	How:
	Acknowledge:
	• It can be scary to make changes to your medications.
	• It seems like you may be worried that starting/stopping [medication name]
	  ○ Means you are dying right now or may cause you to die sooner.
	  ○ would worsen your symptoms of…
	Realign:
	• It sounds like it is important for you to keep taking medications that will help you [manage symptom]. We want to make sure you are safe and comfortable too.
	Reassure:
	• We certainly wouldn't [stop, change, add] a medication if we thought it would
	  ○ Shorten your life.
	  ○ Make your symptoms worse.
	  ○ Cause you harm.

Step 6	Summarize the plan. **Why:** • Ensure that the patient understands and agrees to the plan. **How:** • Would it be OK if we [restart, change, or add medications] now? OR • We need to [restart, change, or add medications] to keep you safe. • We will be here for you and will monitor you very closely to make sure your symptoms are managed and can make changes at any time needed.

patients who have had 5 years of continuous treatment with an oral bisphosphonate, the benefit can persist 5 years after the medication has stopped (with no need for tapering).[36,37]

COMMUNICATING WITH COMPASSION: APPLYING A GOALS-OF-CARE APPROACH TO DISCUSSING MEDICATION CHANGES

To effectively manage polypharmacy, health care providers must not only possess the evidence-based pharmacologic knowledge to make recommendations for or against medications in advanced illness, but must also use compassionate communication skills to share these data successfully. Multiple studies have demonstrated that focusing only on data and information when attempting to educate patients can backfire, so that individuals become more entrenched in their own misperceptions,[38–40] whereas using compassionate communication skills can build trust and adherence.[41] Clinicians can apply communication skills to discussions about medication changes to create a therapeutic alliance with patients and caregivers. These skills include the ask-tell-ask technique and responding to emotions using naming, understanding, respecting, supporting, and exploring (ie, the NURSE mnemonic).[42] These communication skills can be used in a number of steps to apply a goals-of-care approach to discussing medication changes. **Table 1** defines each step in the conversation, outlines rationale for why the step is important, and provides phrases to demonstrate how to conduct the conversation.

SUMMARY

Older adults, particularly those late in life, are at higher risk for medication misadventure, yet bear the burden of increasing polypharmacy. It is incumbent on practitioners who care for this vulnerable population to use one or more approaches to deprescribe medications that impose a greater burden than benefit, including medically futile medications. It is essential that health care providers use compassionate communication skills when explaining these interventions with patients and families, pointing out that this is a positive, patient-centric intervention.

ACKNOWLEDGMENTS

The authors thank Anna Beck, MD, for her input on phrases in **Table 1**.

REFERENCES

1. Rankin A, Cadogan CA, Patterson SM, et al. Interventions to improve the appropriate use of polypharmacy for older people. Cochrane Database Syst Rev 2018;(9):CD008165.
2. Kantor ED, Rehm CD, Haas JS, et al. Trends in prescription drug use among adults in the United States from 1999-2012. JAMA 2015;314:1818–31.
3. Jokanovic N, Tan ECK, Dooley MJ, et al. Prevalence and factors associated with polypharmacy in long-term care facilities: a systematic review. J Am Med Dir Assoc 2015;16:e1–12.
4. Scott IA, Hilmer SN, Reeve E, et al. Reducing inappropriate polypharmacy: The process of deprescribing. JAMA Intern Med 2015;175(5):827–34.
5. Reeve R, Thompson W, Farrell B. Deprescribing: a narrative review of the evidence and practical recommendations for recognizing opportunities and taking action. Eur J Intern Med 2017;38:3–11.
6. Page AT, Clifford RM, Potter K, et al. The feasibility and effect of deprescribing in older adults on mortality and health: a systematic review and meta-analysis. Br J Clin Pharmacol 2016;82:583–623.
7. Dills H, Shah K, Messinger-Rapport B, et al. Deprescribing medications for chronic diseases management in primary care settings: a systematic review of randomized controlled trials. J Am Med Dir Assoc 2018;19:923–35.
8. Sirois C, Ouellet N, Reeve E. Community-dwelling older people's attitudes towards deprescribing in Canada. Res Social Adm Pharm 2017;13:864–70.

9. Kalogianis MJ, Wimmer BC, Turner JP, et al. Are residents of aged care facilities willing to have their medications deprescribed? Res Social Adm Pharm 2016;12:784–8.
10. Qi K, Reeve E, Hilmer SN, et al. Older peoples' attitudes regarding polypharmacy, statin use and willingness to have statins deprescribed in Australia. Int J Clin Pharm 2015;37:949–57.
11. Reeve E, Wolff JL, Skehan M, et al. Assessment of attitudes toward deprescribing in older Medicare beneficiaries in the United States. JAMA Intern Med 2018;178(12):167301680.
12. Djatche L, Singer D, Hegarty SE, et al. How confident are physicians in deprescribing for the elderly and what barriers prevent deprescribing? J Clin Pharm Ther 2018;43:550–5.
13. Morin L, Vetrano DL, Rizzuto D, et al. Choosing wisely? Measuring the burden of medications in older adults near the end of life: nationwide, longitudinal cohort study. Am J Med 2017;130(8):927–36.
14. Morin L, Todd A, Barclay S, et al. Preventive drugs in the last year of life of older adults with cancer: Is there room for deprescribing? Cancer 2019. [Epub ahead of print].
15. Morin L, Wastesson JW, Laroche ML, et al. How many older adults receive drugs of questionable clinical benefit near the end of life? A cohort study. Palliat Med 2019;33(8):1080–90.
16. Arevalo JJ, Geijteman ECT, Huisman BAA, et al. Medication use in the last days of life in hospital, hospice, and home settings in the Netherlands. J Palliat Med 2018;21(2):149–55.
17. Schenker Y, Park SY, Jeong K, et al. Associations between polypharmacy, symptom burden, and quality of life in patients with advanced, life-limiting illness. J Gen Intern Med 2019;34:559.
18. Thompson W, Lundby C, Graacaek T, et al. Tools for deprescribing in frail older persons and those with limited life expectancy: a systematic review. J Am Geriatr Soc 2018;67(1):172–80.
19. Holmes HM, Hayley DC, Alexander GC, et al. Reconsidering medication appropriateness for patients late in life. Arch Intern Med 2006;166:605–9.
20. Garfinkle D, Ma SZ, Ben-Israel J. The war against polypharmacy: a new cost-effective geriatric-palliative approach for improving drug therapy in disabled elderly people. Isr Med Assoc J 2007;9:430–4.
21. Lavan AH, Gallagher P, Parson CA, et al. STOPPFrail (Screening Tool of Older Persons Prescriptions in Frail adults with limited life expectancy): consensus validation. Age Ageing 2017;46:600–7.
22. American Geriatrics Society 2019 Updated AGS beer criteria for potentially inappropriate medications use in older adults. J Am Geriatr Soc 2019;67(4):674–94.
23. Hill-Taylor B, Walsh KA, Stewart S, et al. Effectiveness of the STOPP/START (screening tool of older persons' potentially inappropriate prescriptions/ screening tool to alert doctors to the right treatment) criteria: systematic review and meta-analysis of randomized controlled studies). J Clin Pharm Ther 2016;41(2):158–60.
24. Bruyère deprescribing guidelines research team. Available at: www.deprescribing.org. Accessed October 14, 2019.
25. Lee SJ, Kim CM. Individualizing prevention for older adults. J Am Geriatr Soc 2018;66(2):229–34.

26. Hawley CE, Roefaro J, Forman DE, et al. Statins for primary prevention in those aged 70 years and older: a critical review of recent cholesterol guidelines. Drugs Aging 2019;36(8):687–99.

27. Barter PJ, Waters DD. Variations in time to benefit among clinical trials of cholesterol-lowering drugs. J Clin Lipidol 2018;12(4):857–62.

28. A guide to deprescribing statins. 2019. Available at: https://www.primaryhealthtas. com.au/wp-content/uploads/2018/09/A-Guide-to-Deprescribing-Statins-2019.pdf. Accessed October 10, 2019.

29. Kutner S, Blatchford PJ, Taylor DH Jr, et al. Safety and benefit of discontinuing statin therapy in the setting of advanced, life-limiting illness: A randomised clinical trial. JAMA Intern Med 2015;175(5):691–700.

30. Sue Kirkman M, Briscoe VJ, Clark N, et al. Diabetes in older adults: a consensus report. J Am Geriatr Soc 2012;60:2342–56.

31. Yau CK, Eng C, Cenzer IS, et al. Glycosylated hemoglobin and functional decline in community-dwelling nursing home-eligible elderly adults with diabetes mellitus. J Am Geriatr Soc 2012;60:1215–21.

32. A guide to deprescribing antIhyperglycaemic agents. 2019. Available at: https://www.primaryhealthtas.com.au/wp-content/uploads/2018/09/A-Guide-to-Deprescribing-Anthyperglycaemics-2019.pdf. Accessed October 10, 2019.

33. Choosing wisely American Geriatrics Society ten things clinicians and patients should question. 2015. Available at: https://www.choosingwisely.org/societies/american-geriatrics-society/. Accessed October 10, 2019.

34. A guide to deprescribing cholinesterase inhibitors. 2019. Available at: https://www.primaryhealthtas.com.au/wp-content/uploads/2018/09/A-Guide-to-Deprescribing-Cholinesterase-Inhibitors-2019.pdf. Accessed October 10, 2019.

35. Crandall CJ, Newberry SJ, Diamant A, et al. Comparative effectiveness of pharmacological treatments to prevent fractures. Ann Intern Med 2014;161:711–23.

36. A guide to deprescribing bisphosphonates. 2019. Available at: https://www.primaryhealthtas.com.au/wp-content/uploads/2018/09/A-Guide-to-Deprescribing-Bisphosphonates-2019.pdf. Accessed October 10, 2019.

37. Schwartz AV, Bauer DC, Cummings SR, et al. Efficacy of continued alendronate for fractures in women with and without prevalent vertebral fracture: the FLEX trial. J Bone Miner Res 2010;25(5):976–82.

38. Carroll AE. Health facts aren't enough. Should persuasion become a priority? New York Times 2019.

39. Nyhan B, Reifler J, Richey S, et al. Effective messages in vaccine promotion: a randomized trial. Pediatrics 2014;133:4.

40. Nyhan B, Reifler J, Ubel PA. The hazards of correcting myths about health care reform. Med Care 2013;51(2):127–32.

41. Back AL, Arnold RM, Baile WF, et al. Approaching difficult communication tasks in oncology. CA Cancer J Clin 2005;55(3):164–77.

42. U.S. Department of Veterans Affairs National Center for Ethics in Health Care. Goals of care conversations training for physicians, advance practice registered nurses, and physician assistants website. 2019. Available at: https://www.ethics.va.gov/goalsofcaretraining/practitioner.asp. Accessed October 10, 2019.

Pain Management in Patients with Serious Illness

Kimberly Angelia Curseen, MD[a],*, Jabeen Taj, MD[b], Quintesia Grant, MD, PhD[c,d]

KEYWORDS

- Pain management • Pain assessment • Total pain • Opioids • Nonmalignant pain

KEY POINTS

- Pain management for patient with serious illness is a dynamic process that changes with patients as their illnesses progress.
- Providers need to be skilled at pain assessments to provide the best care and make appropriate choices for patient safety.
- Safe opioid prescribing should be a priority for all patients on opioid therapy.
- Providers should be skilled in assessing for total pain, which can affect the ability of patients to cope serious illness.
- Providers should use a multimodal and interprofessional approach to pain management.

Management of pain in any patient with serious illness is based on a few general principles:

Categorization of pain:

1. Acute versus chronic
2. Cause
3. Characteristics

Acute pain is generally traced back to a noxious stimulus and has a clearly defined onset, pattern, and exacerbating/relieving factors. Chronic pain is more ill-defined, usually more than 6 months in duration, of fluctuating intensity, and not linearly related to the inciting event. Management of chronic pain is therefore more challenging and requires a careful pain assessment and targeted pain relief with

[a] Internal Medicine, Division of Palliative Medicine, Family and Preventive Medicine Emory School of Medicine, Emory Palliative Care Center, 1821 Clifton Road, Northeast, Suite 1017, Atlanta, GA 30329, USA; [b] Hospice and Palliative Medicine, Cardiac Palliative Care, Medicine, Division of Palliative Medicine, Family and Preventive Medicine Emory School of Medicine, Emory University Hospital, 1821 Clifton Road, Northeast, Suite 1017, Atlanta, GA 30329, USA; [c] Palliative and Supportive Care, Grady Memorial Hospital, Harbor Grace Hospice, Atlanta, GA, USA; [d] Medicine, Division of Palliative Medicine, Family and Preventive Medicine Emory School of Medicine, 1821 Clifton Road, Northeast, Suite 1017, Atlanta, GA 30329, USA
* Corresponding author.
E-mail address: kacurseen@emory.edu
Twitter: @curseen (K.A.C.)

Med Clin N Am 104 (2020) 415–438
https://doi.org/10.1016/j.mcna.2020.01.005
0025-7125/20/© 2020 Elsevier Inc. All rights reserved.

achievable goals.[1] Determining the cause of pain in serious illness is extremely important because it aids in choosing the right analgesic. Although opioids treat pain universally, they are not the best medications for psychosomatic or neuropathic pain, which may be best treated with a nonopioid approach. Characteristics of pain lead to further differentiation of the pain symptom and help in completing a comprehensive pain assessment and effective management. This article explores pain management principles that are universally important when managing patients with serious illness.

PAIN ASSESSMENT

The goal of a comprehensive pain assessment is to determine the cause of the pain and to determine the best modality to manage the pain (**Box 1**). The key to achieving this goal is to take a thorough pain history. One of the key objectives is to consider the patient's previous experience with pain, including pain regimens, duration of pain, and description of pain.[2,3] Obtaining as much information as possible during a pain history allows optimal pain management and improvement in function. There have been several tools that have been created to help with important considerations in the

---

Box 1
Comprehensive pain assessment

Location

Radiation

Severity

Character/quality: complains of pain that is continuous, frequent, occasional, fluctuating, aching, nagging, miserable, sharp, tiring, penetrating, exhausting, gnawing, shooting, stabbing, burning, throbbing, numb, tender, and unbearable.

Timing: constant/continuous fluctuating/intermittent

Associated symptoms: it is associated with numbness and/or weakness

Alleviating factors: lifting, standing, walking, bending, sitting, turning, lying, heat, ice, weather changes, stress, cough, rest, medications, and massage

Exacerbating factors: lifting, standing, walking, bending, sitting, turning, lying, heat, ice, weather changes, stress, cough, rest, medications, and massage

Length of time pain has been present/duration:

Inciting event/injury

History of intervention: imaging, surgery and injections with significant/some/minimal/no benefit from the last injection lasting for weeks/months/years

Bowel/bladder incontinence

Weakness/falls

Sleep: pain does/does not interfere with sleep

Smoker: yes/no

Physical therapy/home exercises: with/without benefit

Patient's current pain medications as stated in medication list are providing significant/some/minimal/no benefit

Medication cause side effects: yes/no

Data from McGuire DB. Comprehensive and multidimensional assessment and measurement of pain. J Pain Symptom Manage 1992;7(5):312-9.

pain assessment. One common tool is the PQRST mnemonic, which prompts clinicians to focus on ameliorating factors, exacerbating factors, pain quality, radiation, severity, and timing[4,5] **(Table 1)**.

There are key considerations when asking a patient to indicate the severity of pain, including establishing the pain intensity pattern with the patient.[4,5] For example, asking the patient to give an average pain score over a period of 24 hours versus the current pain level.[5] In addition, make sure to use terms that the patient uses. Some patients tend to state that they are not in pain but are uncomfortable.[6,7] These considerations are critical because the severity of a patient's reported pain often drives the type of modality that is suggested for pain relief.[8] There are both unidimensional and multidimensional models that can be used to determine and describe the severity of a patient's pain.[9] Examples of a unidimensional pain scale include a numerical scale (from 1 to 10) or descriptors (mild, moderate, or severe). Multidimensional scales assess intensity, location, nature, and how pain is affecting functionality or mood of the patient. These scales may require assistance from a care provider to complete. Examples of a multidimensional scale include the Wong-Baker FACES Pain Rating Scale, which is commonly used for pediatric patients, or the Iowa Pain Thermostat.[10–12] Multidimensional scales should be considered in patients who speak different languages or who have speech impairment.

PAIN QUALITY

The common types of pain include nociceptive and neuropathic **(Table 2)**. Nociceptive pain is a result of tissue damage. This type of pain is recognized by nociceptors whose function is to recognize stimuli that can be harmful to the body. Furthermore, nociceptive pain can be divided into visceral and somatic pain. Somatic pain originates from skin, tissue, or muscles, whereas visceral pain originates from internal organs. Neuropathic pain is the result of nerve damage or an improperly working nervous system.[13] It can develop over time as a result of several chronic illnesses, including diabetes, stroke, cancer, or multiple sclerosis. Also, psychological pain is component of pain that is often overlooked but has specific characteristics that can be identified and managed appropriately. The adjectives that a patient uses can be used to determine the type of pain that is being experienced, and this can also help guide the type of analgesic that is most appropriate. Most patients with serious illness have mixed causes of pain, which can make management challenging.

Table 1 PQRST mnemonic		
P	Provocative or palliative factors	What makes your pain better or worse?
Q	Quality	Can you describe your pain? Is it sharp or dull?
R	Region or radiation	Where is your pain located? Does it stay in 1 place or does it move?
S	Severity	On a scale of 1–10, how bad is your pain?
T	Timing	Is your pain constant or does it come and go?

Adapted from Fink RM, Gallagher E. Cancer Pain Assessment and Measurement. Semin Oncol Nurs 2019;35(3):232; with permission.

Table 2
Pain categories

Nociceptive	Somatic	Visceral	Neuropathic	Psychological
Pain pathway activation following a noxious stimulus >> nociceptive afferent fibers >> spinal cord >> thalamus >> cerebral cortex	Afferent sensory pain fibers	Sympathetic fibers	Activation of excitatory neurotransmitters (aspartate and glutamate) involving the nerve fibers of the central and/or peripheral nervous system	Emotional distress, depression, chemical coping
Stabbing, piercing, hurting, burning, superficial, or deep, associated with noxious stimulus	Like nociceptive, aching, sharp, deep, well described	Vague, deep, ill-defined, cramping, difficult to quantify	Burning, stabbing, ice cold, hot pricking, electric shock, shooting, numbness, pins and needles	Emotional upset, pain medicines generally do not provide relief, amplifies physical pain

From Arthur J, Yennurajalingam S, Nguyen, L., et al. The routine use of the Edmonton Classification System for Cancer Pain in an outpatient supportive care center. Palliat Support Care. 2015;13(5):1185-92; with permission.

TEMPORAL FEATURES

Initial questions should focus on the duration of the patient's pain.[8,14] Specifically, whether the patient's pain is constant or intermittent. Patients with chronic illnesses often report having constant pain that has episodes of worsening or breakthrough pain. Intermittent pain can be attributed to activity or can be spontaneous. It is important to elicit the frequency, duration, associated factors, and impact of the pain.

ALLEVIATING AND EXACERBATING FACTORS

Before presenting to a clinician, patients often try different modalities for pain improvement. This approach may include medications in addition to physical stimuli such as use of heat, cold, massage, stretching, chiropractic maneuvers, as well as over-the-counter medications.[3,9] Similarly, asking about exacerbating factors is critical. Patients may report increased headache or back pain with Valsalva movements, which could indicate increased intracranial pressure or spine metastases, respectively. Reports of pleuritic pain could indicate irritation of the diaphragm.[3]

EFFECT OF PAIN ON FUNCTION

At the core of pain management is the goal of assisting the patient to maintain independence and to perform activities of daily living. It is imperative to ascertain what effect the pain is having on the patient's performance status.[15] An effective tool that focuses on the effect of a pain on a patient's function is the Brief Pain Inventory, which was developed by the Pain Research Group of the World Health Organization (WHO) Collaborating Centre for Symptom Evaluation in Cancer Care.[16,17] In addition to asking questions that focus on the patient's pain severity and relief in the past 24 hours, there are questions that focus on how the patient's pain is experienced. The questionnaire uses a numerical scale ranging from 1 to 10 to ask patients to describe how their pain interferes with the following: general activity, mood, walking ability, normal work, relation with other people, sleep, and enjoyment of life. Although thorough, the Brief Pain Inventory may be difficult to administer in the ambulatory care setting.

SPECIAL CONSIDERATIONS

It is important to remember that pain assessment includes more than exploring the patient's pain severity or previously used medications. It also important to determine how a patient views pain as well as additional factors that may exacerbate pain.[14,15] Principles of management of chronic pain include multidisciplinary management, including nonpharmacologic interventions, medications, and treatment of the underlying cause. Often patients have existential or spiritual pain that must be addressed in addition to physical pain. Patients who have chronic pain or who are seriously ill and experience pain may have other symptoms, such as anxiety or depression, that contribute to the pain experience.[11,18] Modalities such as cognitive behavior therapy, mindfulness, imagery, and pain journals are helpful nonpharmacologic tools that help to positively manage pain (**Table 3**).

Nonopioid Pain Management

The key to effective pain management is to determine the cause of the patient's pain and to proceed with the most appropriate modality for pain relief. Opioids are an important tool for pain relief in patients with serious illnesses. However, it is important to also consider other modalities, both nonopioid and nonpharmacologic, that will

| Table 3 | |
| Management of chronic pain in serious illness | |
Pharmacologic	Nonpharmacologic

WHO stepwise pain ladder approach:
Acetaminophen
NSAIDs
Opioids
Adjuvants
Interventions: injections, radiofrequency
   ablation, spinal cord stimulators,
   intrathecal/epidural pain pumps
	Physical therapy: aqua therapy, massage,
	   TENS
	Scrambler therapy
	Music therapy
	Pain psychology: guided imagery, cognitive
	   behavior therapy, biofeedback
	Exercise

Abbreviations: NSAIDs, nonsteroidal antiinflammatory drugs; TENS, transcutaneous electrical nerve stimulation.

more specifically target the pain stimulus. Nonopioid therapies include nonsteroidal antiinflammatory drugs (NSAIDs), acetaminophen, antidepressants, anticonvulsants, steroids, and topical agents. Nonpharmacologic interventional therapies include rehabilitative efforts, psychoeducational therapies, and alternative therapies.

World Health Organization pain ladder

The WHO developed the analgesic ladder to provide a framework for treating cancer pain.[19–21] The pain ladder was created because of the belief that uncontrolled cancer pain had become a public health concern and on the premise that health care providers could be taught to administer effective, available, and cost-effective medicines to adequately treat the cancer pain population.[20] However, the management of chronic pain syndromes requires a multipronged approach and the major critique for the WHO stepladder is its oversimplification of the complex pharmacologic strategies applied to chronic pain management and concerns around opioid dependence with limited analgesic benefits.[22] Please refer to **Box 2**.

Originally, the ladder consisted of 3 steps divided into mild, moderate, and severe pain. There is now a fourth step for interventional pain. Recommendation is for mild pain (rated 0–3) to be treated with acetaminophen, NSAIDs, or an adjuvant.[19–21] Opioid therapy is recommended starting at step 2 and 3, which are described as mild to moderate and moderate to severe pain, respectively. Adjuvant pain medications can be used at any step of the treatment ladder.[21] Interventional pain should be considered when pain medications have proved to be ineffective or if a patient has a specific structural area that can be targeted, thereby decreasing the need for oral pain medication.

| Box 2 |
World Health Organization analgesic ladder
Step 1: for mild pain, start with nonsteroidal antiinflammatories and acetaminophen ± adjuvants
Step 2: for mild to moderate pain, adding a weak opioid, which is defined as codeine, tramadol, hydrocodone ± adjuvants
Step 3: for moderate to severe pain, add a strong opioid such as morphine or fentanyl ± adjuvants
From Ballantyne JC, Kalso E, Stannard C. WHO analgesic ladder: a good concept gone astray. BMJ 2016;352:i20; with permission.

ACETAMINOPHEN AND NONSTEROIDAL ANTIINFLAMMATORY DRUGS

As discussed earlier, the recommendation for pain that is mild (rated 0–3 usually) is to begin with either acetaminophen or NSAIDs as first-line pharmacotherapy. Considerations for choosing between acetaminophen and an NSAID as the initial agent can be made by considering the patient's comorbid conditions, possible medication interactions, and previous treatment regimens. Acetaminophen is the drug of choice in patients that cannot be treated with NSAIDs because of comorbidities such as peptic ulcer disease, specific blood disorders (ie, hemophilia), or bronchial disease.[23,24] In addition, NSAIDs should be avoided in pregnancy and women who are breast feeding. Acetaminophen can be considered for long-term treatment of mild pain. The mechanism of action is not clearly known but is thought to be a result of prostaglandin inhibition in the central nervous system. The recommendation would be to schedule the chosen analgesic with allotment for breakthrough dosing if needed. Because of its ceiling effect, the maximum amount of acetaminophen given in 1 dose is 1 g. Prescribing more than this amount does not provide additional analgesia but increases associated toxicities. It is also important to remember that the maximum daily dose of acetaminophen is 4 g. However, the total daily dose should be decreased to 2 to 3 g in patients with liver disease and avoided in patients who abuse alcohol.[25,26]

NSAIDs provide pain relief by the inhibition of cyclooxygenase (COX) enzyme in the peripheral and central nervous systems[24] (Table 4). Additional functions include fever reduction, prevention of blood clots, and reduction of inflammation. NSAIDs have several benefits, including easy availability, several treatment indications, and additive relief if given with opioids. Common side effects from NSAID administration include gastrointestinal effects, acute renal injury, and bleeding.[25] NSAIDs can be classified into different categories based on their chemical structures in addition to whether they inhibit both types of COX enzymes or there is specific inhibition of the COX 2 enzyme.[24,27]

The National Comprehensive Cancer Network (NCCN) has also developed guidelines for cancer pain that provide specific recommendations for the use of NSAIDs for pain relief.[18] The first step is always to determine whether the patient has used a drug before with desired analgesic effect. If the patient has no prior history of NSAID use or no stated preference, NCCN advises using ibuprofen as the drug of choice. The starting dosage should be 400 mg every 8 hours, with consideration for a maximum daily dose of 3200 mg.[14,18] The maximum single dose of ibuprofen that should be administered is 800 mg. As noted earlier, there are intravenous (IV) formulations, such as ketorolac and indomethacin. Note that IV ketorolac is more common in the United States. It is recommended for acute, severe pain rather than only mild pain because the onset of action is within 10 minutes. Because of concerns for acute renal

Table 4				
Classes of nonsteroidal antiinflammatory drugs				
Salicylates	**Propionic Acids**	**Acetic Acids**	**Enolic Acids**	**Selective COX-2**
Aspirin	Ibuprofen	Etodolac	Piroxicam	Celecoxib
Salsalate	Ketoprofen	Ketorolac[a]	Meloxicam	
	Naproxen sodium	Indomethacin[a]		
		Sulindac		
		Diclofenac		
		Nabumetone		

[a] Drugs with intravenous formulations.
Data from Refs.[18,23,26]

failure, ketorolac is typically used for a maximum of 5 consecutive days.[28] Advised dosing is every 6 hours scheduled or as needed with maximum dose of 30 mg at once.

ADJUVANT MEDICATIONS

Adjuvant analgesics are indicated for pain that may be poorly responsive to opioids or, conversely, may be used in addition to prescribed opioids with the goal of decreasing the dose of opioids that a patient requires (**Table 5**). There are several classes of medications, including corticosteroids, bisphosphonates, tricyclic antidepressants, selective serotonin and norepinephrine uptake inhibitors, anticonvulsants, and topical analgesics.[14,18,28] The choice of adjuvant is based on the type of pain the patient reports. Somatic pain includes arthritis, bone pain secondary to metastasis, and wound pain. This pain is often described as throbbing, aching, or stabbing. Medications that are indicated for somatic pain include corticosteroids, NSAIDs, acetaminophen, and bisphosphonates.[14,28] Specifically, bone pain can be addressed with bisphosphonates and corticosteroids.[29,30] Visceral pain is often described as crampy, colicky pain that is well defined. Anticholinergics are helpful with addressing this type of pain; however, it is important to monitor for adverse effects such as delirium, constipation, and urinary retention.[28]

Neuropathic pain is the result of diseases as well as treatment. Diseases that result in neuropathic pain include diabetes mellitus, herpetic neuralgia, radiculopathy, spinal cord lesions, storage disorders, renal failure, mononeuritis multiplex (diabetes, leprosy), and demyelinating diseases. Alternatively, neuropathy can be the side effect of treatment such as chemotherapy. Neuropathic pain often has inadequate response to opiates alone because of atypical pathophysiology compared with nociceptive pain. Adjuvants are well studied and effective in managing a variety of neuropathic pain and should be first line in many cases to optimize pain regimens. It is appropriate to add opioid therapy for refractory pain, and they have shown efficacy in neuropathic pain.[31,32]

Neuropathic pain is characterized as burning, tingling, lightninglike, and needlelike. Some patients also report debilitating pain that interferes with the ability to perform activities of daily living. Additional symptoms that are associated with neuropathic pain include anxiety, depression, sleep disturbances, and increased debility.[32,33] First-line therapy for neuropathic pain includes pregabalin, gabapentin, duloxetine, and some tricyclic antidepressants.[32–34] Gabapentin and pregabalin require dose adjustment

Table 5 Adjuvant pain medications		
Type of Pain	**Medication Class**	**Specific Medications**
Somatic	Corticosteroids	Decadron, prednisone
	Bisphosphonates	Pamidronate, zoledronate
	NSAIDs	See **Box 1**
	Para-aminophenol	Acetaminophen
Visceral	Anticholinergics	Scopolamine, glycopyrrolate, hyoscyamine
Neuropathic	TCAs	Nortriptyline, amitriptyline, desipramine
	SNRIs	Duloxetine, venlafaxine gabapentin, pregabalin,
	Anticonvulsants	carbamazepine, oxcarbazepine
	Topical	Capsaicin, topical lidocaine
	Other agents	Ketamine, dexmedetomidine, lidocaine IV

Abbreviations: SNRIs, serotonin norepinephrine reuptake inhibitors; TCAs, tricyclic antidepressants.
Data from Refs.[28–30]

in chronic kidney disease, and usually the titration is based on glomerular filtration rate. For patients with end-stage renal disease on dialysis, it is recommended to dose gabapentin on dialysis days after treatment, in order to maximize benefit of analgesia and reduce the risk of side effects.[32,35] Methadone is also very effective in management of neuropathic pain, but, because of its multiple drug interactions and adverse effects profile, its risks may outweigh benefits for chronic neuropathic pain in patients with renal disease. There is a growing body of literature showing effectiveness of supplement alpha lipoic acid in peripheral neuropathy, but more research is needed. It may be an appropriate adjuvant with a low side effect profile.[33,35]

Topical agents such as capsaicin and lidocaine patches are second-line therapies (**Table 5**).

INTERVENTIONAL PAIN

Approximately 10% to 20% of patients with a serious illness do not experience pain relief with the first 3 steps of the WHO pain ladder.[19,20] These patients are candidates for therapeutic nerve blocks. The goal of a nerve block is to disrupt the pain impulse and to remodel the nerve response to pain. The types of nerve blocks include nonneurolytic pain blocks and neurolytic nerve blocks[35,36] (**Table 6**). Nonneurolytic blocks are performed with a combination of a local anesthetic, such as lidocaine or bupivacaine, and a corticosteroid, although neurolytic blocks are performed with an agent that kills the nerve root, such as ethanol.[36] The key to successful nerve blocks is to implement the treatment early rather than using it as a last resort.

Opioid Pain Management

There is increasing literature to suggest that use of long-term opioid therapy may not be beneficial and is possibly harmful for patients with chronic nonmalignant pain.[22,37]

Table 6
Interventional pain block indications

Type of Block	Type of Pain	Indication
Celiac plexus	Deep visceral pain	Pancreatic cancer Pancreatitis
Superior hypogastric	Pelvic pain	Rectal cancer Bladder cancer Uterine cancer Cervical cancer
Stellate ganglion	Deep visceral pain	Diffuse metastasis Ulcerative colitis
Brachial plexus	Neuropathic pain Associated symptoms include weakness, numbness, or paralysis	Upper extremity pain caused by: Cancer Trauma Scar Radiation
Lumbar sympathetic	Neuropathic pain	LE pain from cancer Phantom pain Complex regional pain syndrome
Peroneal or popliteal nerve	Neuropathic	Ischemia Cancer

Abbreviation: LE, lower extremity.

Adapted from Brogan S, Junkins S. Interventional therapies for the management of cancer pain. J Support Oncol 2010;8(2):52-59; and Sindt JE, Brogan SE. Interventional treatments of cancer pain. Anesthesiol Clin 2016;34(2):317-339; with permission.

According to the recent Centers for Disease Control and Prevention guideline, patients on greater than 90 oral morphine milligram equivalents per day for chronic pain are at increased risk for accidental overdose and death.[37] Current literature has shown that patients on long-term opioid therapy have not shown long-term improved quality of life or sustained improvement in function. Long-term opioid therapy places patients at risk for mood disorders, development of opioid misuse disorder, hyperalgesia, hypogonadism, cognitive impairment, and osteoporosis.[38–40] Physical dependence can develop after a few days of opioid use. However, as discussed earlier, they are still a useful tool for management of pain for patients with serious illness as a part of a multimodal strategies. Although the literature does not support improved quality-of-life scores with long-term opioid use alone as a pain management plan, it does show evidence of pain reduction.[37] Using opioids for pain management for patients with serious illness is a clinical decision based on a variety of factors specific to the patient. Using harm reduction strategies, opioids can be used safely and may be the medication of choice for patients with a serious illness.[41] Clinical guidelines of opioid use currently exclude patients who are on hospice, have cancer, or are being managed by palliative care.[37] There is no clear clinical evidence for these exclusions, but it is recognized that seriously ill patients have complex clinical needs that must be considered when developing symptom management plans of care. If used properly, studies have shown that using opioids for symptom management does not significantly hasten death, with effects being none to minor for patients who are at end of life.[42]

As with any medication that has significant potential side effects, patient education and informed consent focusing on risk versus benefits should be provided for patients who will be treated with opioid therapy. Controlled substance agreements are part of the standard of care because they provide education, safety instructions, and parameters for treatment. Random urine toxicology screens should be a part of the safety plan when appropriate. If patients are on greater than 50 morphine milligram equivalents or on current opioids and benzodiazepines, they should be prescribed naloxone (intranasal/intramuscular), which is the agent used to treat an accidental opioid overdose. Naloxone can be administered by a caregiver or third party while awaiting emergency management services and is potentially lifesaving. Patients and caregivers require education on how and when to use it appropriately.[37,43] Many states have prescription drug monitoring programs that allow providers to see whether patients are receiving prescriptions from different provider and for other controlled substances. If available, providers should monitor their patients using this tool for safety regardless of the seriousness of the illness. There is still a risk of opioid/controlled substance misuse or diversion in the seriously ill population, and it is a matter of patient and public safety.

When using opioids for pain management, it important to assess and document the 4 As to determine whether the current opioid plan is appropriate or effective (**Table 7**).

For patients with serious illness, it is important also to consider the status of clinical illness and goals of care. Treating a patient's pain who has serious illness with a prognosis of days to weeks versus months to years has different treatment paradigms based on goals. However, safe practice principles still apply. As serious illness progresses, drug metabolism is affected for both opioid and nonopioid medications. Tolerance to side effects of both opioid and nonopioid analgesics also changes as serious illness progresses, usually caused by progression of organ dysfunction.

The management of pain in the seriously ill is dynamic. Choosing which opioid to use may depend on several factors, which include pharmacokinetics, available preparation, cost, availability, patient and provider comfort, and patient tolerance (**Table 8**).

Table 7 Assessing opioid efficacy: the 4 As	
Analgesia	Assessment of effectiveness of pain control
Activities	Is the patient engaging in the activities that provide acceptable quality of life?
Adverse effects	Is the patient experiencing side effects, and, if so, how are they affecting quality of life? Have side effects been managed?
Aberrant drug behaviors	Are there signs of opioid misuse disorder

Data from Passik SD, Kirsh KL, Whitcomb L, et al. A new tool to assess and document pain outcomes in chronic pain patients receiving opioid therapy. Clin Ther 2004;26(4):552-61.

There are limited data using head-to-head comparisons of opioids for effectiveness.[44,45] Seriously ill patients require frequent reassessment including laboratory values, physical evaluations, and chart reviews to determine the safety of treatment plans and to anticipate changes.

When choosing opioid therapy, providers often consider using long-acting preparations with short-acting preparations for breakthrough pain if patients are requiring frequent dosing of opioid or have persistent pain throughout the day. Although providers have been educated to prescribe opioids in this manner, there are few data to support this practice. Pharmacologically and logistically, this approach seems like a reasonable way to provide patients with more consistent pain control and reduce the peak-and-valley effect that can be seen with frequent daily dosing of immediate-release opioid therapy.

Long-acting opioids are not appropriate for acute pain and should be avoided in opioid-naive patients.[37] More recent scrutiny has been placed on appropriate

Table 8 Opioid analgesics: cost, clearance, and route of administration			
Name	Primary Metabolism and Excretion	Preparation	Cost of Oral Outpatient Preparations
Methadone	Hepatic	Parental/oral/SL	$–$$
Morphine	Renal/hepatic	Parental/oral/SL	$$
Hydrocodone	Hepatic/renal	Oral	IR $; ER $$$
Oxycodone	Hepatic	Oral	IR $; ER $$$–$$$$
Hydromorphone	Hepatic	Parental/oral	IR $$; ER $$$
Buprenorphine	Hepatic	Parental/transdermal/buccal	$$–$$$
Fentanyl	Hepatic	Parental/transdermal/buccal/oral	$$$
Oxymorphone	Hepatic	Oral/parental	$$$
Tapentadol	Hepatic/renal	Oral	$$$$
Tramadol	Renal/hepatic	Oral (only available in United States)	IR $; ER $$$

$, <$10; $$, $10–$50; $$$, $100–$200; $$$$, >$200/mo.
Abbreviations: ER, extended release; IR, immediate release; SL, sublingual.
Adapted from Motov SM. Tarascon Pain Pocketbook, 1st edition. Burlington: Jones & Bartlett Learning; 2019; and Hamilton RJ. Tarascon Pharmacopoeia 2017 Professional Desk Reference Edition, 7th edition. Burlington: Jones & Bartlett Learning; 2017; with permission.

Table 9 Morphine milligram equivalent required to transition to long-acting opioid	
Morphine	60 mg daily
Oxycodone	40 mg daily
Hydromorphone	8 mg daily
Fentanyl	25 µg daily

Adapted from Dowell D, Haegerich TM, Chou R. CDC guideline for prescribing opioids for chronic pain—United States, 2016. JAMA 2016;315(15):1624-1645; with permission.

prescribing and the risk of long-acting opioid and immediate-release fentanyl therapy. The US Food and Drug Administration has approved risk evaluation and mitigation strategies (REMSs) to reinforce education to providers concerning safe opioid prescribing, which can be accessed at www.fda.gov. Transmucosal immediate-release fentanyl (TIRF) has a restricted use for opioid-tolerant patients with cancer and requires prescribing providers to participate in a REMS TIRF program.[46]

In order to safely transition a patient to long-acting opioid preparation, the patient must be on at least 60 mg of oral morphine daily or oral morphine equivalent for 1 week or longer (**Table 9**).

Once long-acting medication is prescribed for breakthrough pain, it is reasonable for breakthrough dosing to be at least 10% to 15% of the 24-hour long-acting requirement. If taking an oral preparation, the dosing could be 1 to 2 hours apart; however, more conservatively, dosing could be every 4 hours. Patients with organ dysfunction; particularly the elderly, receiving opioids maybe may have fewer side effects with less frequent breakthrough dosing. These patient can achieve good analgesic control with less frequent dosing secondary to decreased opioid clearance. In patients on parental preparations, breakthrough dosing may reasonably be spaced 10 to 15 minutes apart. There is no evidence that parental medication provides better analgesic control than oral medication. The difference lies in the onset of action. Understanding the pharmacokinetics of the opioid being used and the route of administration is helpful when deciding on dosing intervals. Sublingual preparations are absorbed rapidly when the drug is more lipophilic; hence maximum serum concentration (C-max) varies based on the choice of opioid and its lipophilicity[47,48] (**Table 10**).

There are several key reasons for rotating opioid therapy, which include intolerable side effects, development of hyperalgesia, and ineffective analgesia (**Tables 11–14**). Opioid-induced hyperalgesia is a paradoxic response that results in nociceptive sensitization caused by increasing exposure to an opioid usually at escalating doses. The result is that the opioid treatment causes increased sensitization to painful and nonpainful stimuli.[49,50]

Table 10 Time to maximum concentrate based on route of administration for opioid analgesia	
Route of Administration: Short Acting	**C-max (min)**
Oral/per rectum	60
SC	30
IV	10–15

Data from Rennick A, Atkinson T, Cimino NM, et al. Variability in opioid equivalence calculations. Pain Med 2016;17(5):892-898.

Table 11
Opioid-related side effect management

Opioid-Related Side Effect	Symptom Duration	Management
Constipation	Indefinite	Start stimulant laxative, and osmotic laxative (senna/polyethylene glycol)
Nausea/vomiting	7–10 d	Premedicate with antiemetic, opioid rotation, manage constipation
Sedation	2–3 d	Opioid reduction, opioid rotation, avoid CNS depressants, may consider psychostimulant if symptom persist, hydration
Pruritus	7–10 d	Opioid rotation, antihistamines, severe cases naltrexone
Respiratory depression	Rare	Naloxone Avoid combining opioid therapy with another CNS depressant Use opioid cautiously in patients with underlying restrictive/obstructive pulmonary illness second to increased risk of respiratory depression and development of hypercapnia/hypoxic respiratory failure
Hyperalgesia	Occurs later in treatment	Opioid reduction, rotation
Myoclonus	Variable, occurs with progressive organ dysfunction affecting medication clearance	Opioid reduction, rotation, hydration, benzodiazepines

Abbreviation: CNS, central nervous system.

Data from Gregorian RS, Gasik A, Kwong WJ, et al. Importance of side effects in opioid treatment: a trade-off analysis with patients and physicians. The Journal of Pain 2010;11(11):1095-1108; and Goldstein NE, Morrison RS. Evidence-Based Practice of Palliative Medicine. Philadelphia: Saunders; 2013.

Table 12
Example opioid conversion

Opioid	Oral	Parenteral (mg)
Morphine	30	10
Oxycodone	20	10
Hydromorphone	7.5	1.5
Buprenorphine	0.4	0.3
Codeine	200	100
Tramadol	120	NA; not available in United States
Tapentadol	100	NA
Hydrocodone	30	NA
Fentanyl	NA	0.1

Abbreviation: NA, not applicable.

Adapted from McPherson ML. Demystifying Opioid Conversion Calculations: A guide for effective dosing, 1st edition. Bethesda: American Society of Health-System Pharmacists; 2010; with permission.

Table 13 Methadone conversion	
Morphine Oral Equivalents (mg)	**Oral Morphine/Methadone Ratio**
<100	3:1
100–300	5:1
300–600	10:1
600–800	12:1
800–1000	15:1
>1000	20:1

Adapted from Goldstein NE, Morrison RS. Evidence-Based Practice of Palliative Medicine. Philadelphia: Saunders; 2013; and Lukin B, Greenslade J, Kearney AM, et al. Conversion of other opioids to methadone: a retrospective comparison of two methods. BMJ Support Palliat Care 2019;pii: bmjspcare-2018-001645; with permission.

When rotating from one opioid to another, there are several opioid conversion tables available that use various methodologies but are similar (**Tables 10** and **11**). Most important when making an opioid rotation is to keep clinical judgment central to decision making. When making an opioid rotation, it is important to reduce the dose of the new opioid by 25% to 50% to account for incomplete cross-tolerance. Although many opioids/opiates have similar chemical structures and affinity for the same mu receptors, incomplete cross-tolerance happens because tolerance to one opioid does not mean that there will be complete tolerance to another during rotation. Rotating without taking this concept into account may lead to accidental sedation or unintended overdose.[48]

Morphine for cost-effectiveness and access remains usual first-line opioid of choice. Morphine in patients with renal failure can cause an increase in morphine metabolites leading to neurotoxicity and increased risk of accidental overdose.[44] Oxycodone use has been increasing associated with the opioid crisis, with long-acting and short-acting preparation being misused intranasal and intravenously. Oxycodone is metabolized in the liver, and liver failure or cachexia may increase the half-life of the medication. Transdermal fentanyl may have decreased absorption in patients with cachexia. Codeine requires that patients be genetically able to metabolize codeine to morphine to have an analgesic effect.[47,49]

Methadone has a long and variable half-life of 8 to 59 hours, and even up to 190 hours. Methadone titration requires expertise and careful monitoring because the titration is slow, over 5 to 7 days, to avoid sedation and accidental overdose (see **Table 11**). Methadone is primarily metabolized and eliminated by the cytochrome P450 enzyme system in the liver (cytochrome P450 3A4, 2B6, and 2D6). It has a high bioavailability (40%–99%) and potent analgesic properties caused by its blockade of the N-methyl-D-aspartate receptors, which are known to be more widespread than mu, kappa, and delta receptors. Because of its hepatic pharmacokinetics, methadone has significant interactions with other medications cleared by cytochrome P450, inducers of the enzymatic pathway (phenytoin, barbiturates, rifampicin, haloperidol, carbamazepine) speed up elimination, and inhibitors (fluoroquinolones, macrolide antibiotics, selective serotonin reuptake inhibitors) cause the drug to accumulate and precipitate toxicity. Before starting methadone, a baseline corrected QT (QTc) should be obtained; if the QTc is greater than 500 milliseconds, then that should be consider a contraindication, and greater than 45 milliseconds a relative contraindication. It is generally recommended and practiced that repeat QTc is obtained with dose

Table 14

Pain Assessment in Advanced Dementia pain assessment scale in advanced dementia

	0	1	2	None
Breathing independent of vocalization	Normal	Occasional labored breathing. Short period of hyperventilation	Noisy, labored breathing. Long period of hyperventilation. Cheyne-Stokes respiration	—
Negative vocalization	None	Occasional moan or groan. Low-level speech with a negative or disapproving quality	Repeated troubled calling out. Loud moaning or groaning. Crying	—
Facial expression	Smiling or expressive	Sad, frightened, frowning	Facial grimacing	—
Body language	Relaxed	Tense, distressed pacing, fidgeting	Rigid. Fists clenched; knees pulled up. Pulling or pushing away. Striking out	—
Consolability	No need to console	Distracted or reassured by voice or touch	Unable to console, distract or reassure	—

Data adapted from (1) Carr DB, Jacox AK, Chapman CR, et al. "Acute Pain Management: Operative or Medical Procedures and Trauma. Clinical Practice Guideline No. 1." AHCPR Pub. No. 92-0032. Rockville, MD: Agency for Health Care Policy and Research, Public Health Service, U.S. Department of Health and Human Services. Feb. 1992; and (2) Jacox A, Carr DB, Payne R, et al. Management of Cancer Pain. Clinical Practice Guideline No. 9. AHCPR Publication No. 94-0592. Rockville, MD. Agency for Health Care Policy and Research, U.S. Department of Health and Human Services, Public Health Service, March 1994.

titrations, but the literature on how often and the clinical relevance is inconclusive. A Cochrane Review reported that "No evidence has been found to support the use of the electrocardiogram (ECG) for preventing cardiac arrhythmias in methadone-treated opioid dependents."[51] If a patient's QTc is increasing, it is important to review the medication list for other QTc-prolonging medications that could be contributing to the increase if continuing methadone is the preferred treatment. High-dosage methadone (>200 mg/d) has a possible association with arrhythmia (torsades de pointes) in patients with risk factors for arrhythmia.[52]

Fentanyl and buprenorphine also can prolong QTc. Methadone, fentanyl, buprenorphine, tramadol, and tapentadol should be used with caution with other serotonergic medications.[47,50]

Buprenorphine is an opioid agonist/antagonist that is used for opioid replacement therapy for patients with opioid addiction. It is also an effective medication for pain and it may have several advantages as a first-line agent. It comes in transdermal and buccal mucosa preparations. It has been shown to have fewer adverse side effects, including constipation and respiratory depression, to be better tolerated in the elderly and in end-stage renal disease, and to have fewer withdrawal symptoms. The transdermal preparation (5 μg/h) can be initiated in opioid-naive patients. However, rotation from another opioid to buprenorphine must be done carefully because it can precipitate withdrawal. Patients should not be on greater than 30 mg of morphine equivalent for at least 7 days before rotation.[8,53]

It is appropriate before starting a patient on opioid therapy to assess the risk for misuse. Risk factors for opioid misuse disorder are personal or family history of drug/alcohol misuse, mental illness, history of incarceration, and male sex. If it will be necessary to prescribe opioids, it is recommended to assess for the risk of potential opioid abuse using the Opioid Risk Assessment Tool before beginning opioid therapy for pain management.[47,54] Scores of 0 to 3 indicate low risk for future opioid abuse, scores of 4 to 7 indicate moderate risk for opioid abuse, and scores of 8 or higher indicate a high risk for opioid abuse.[54]

In addition to the Opioid Risk Assessment Tool before starting opioid therapy, it may be beneficial to consider monitoring the patient with the Current Opioid Misuse Measure, which is a self-report measure of risk for aberrant behavior for patients being treated with chronic opioids. It is validated screen tool that helps patients to identify at-risk behavior in themselves, allowing better provider and patient communication.[55,56] Patients with serious illness and a history or current substance use disorders present special challenges to management. They may have developed tolerance, which means they may also require higher doses of opioid therapy to achieve analgesia.[56,57] Buprenorphine may be an appropriate first-line therapy to consider for patients with a history of misuse disorder. Avoiding concurrent benzodiazepine use is appropriate for all patients on chronic opioid therapy but more so for patients with a history or current substance use.[37] These patients require frequent monitoring, urine toxicology screen, access to mental health resources, and clear boundaries.[58,59] Managing them with the assistance of an addiction specialist is an ideal approach. Some patients may be afraid to report an increase in pain because of fear about disease progression or fear that they will be prescribed opioids secondary to concern for relapse or stigma.[57]

When tapering a patient on chronic opioid therapy with serious illness, efforts should be made to prevent withdrawal symptoms, which can be confused depending on the diagnosis and exacerbation of the serious illness. The dehydration, tachycardia, insomnia, pain, and mental agitation can have serious medical consequences for medically fragile patients. Patients should be educated not to stop their opioid regimens abruptly on their own. There is no evidence to support rapid tapering for patients on chronic opioid therapy. Tapers can range from a 10% reduction per week to 10% reduction per month, and slower if needed.[60,61] Management of withdrawal with antiemetic, antidiarrheal, α-blockers, and anticholinergic medications may be required with careful monitoring.

Pain Management: Serious Illness

Liver disease

Patients may experience pain secondary to diseased liver or may have pain of other causes in the setting of decompensated liver disease, thereby requiring fine tuning of analgesics to avoid side effects and toxicity. Pain is often associated with common liver diseases such as polycystic liver disease, alcoholic steatohepatitis, congestive hepatopathy, and nonalcoholic fatty liver disease (NAFLD). In almost all these conditions, treatment of the primary liver disease effectively controls the symptom of abdominal pain. For example, NAFLD improves significantly with weight loss.

Conditions such as malignancy, diabetes, complex regional pain syndrome, and fibromyalgia may cause complex pain in patients with chronic liver disease and require careful titration of pain medications to maintain comfort and avoid drug accumulation and toxicity. When discussing liver disease, it is extremely important to mention acetaminophen because it undergoes complex pharmacokinetics primarily in the liver (sulfation and glucuronidation), with a very small amount being excreted by the kidneys. In severe liver disease, despite the enormous reserves, higher dosages of acetaminophen (close to 4 g/d) can stress the already decompensated liver. Acetaminophen is the leading cause of acute liver failure in the United States, accounting for 50% of cases. Low-dose acetaminophen in liver disease can be used for pain management when used judiciously and considering patient-specific factors. For management of mild to moderate pain, the recommended dosage of acetaminophen in patients with decompensated liver disease is less than 2 g/d. NSAIDs are not recommended in cirrhosis and ascites because of increased incidence of hepatorenal syndrome.[62]

Adjuvants such as gabapentin and pregabalin that are mainly excreted through the kidney do not require adjustment in dosage in mild to moderate liver disease. Active and inactive metabolites of morphine, hydromorphone, oxymorphone, and oxycodone are primarily excreted by the kidneys (40%–70%). About 30% is excreted by the liver. No dosage adjustments are necessary in mild liver disease (normal transaminase levels). However, as liver disease worsens and hepatorenal syndrome develops, dosage adjustment and spacing of doses is warranted to prevent drug accumulation and systemic toxicity.

Methadone can be used in liver disease but is contraindicated in severe liver dysfunction secondary to its metabolism through the cytochrome P450 enzyme system in the liver.[63]

End-stage renal disease

Pain is a common symptom in severe renal disease because, as the body ages, frailty and comorbidities can cause pain in the setting of disease or age-related nephron loss. Pain caused by primary renal disorders include adult polycystic kidney disease, renal and ureteral calculi, and mononeuropathy in renal vein thrombosis or lymphadenopathy. The common secondary causes of pain in patients with renal disease include diabetes, pathologic fractures from renal osteodystrophy, and peripheral neuropathy.[64]

Most of the routinely used pain medications, such as NSAIDs, opioids, and adjuvants (except for acetaminophen, methadone, and fentanyl), are mainly excreted by the kidney (70%–80%); hence, it is important to adjust doses early and often. NSAIDs are nephrotoxic and so should be avoided in renal insufficiency of any kind, whether acute or chronic. Of the opioid analgesics, morphine is least preferable in patients with renal failure, particularly oral morphine, because it has poor bioavailability (20%) and high tolerance. In order to achieve adequate analgesia, this setting can therefore compromise patient care quickly with higher chances of side effects caused by buildup of active metabolites.[47]

Codeine is a prodrug requiring activation to morphine in the liver; hence, it is a less potent analgesic compared with purer opioids such as morphine and hydromorphone and has a higher burden of side effects caused by accumulation of active and inactive metabolites that are eventually eliminated renally. Although oxycodone and hydrocodone are not prodrugs, they are metabolized to oxymorphone and hydromorphone in vivo, so their pharmacokinetic profile can be altered in hepatic and renal dysfunction. Oxycodone has 19% renal clearance, and long-acting preparations can also pose difficulty in patients with severe renal dysfunction. For select patients showing signs of sedation or neurotoxicity, once-daily dosing, as opposed to multiday dosing, with concurrent use of an immediate-release preparation can be an appropriate alternate strategy.[47,48,50]

Hydromorphone is excreted by the liver and kidney (70% and 30% respectively) and it is more potent compared with morphine in patients with moderate or severe pain. Although the risk for neurotoxicity is a dose-dependent effect with all opioids, this adverse effect is more common with hydromorphone because of higher saturation of the kappa receptors in the central nervous system by hydromorphone and its metabolites. Buprenorphine is becoming a more popular option secondary to its better side effect profile. Methadone is safer to use in patients with kidney failure because it is excreted by the liver. In patients who have liver and kidney disease, fentanyl is a potent opioid and is safer to use in renal failure because it is neither eliminated nor activated (1 inactive metabolite [norfentanyl]) in the liver or kidney.[65]

Heart disease

Pain is mainly a symptom of ischemic heart disease and peripheral vascular disease. Pain management strategies require a stepwise approach tailored to this population. In patients with congestive heart failure, pain is seen closer to stage D/E (advanced/end-stage/refractory) heart failure, with an incidence of 40% to 75% of patients. When it occurs, pain in advanced heart failure is most commonly described in the legs and knees, back and major joints, abdomen (hepatic congestion), and chest.[66] NSAIDs are contraindicated secondary to patients' impaired renal function, sodium and fluid retention, and worsening heart failure, thereby increasing the risk of rehospitalization. A multidisciplinary approach to complex pain syndromes in organ failure includes localized heat/cold therapy, topical NSAIDs/capsaicin (weak recommendation, low evidence), and acupuncture in addition to systemic pain medications. Opioids are helpful in managing symptom clusters such as pain, dyspnea, and anxiety. They may worsen fatigue. For patients with left ventricular assist devices, driveline-related pain is common and this can be either neuropathic or psychosomatic depending on the cause (irritation vs infection).[47,66,67]

Cancer pain

Management of cancer pain can be complex. Patient with malignancies can have primary pain secondary to malignancy, such as bone, or visceral pain secondary to metastatic disease. They may also have pain secondary to treatment, such as chemotherapy-induced neuropathy, or myalgia/arthralgias. Most cancer pain is mixed somatic and neuropathic. Opioids remain the mainstay of treatment of cancer pain, with adjuvants to control neuropathic pain (tricyclic antidepressant, anticonvulsants, serotonin norepinephrine reuptake inhibitors) and inflammation (NSAIDs, steroids). However, there are treatment-specific pain syndromes that providers should be familiar with when evaluating and treating pain in patients with cancer. For example, use of the antihistamine loratadine can help with pain from pegfilgrastim. Use of opioids and NSAIDs can be helpful for these patients, but use of loratadine has a better side effect profile and is opioid sparing for these patients. Interventional pain management procedures for localized pain from metastatic disease are increasingly gaining popularity. Interventional pain management referrals should be considered when developing a cancer pain plan.[68] Also, nonpharmacologic complementary techniques such as acupuncture, medical massage, reiki therapy, moderate activity, and mindfulness can also play a meaningful role in helping patients manage pain, promote well-being, and limit the pharmacologic therapy that often has unintended side effects. Side effects of opioid and nonopioid therapy can include sedation, constipation, mental clouding, and depression, which leads to decreased quality of life. Herbal supplements such as turmeric for inflammation and cannabidiols should be evaluated by an oncology pharmacist before using to rule out any drug interactions that could affect therapy.[47,50,68]

PAIN MANAGEMENT IN THE ELDERLY

Nonmalignant pain syndromes in elderly patients are mostly caused by musculoskeletal disorders, immobility, contractures, and psychosomatic conditions such as depression. Common geriatric conditions causing pain include gait instability and frailty resulting in falls and fractures, osteoarthritis, rheumatoid arthritis, low back pain secondary to degenerative joint disease and spinal canal stenosis, depression, and Parkinson disease. Careful pain assessment and minimizing polypharmacy are key components to safe and effective analgesia in the elderly.

Pain assessment can be challenging in patients with advanced dementia because they may show more behavioral changes, such as withdrawal or aggression, particularly as their ability to communicate verbally declines.[69–71] Because of limitations in ability to self-report pain, objective scales such as Pain Assessment in Advanced Dementia Scale (PAINAD) have been developed to provide a true assessment of pain in the dementia population.

Osteoarthritis and Degenerative Joint Disease

These are perhaps the commonest causes of pain in the joints and back in patients more than 65 years of age. Acetaminophen remains the mainstay of management of arthritis pain in the elderly. Doses typically start at 650 to 1000 mg, 2 to 3 times daily on a scheduled basis rather than as needed. NSAIDs are best avoided for chronic arthritis pain because of the risk of bleeding and renal impairment.[69]

Older adults frequently need dose adjustment for hepatic and renal impairment caused by comorbidities and/or aging. Screening liver and renal function tests are beneficial before initiating a chronic pain regimen in the elderly. Starting doses are usually 50% lower than the recommended starting dose (eg, 2.5 mg of morphine or oxycodone, 12.5 μg fentanyl).[72]

Medications that are best avoided in the elderly include tramadol, and NSAIDs secondary to the side effect profile. Predictable pain control with the least amount of side effects and drug interactions are the goal for pain management in this special population. Although some of these medications (such as methadone) can be used for management of complex unrelenting pain in the elderly, synthetic opioids such as tramadol have a high risk/benefit ratio and weak potency as analgesics. NSAIDs are largely undesirable in the elderly population because of nephrotoxicity, fluid retention, and mucositis/bleeding.

Polypharmacy is a significant problem in elderly patients. It is pertinent to have accurate medical reconciliation during the patient's admission and discharge process to ensure safe and effective pain and symptom management strategies. Certain medications, such as extended-release morphine and fentanyl patches, may need to be held in the immediate perioperative period (because the patient may be receiving parenteral pain medications), whereas others, such as antidepressants, should be resumed as soon as possible to prevent rebound anxiety and headaches.[47,73] Strategies in preventing polypharmacy include fluidity in pain medication prescribing and deprescribing, as medically appropriate.

Postoperative Pain

Traumatic falls and fractures (hip, wrist) are common in elderly people. Most patients do well with operative interventions such as open reduction and fixation. Joint replacement in severe debilitating osteoarthritis has a good prognosis with early physical therapy made possible by meticulous pain control. Most patients respond well to IV acetaminophen in the immediate postoperative period with transition to limited courses of oral pure opioids such as morphine, oxycodone, and fentanyl. Hydromorphone has a higher incidence of neurotoxicity compared with other opioids and is generally not the first choice in patients more than 75 years old.[47,49]

Total Pain

Total pain was defined by Dame Cicely Saunders as the suffering that encompasses all of a person's physical, psychological, social, spiritual, and practical struggles. The concept of total pain explains this complex phenomenon In patients with serious illness and highlights the holistic aspects of pain management.[74]

Physical pain gets worse when patients experience psychosocial and existential suffering. Chaplains have gleaned from patients and families how total pain causes suffering in more than 1 domain, and the interrelatedness of this phenomenon makes it impossible for pain to be managed effectively without addressing all the domains with a holistic approach.

Palliative care is centered in the management of total pain and suffering primarily by providing holistic multidimensional pain and symptom management with a transdisciplinary team spanning physicians, nurses, chaplains, and social workers. The role of caregivers cannot be ignored in the management of total pain because they spend the most time with the patients and experience their own suffering in the form of physical and emotional fatigue and anticipatory grief.

Management of total pain includes pharmacologic and nonpharmacologic interventions, as discussed previously. The nonpharmacologic interventions account for a significant portion of the therapeutic plan in the form of active listening, motivational interviewing, and allowing patients and families the space and security to share their feelings. Most patients feel a sense of helplessness in the throes of total pain and suffering and are unable to think cognitively. Hence, the management of total pain involves a careful balance of potent pain medications combined with psychotherapy and family support.

Spiritual health clinicians (SHCs) play a vital role in easing existential distress and exploring positive coping strategies. A study published in the *Journal of General Internal Medicine* in 2007 showed this phenomenon by having SHCs explore spiritual and existential crises in seriously ill patients. Patients who were able to identify peace and meaning in the journey of their serious illness were found to have a greater sense of well-being and less depression compared with patients who identified faith alone.[75,76] Chaplains and SHCs are trained to provide spiritual care assessment and grief counseling. However, the screening for spiritual distress is the responsibility of the multidisciplinary team. The screening can often be completed with just a couple of open-ended questions such as "How are you feeling within yourself?" or "Tell me how you cope." The FICA screening tool developed by Puchalski and Romer[77] provides standardized tools in the form of a simple questionnaire to allow any health care professional to provide screening for spiritual and existential distress.

DISCLOSURE

The authors have nothing to disclose.

REFERENCES

1. Benzon H, Raja SN, Fishman SE, et al. Essentials of pain medicine E-book. Philadelphia, PA: Elsevier Health Sciences; 2011.
2. Fernandez VE, Rozanski MJ, Rothmell JP, et al. Quality Assessment and Improvement and Patient Safety in the Pain Clinic. In: Practical management of pain. Philadelphia, PA: Mosby; 2014. p. 56–77.
3. Mercadante S, Radbruch L, Caraceni A, et al, Steering Committee of the European Association for Palliative Care (EAPC) Research Network. Episodic (breakthrough) pain: consensus conference of an expert working group of the European Association for Palliative Care. Cancer 2002;94(3):832–9.
4. Mearis M, Shega JW, Knoebel RW. Does adherence to National Comprehensive Cancer Network guidelines improve pain-related outcomes? An evaluation of inpatient cancer pain management at an academic medical center. J Pain Symptom Manage 2014;48(3):451–8.
5. Fink RM, Gallagher E. Cancer pain assessment and measurement. In: Seminars in oncology nursing. WB Saunders; 2019;35(3):229-34.
6. Magnusson JE, Fennell JA. Understanding the role of culture in pain: Māori practitioner perspectives relating to the experience of pain. Clinical Correspondence 2011;5(6):41–143.
7. Holt S, Waterfield J. Cultural aspects of pain: a study of Indian Asian women in the UK. Musculoskelet Care 2018;16(2):260–8.
8. Green E, Zwaal C, Beals C, et al. Cancer-related pain management: a report of evidence-based recommendations to guide practice. Clin J Pain 2010;26(6): 449–62.
9. Mcafferty E, Farley A. Assessing pain in patients. Nurs Stand 2008;22(25):42–6.
10. Hicks CL, von Baeyer CL, Spafford PA, et al. The Faces Pain Scale–Revised: toward a common metric in pediatric pain measurement. Pain 2001;93(2):173–83.
11. Hølen JC, Hjermstad MJ, Loge JH, et al. Pain assessment tools: is the content appropriate for use in palliative care? J Pain Symptom Manage 2006;32(6): 567–80.
12. Hockenberry MJ, Wilson D. Wong's essentials of pediatric nursing9: Wong's essentials of pediatric nursing. St. Louis (MO): Elsevier Health Sciences; 2013.
13. Haanpää ML, Backonja MM, Bennett MI, et al. Assessment of neuropathic pain in primary care. Am J Med 2009;122(10):S13–21.
14. Swarm RA, Abernethy AP, Anghelescu DL, et al. Adult cancer pain. J Natl Compr Canc Netw 2013;11(8):992–1022.

15. Gordon DB. Acute pain assessment tools: let us move beyond simple pain ratings. Curr Opin Anesthesiol 2015;28(5):565–9.
16. Pelayo-Alvarez M, Perez-Hoyos S, Agra-Varela Y. Reliability and concurrent validity of the palliative outcome scale, the rotterdam symptom checklist, and the brief pain inventory. J Palliat Med 2013;16(8):867–74.
17. Lorenz KA, Lynn J, Dy SM, et al. Evidence for improving palliative care at the end of life: a systematic review. Ann Intern Med 2008;148:7.
18. Swarm RA. The management of pain in patients with cancer. J Natl Compr Canc Netw 2013;11(5S):702–4.
19. Jadad AR, Browman GP. The WHO analgesic ladder for cancer pain management: stepping up the quality of its evaluation. JAMA 1995;274(23):1870–3.
20. Maltoni M, Scarpi E, Modonesi C, et al. A validation study of the WHO analgesic ladder: a two-step vs three-step strategy. Support Care Cancer 2005;13(11):888–94.
21. Azevedo Sao Ferreira K, Kimura K, Jacobsen T. The WHO analgesic ladder for cancer pain control, twenty years of use. How much Pain relied does one get from using it? Support Care Cancer 2006;14(11):1086–93.
22. Ballantyne JC, Kalso E, Stannard C. WHO analgesic ladder: a good concept gone astray. BMJ 2016;352:i20.
23. Lanza FL, Chan FK, Quigley EM. Guidelines for prevention of NSAID-related ulcer complications. Am J Gastroenterol 2009;104(3):728.
24. Mercadante S, Casuccio A, Agnello A, et al. Analgesic effects of nonsteroidal anti-inflammatory drugs in cancer pain due to somatic or visceral mechanisms. J Pain Symptom Manage 1999;17(5):351–6.
25. Manchanda A, Cameron C, Robinson G. Beware of paracetamol use in alcohol abusers: a potential cause of acute liver injury. N Z Med J 2013;126:80–4.
26. Bosilkovska M, Walder B, Besson M, et al. Analgesics in patients with hepatic impairment. Drugs 2012;72(12):1645–69.
27. Taruc-Uy RL, Lynch SA. Diagnosis and treatment of osteoarthritis. Prim Care 2013;40(4):821–36.
28. Abrahm JL. A physician's guide to pain and symptom management in cancer patients. JHU Press; 2014.
29. Mercadante SL, Berchovich M, Casuccio A, et al. A prospective randomized study of corticosteroids as adjuvant drugs to opioids in advanced cancer patients. Am J Hosp Palliat Med 2007;24(1):13–9.
30. Porta-Sales J, Garzón-Rodríguez C, Llorens-Torromé S, et al. Evidence on the analgesic role of bisphosphonates and denosumab in the treatment of pain due to bone metastases: a systematic review within the European Association for Palliative Care guidelines project. Palliat Med 2017;31(1):5–25.
31. Colloca L, Ludman T, Bouhassira D, et al. Neuropathic pain. Nat Rev Dis Primers 2017;3:17002.
32. Smith ESJ. Advances in understanding nociception and neuropathic pain. J Neurol 2018;265(2):231–8.
33. Dworkin RH, O'Connor AB, Backonja M, et al. Pharmacologic management of neuropathic pain: evidence based recommendations. Pain 2007;132(3):237–51.
34. Derry S, Wiffen PJ, Aldington D, et al. Nortriptyline for neuropathic pain in adults. Cochrane Database Syst Rev 2015;(1):CD011209.
35. Brogan S, Junkins S. Interventional therapies for the management of cancer pain. J Support Oncol 2010;8(2):52–9.
36. Sindt JE, Brogan SE. Interventional treatments of cancer pain. Anesthesiol Clin 2016;34(2):317–39.

37. Dowell D, Haegerich TM, Chou R. CDC guideline for prescribing opioids for chronic pain—United States, 2016. JAMA 2016;315(15):1624–45.
38. Moss C, Bossano C, Patel S, et al. Weaning from long-term opioid therapy. Clin Obstet Gynecol 2019;62(1):98–109.
39. Ballantyne JC. Opioid therapy in chronic pain. Phys Med Rehabil Clin 2015;26(2): 201–18.
40. Gregorian RS Jr, Gasik A, Kwong WJ, et al. Importance of side effects in opioid treatment: a trade-off analysis with patients and physicians. J Pain 2010;11(11): 1095–108.
41. Hallinan R, Osborn M, Cohen M, et al. Increasing the benefits and reducing the harms of prescription opioid analgesics. Drug Alcohol Rev 2011;30(3):315–23.
42. Morita T, Tsunoda J, Inoue S, et al. Effects of high dose opioids and sedatives on survival in terminally ill cancer patients. J Pain Symptom Manage 2001;21(4): 282–9.
43. Tobin DG, Keough Forte K, Johnson McGee S. Breaking the pain contract: A better controlled-substance agreement for patients on chronic opioid therapy. Cleve Clin J Med 2016;83(11):827–35.
44. Caraceni A, Pigni A, Brunelli C. Is oral morphine still the first choice opioid for moderate to severe cancer pain? A systematic review within the European Palliative Care Research Collaborative guidelines project. Palliat Med 2011;25(5): 402–9.
45. Motov SM. Tarascon pain pocketbook. Jones & Bartlett Learning; 2018.
46. Available at: https://ce.opioidanalgesicrems.com.
47. Goldstein NE, Morrison RS. Evidence-based practice of palliative medicine E-book: expert consult: online and print. Elsevier Health Sciences; 2012.
48. Rennick A, Atkinson T, Cimino NM, et al. Variability in opioid equivalence calculations. Pain Med 2015;17(5):892–8.
49. Mitra S. Opioid-induced hyperalgesia: pathophysiology and clinical implications. J Opioid Manag 2018;4(3):123–30.
50. Mcpherson M. Demystifying opioid conversion calculations, a guide for effective dosing. 1st edition 2010.
51. Pani PP, Trogu E, Maremmani I, et al. QTc interval screening for cardiac risk in methadone treatment of opioid dependence. Cochrane Database Syst Rev 2013;(6):CD008939.
52. Hamilton RJ. Tarascon Pharmacopoeia 2017 professional desk reference edition. Burlington, MA: Jones & Bartlett Learning; 2016.
53. Mcpherson M. Demystifying opioid conversion calculations, a guide for effective dosing. 2st edition 2018.
54. Cheatle MD, Compton PA, Dhingra L, et al. Development of the revised opioid risk tool to predict opioid use disorder in patients with chronic nonmalignant pain. J Pain 2019;20(7):842–51.
55. Morris C, Green KE, Chimuma LL. A Rasch analysis of the Current Opioid Misuse Measure for patients with chronic pain. J Opioid Manag 2018;14(1):9–14.
56. Ebenau A, Dijkstra B, Stal-Klapwijk M, et al. Palliative care for patients with a substance use disorder and multiple problems: a study protocol. BMC Palliat Care 2018;17(1):97.
57. Kirsh KL, Passik SD. Palliative care of the terminally ill drug addict. Cancer Invest 2006;24(4):425–31.
58. Payne R, Anderson E, Arnold R, et al. A rose by any other name: pain contracts/ agreements. Am J Bioeth 2010;10(11):5–12.

59. Penko J, Mattson J, Miaskowski C, et al. Do patients know they are on pain medication agreements? Results from a sample of high-risk patients on chronic opioid therapy. Pain Med 2012;13(9):1174–80.
60. Matthias MS, Johnson NL, Shields CG, et al. "I'm not gonna pull the rug out from under you": patient-provider communication about opioid tapering. J Pain 2017; 18(11):1365–73.
61. Vanderlip ER, Sullivan MD, Edlund MJ, et al. National study of discontinuation of long-term opioid therapy among veterans. Pain 2014;155(12):2673–9.
62. Schweighardt AE, Juba KM. A systematic review of the evidence behind use of reduced doses of acetaminophen in chronic liver disease. J Pain Palliat Care Pharmacother 2018;32(4):226–39.
63. Craig DGN, Lee A, Hayes PC, et al. The current management of acute liver failure. Aliment Pharmacol Ther 2010;31(3):345–58.
64. Davison SN. Chronic pain in end-stage renal disease. Adv Chronic kidney Dis 2005;12(3):326–34.
65. Furlan V, Hafi A, Dessalles MC, et al. Methadone is poorly removed by haemodialysis. Nephrol Dial Transplant 1999;14(1):254–5.
66. Yu DS, Chan HY, Leung DY, et al. Symptom clusters and quality of life among patients with advanced heart failure. J Geriatr Cardiol 2016;13(5):408.
67. Maciver J, Ross HJ. A palliative approach for heart failure end-of-life care. Curr Opin Cardiol 2018;33(2):202.
68. Yu DS, Chan HY, Leung DY, et al. Symptom clusters and quality of life among patients with advanced heart failure. Journal of geriatric cardiology 2016;13(5):408.
69. Schofield P. The assessment of pain in older people: UK national guidelines. Age Ageing 2018;47(suppl_1):i1–22.
70. Pieper MJ, van der Steen JT, Francke AL, et al. Effects on pain of a stepwise multidisciplinary intervention (STA OP!) that targets pain and behavior in advanced dementia: A cluster randomized controlled trial. Palliat Med 2018; 32(3):682–92.
71. Tapp D, Chenacher S, Gérard NPA, et al. Observational pain assessment instruments for use with nonverbal patients at the end-of-life: a systematic review. J Palliat Care 2019. 0825859718816073 [Epub ahead of print].
72. Pepersack T. Nutritional problems in the elderly. Acta Clin Belg 2009;64(2):85–91.
73. Morio K, Maeda I, Yokota I, et al. Risk factors for polypharmacy in elderly patients with cancer pain. Am J Hosp Palliat Med 2019;36(7):598–602.
74. Ong CK, Forbes D. Embracing Cicely Saunders's concept of total pain. BMJ 2005;331(7516):576–7.
75. Rodrigues P, Crokaert J, Gastmans C. Palliative sedation for existential suffering: a systematic review of argument-based ethics literature. J Pain Symptom Manage 2018;55(6):1577–90.
76. Balducci L. Geriatric oncology, spirituality, and palliative care. J Pain Symptom Manage 2019;57(1):171–5.
77. Puchalski C, Romer AL. Taking a spiritual history allows clinicians to understand patients more fully. J Palliat Med 2000;3(1):129–37.

Management of Gastrointestinal Symptoms (Nausea, Anorexia and Cachexia, Constipation) in Advanced Illness

Monica Malec, MD[a], Joseph W. Shega, MD[b,c],*

KEYWORDS

- Anorexia • Cachexia • Nausea • Vomiting • Constipation • Serious illness

KEY POINTS

- Anorexia and cachexia are catabolic states secondary to inflammation not responsive to nutritional interventions with muscle loss, where multimodal interventions focus on reduction of inflammation, anabolic efforts, and improved nutritional status.
- Treatment of nausea and vomiting benefits from the identification of the predominantly involved pathway with accompanying receptor and neurotransmitters, where the antiemetic chosen blocks transmission of implicated neurotransmitters at the receptor level.
- Constipation commonly occurs with serious illness secondary to alterations in peristalsis, changes in fluid secretion and absorption, and dysfunction of the anal sphincter, which can typically be managed through lifestyle modifications and over-the-counter laxatives.
- Opioid-induced constipation should be anticipated with initiation of treatment and prophylactically managed by osmotic agents and/or stimulants, with peripherally acting µ-opioid receptor antagonists (PAMORAs) being reserved for refractory cases.

INTRODUCTION

Gastrointestinal symptoms commonly occur in patients with serious illness and can be associated with substantial distress, increased health care use, a poorer prognosis, and a decreased quality of life.[1,2] Symptoms attributed to the gastrointestinal tract may include heartburn and indigestion, dysphagia, early satiety, abdominal pain, anorexia and cachexia, nausea and vomiting, anorectal symptoms, diarrhea, and constipation.[1] The experience of symptoms can be a manifestation of the underlying disease itself, such as nausea and vomiting from a gastric cancer or secondary to

[a] Section of Geriatrics and Palliative Medicine, Department of Medicine, University of Chicago, 5841 South Maryland Avenue (MC 6098), Chicago, IL 60637, USA; [b] Vitas Healthcare, Miami, FL, USA; [c] University of Central Florida, Orlando, FL, USA
* Corresponding author. VITAS Healthcare, 2201 Lucien Way, Maitland, FL 32759.
E-mail address: jshega@gmail.com

Med Clin N Am 104 (2020) 439–454
https://doi.org/10.1016/j.mcna.2019.12.005
0025-7125/20/© 2019 Elsevier Inc. All rights reserved.

treatments of the underlying disease or symptoms associated with it. For example, a patient with cancer who has metastatic disease to the lower thoracic spine contributing to substantial pain can develop nausea secondary to radiation and/or opioid treatments. The goal of this article is to describe the pathophysiology, assessment, and management of the more common gastrointestinal symptoms in serious illness—anorexia and cachexia, nausea and vomiting, and constipation—to improve clinical management and patient-related outcomes.

ANOREXIA AND CACHEXIA

Serious illness is often associated with poor appetite, nutritional decline, and loss of muscle mass resulting in poorer response to treatment and greater treatment-related toxicities, weakness and fatigue, functional deterioration, and mortality.[3] Such appetite, nutrition, and muscle changes manifest as sarcopenia and/or cachexia. Sarcopenia is age-related muscle loss defined by low muscle mass resulting in impaired functional status. Cachexia, on the other hand, is skeletal muscle loss predominately through inflammation and metabolic changes that cannot be reversed with nutritional support alone. Key differentiators between sarcopenia and cachexia are that cachexia has underlying inflammation and an increased basal metabolic rate, whereas sarcopenia does not have an increase in inflammation and the basal metabolic rate is either unchanged or decreased.[4]

Pathophysiology

Conditions commonly associated with cachexia include cancer, particularly gastrointestinal, heart disease, lung disease, renal disease, and liver disease, with its development generally reflective of progressive serious illness. Prevalence rates vary by condition and disease severity, with 50% to 80% of patients with advanced cancer experiencing cachexia, compared with 5% to 15% in end-stage heart failure.[5] Cachexia results from a catabolic state due to underlying inflammation with an imbalance of pro-inflammatory and anti-inflammatory cytokines along with metabolic changes that increase energy expenditure, contribute to anorexia, and reduced food intake.[6] At the system level, inflammation and associated mediators result in immune, endocrine (including insulin resistance), and metabolic alterations. Such alterations produce a catabolic milieu with tissue loss, predominantly muscle, secondary to proteolysis and autophagy.

Assessment

The identification of the presence and stage of cachexia is paramount along with the determination of other clinical conditions that might be contributing to a worsening of the condition. An agreed definition of cachexia is lacking due in part to the heterogeneity of expression with several definitions being advocated and in varying levels of validation. The 3 consensus-based definitions include Fearon and colleagues,[7] Evans and colleagues,[8] and EPCRC (European Palliative Care Research Collaborative) with the Evans criteria being applicable to all conditions and the other 2 being specifically developed for cancer cachexia. Weight loss is a component of all criteria, but relatively deemphasized with the Evans criteria, which also incorporate inflammation, metabolic alterations, and symptoms. The EPCRC undertook a large validation study leveraging an international population of 1070 patients with advanced cancer, and found that cachexia was associated with significantly higher levels of inflammation, lower nutritional intake and performance status, and shorter survival.[9] The study also examined the validity of the proposed stratification of no cachexia, precachexia, cachexia, and refractory cachexia, which is commonly used clinically to better categorize patients. Cachexia and precachexia were difficult to distinguish, likely secondary to small amounts of weight loss not necessarily being muscle, but did differentiate among the other groups when comparing by mortality. The framework remains very relevant as we try to identify patients earlier, incorporate multimodal interventions, and quantify their impact across the spectrum of cachexia.

A more recent definition that was proposed and being evaluated is the CASCO (cachexia score), which summarizes 5 contributors to the syndrome and its manifestation—body weight and lean body mass loss; anorexia; inflammatory, immunologic, and metabolic disturbances; physical performance; and quality of life.[10] Total score is the summation of scores derived from each of the 5 components that are uniquely weighted where scores range from 0 to 100, with higher scores indicating greater cachexia. Cutoffs exist within the 0 to 100 range to identify the stage of cachexia. The methodology benefits from a broad approach incorporating the many facets of cachexia and the continued emphasis to categorize cachexia into stages to facilitate earlier identification and treatments. However, additional research is needed to better understand how this tool fits in with the others because limitations include its cancer-only focus and the efforts needed to assess each of the 5 domains to generate a total score.

With the identification of cachexia, a multidimensional history and targeted physical examination ensues, including the identification and management of secondary contributors. The assessment incorporates nutritional intake and weight changes, muscle mass determination, physical function, psychosocial and quality of life evaluation, and potential biomarkers, particularly inflammation, focusing on acute phase response proteins. Important contributors to be considered include the following:

- Oral/swallowing issues (dentures, mouth sores, thrush, dry mouth, and dysphagia)
- Digestive problems (early satiety, nausea/vomiting, constipation, and bowel obstruction)
- Malabsorption
- Psychological factors (anxiety, depression, family distress, and spiritual distress)
- Alterations in the sense of smell and taste
- Other symptoms (pain, delirium, and fatigue)
- Metabolic disorders (diabetes, hypogonadism, adrenal insufficiency, and thyroid insufficiency)

At the same time, clinicians should evaluate disease-specific and symptom-related treatments that might be exacerbating cachexia, with discontinuation if feasible and appropriate.

Symptom clusters are another important consideration in the assessment of anorexia and cachexia. Three symptom clusters identified for anorexia include:

1. Bloating, dyspepsia, nausea, and early satiety
2. Depression, anxiety, and insomnia
3. Nausea, fatigue, and pain

Each symptom cluster benefits from a unique management approach. Management of the upper gastrointestinal symptom cluster includes prucalopride, which stimulates peristalsis as a serotonin 5-hydroxytryptamine 4 (5-HT$_4$) agonist,[11] or metoclopramide, which is discussed in greater detail in the nausea and vomiting section. The psychological symptom cluster treatment approach focuses on antidepressants that help stimulate appetite, such as mirtazapine and olanzapine, as well as corticosteroids.[12]

Finally, the physical symptom cluster incorporates the management of the contributing symptom, such as pain, along with corticosteroids or methylphenidate for fatigue.

Management

The management of anorexia and cachexia focuses on the reduction of inflammation, anabolic efforts, and improved nutritional status, including appetite stimulation. Most recent interventions are multimodal, incorporating 2 or more approaches focused on specific stages of cachexia and generally include pharmacologic intervention targeting inflammation and/or anabolic efforts, exercise, and nutritional enhancements.[13] Interventions occur within the context of best supportive care and disease-modifying treatment. A large study is currently underway, MENAC (multimodal exercise, nutrition, and anti-inflammatory medication for cachexia) to overcome limitations of previously conducted studies that lacked randomization, adherence to strict protocols, and high dropout rates. One limitation of such proscriptive studies is patient preference, which in advanced serious illness may have a substantial impact on the fidelity of any intervention. In addition, the heterogeneity of anorexia and cachexia potentially results in interventions being incorporated that are not relevant to all participants. Finally, key components of cachexia are subjective, such as fatigue, weakness, and quality of life and occur in the backdrop of progressive illness further complicating outcome determinations.

The cornerstone of nonpharmacologic management is combination of exercise and nutrition. In incurable cancer, the data are limited but do support better physical endurance and lower depression symptoms; however, without much evidence for improvement in nutrition/weight, overall function, fatigue, and quality of life.[14] The predictors of adherence to the protocols and likely better outcomes were higher baseline nutritional and functional status along with lower overall levels of inflammation. In contrast, studies in other less seriously ill populations, such as chronic obstructive pulmonary disease, demonstrate more robust evidence for multimodal exercise and nutritional interventions that can enhance weight, improve physical function, decrease depression, and prolong survival.[15] Taken together, research needs to delineate the ideal time to incorporate exercise and nutrition in patients with serious illness and cachexia.

Pharmacologic management of cachexia has included anti-inflammatory treatments, anabolic agents, and appetite stimulants. Anti-inflammatory agents, such as nonsteroidal anti-inflammatory drugs and omega-3 supplements, as well as minerals and dietary supplements, have not improved cachexia outcomes in patients with cancer.[14] Megestrol acetate is Food and Drug Administration (FDA) approved for AIDS-associated cachexia and considered the most efficacious of available treatments (**Table 1**). Dronabinol is FDA approved for AIDS-related anorexia and chemotherapy-induced nausea, but is not associated with weight gain. For short-term use, corticosteroids demonstrate efficacy for the management of cachexia, but long-term use is hampered by muscle catabolism, insulin resistance, and adrenal insufficiency. Anamorelin remains under investigation for cancer-related cachexia with 2 published phase 3 clinical studies in non-small cell lung cancer demonstrating increased appetite and weight but without improvement in physical function as measured by hand-grip strength.[16]

NAUSEA AND VOMITING

Nausea and vomiting are common, debilitating, and frequently undertreated symptoms in patients with serious illness, occurring in 16% to 78% of patients.[17,18] In

Table 1
Pharmacologic treatment options for cachexia

Generic Name	Drug Category	Adult Dose	Comments
Megestrol acetate	Progestogens	Initiate at 160 mg/d and increase up to 800 mg/d	Improved appetite in 35%–60% of patients within 1 wk, weight gain may take weeks and is fat and fluid, not muscle Side effects: deep venous thrombosis, edema, adrenal insufficiency, and hypogonadism
Prednisone Dexamethasone	Corticosteroids	20–40 mg/d 4 mg/d	Stimulates appetite for several weeks Short-term use only Prolonged use: myopathy, adrenal insufficiency, immunosuppression, osteoporosis, hypertension, and diabetes
Dronabinol	Cannabinoids	5–20 mg/d, use twice daily dosing starting at 2.5 mg	Increased appetite only Central nervous system side effects of hallucinations, confusion, somnolence, and paranoia Tachycardia

patients with cancer, approximately 30% report nausea, with its frequency increasing to 70% in the last week of life.[19] The symptoms result from the disease itself, along with associated treatments, including medications used for supportive care. The overall evidence base for effective treatment outside of chemotherapy-induced nausea and vomiting (CINV) remains limited.[5] Regardless of the underlying cause, these symptoms negatively impact a person's physical, social, emotional, and psychological well-being.

Nausea is a subjective unpleasant sensation that one will vomit, whereas vomiting is the forceful expulsion of gastric contents through the mouth. Although usually thought of as occurring together and on a continuum, nausea can occur both independently of or lead to the action of vomiting, and vomiting can at times occur in the absence of nausea. Because nausea is a subjective sensation, its severity is often mistakenly characterized by the presence of accompanying emesis; however, persistent nausea is often more distressing and debilitating than that accompanied by vomiting.

Pathophysiology

Nausea with or without vomiting results from the interaction of multiple systems, including the central and peripheral nervous system, the endocrine system, and the gastrointestinal tract. Nauseogenic and emetogenic stimuli arise from the visceral and vestibular systems and the chemoreceptor trigger zone. These inputs then project to the vomiting center via the nucleus tractus solitarius to the medulla, which presents as a diffuse neural circuitry.[7] Inputs to the vomiting center arise from the following locations:

1. Gastrointestinal tract via vagal and glossopharyngeal afferents and splenic nerves
2. Motion detectors in the cerebellum and vestibular system
3. Chemoreceptor trigger zone in the area postrema, which detects toxins in the blood in an area not protected by the blood-brain barrier
4. Cerebral cortex and limbic system, which provides emotional and cognitive response. Neurotransmitters serotonin, dopamine, histamine, and acetylcholine mediate the inputs and vary by location

Endocrine system changes also contribute to the symptoms of nausea and vomiting. Vasopressin levels correlate to the intensity of nausea and increase before emesis. Corticotropin-releasing factor stimulates inhibitory motor nerves in the dorsal motor nucleus of the vagus causing delayed gastric emptying and nausea.[20] The resultant gastric dysrhythmia, an upset of the balance of gastric myoelectrical activity, is dictated by intrinsic pacemaker activity of the stomach, smooth muscle, enteric nervous system, the autonomic nervous system, and hormone levels. Gastric electrical rhythms can be abnormally fast or slow, with both conditions leading to the symptom of nausea.[21]

Another influential contributor to the experience of nausea and vomiting is a person's psychological state. Each person has a particular threshold for nausea and vomiting that varies based on the interaction between these systems and their psychological state. The interplay between these systems is a likely explanation for variability of experience both between individuals and even within the same person at different times in the face of the same stimulus.[22]

Assessment

The foundation of evaluation for nausea and vomiting is a detailed history, physical examination, and targeted testing depending on the goals of care. Components of the history include symptom severity, temporal variation, associated symptoms, previous treatments, and factors that improve or worsen symptoms. Details from the history, corroborated with physical examination findings, give clues to the underlying pathophysiology, which in turn is used to both diagnose reversible causes and guide the selection of antiemetic therapy. **Table 2** lists causes of nausea and vomiting commonly encountered in persons with serious illness.

Management

The first step in management of nausea and vomiting incorporates addressing contributing causes, such as constipation, medication-related side effects, electrolyte disturbances, and dehydration. Adrenal insufficiency leading to chronic nausea and vomiting should be considered in persons with serious illness, particularly in patients on chronic steroid or megestrol use with symptoms being exacerbated by abrupt discontinuation.[23] Adrenal insufficiency has also been reported with immunotherapy drugs through an autoimmune mechanism and its evaluation should be considered within the appropriate clinical context.[24]

Nonpharmacologic treatments remain an important consideration and include avoiding known triggers, such as strong smells. If eating is problematic, focus on small frequent meals that meet the patient's preference in taste and texture. Hypnosis has demonstrated effectiveness in preventing anticipatory CINV primarily in children.[25] Relaxation techniques may be helpful for patients who have anxiety as a factor contributing to symptoms. Benefit from acupuncture and acupressure arises from stimulation of the P6 acupoint and has demonstrated efficacy in multiple randomized controlled trials for postoperative nausea and vomiting, postsurgical gastroparesis, and CINV.[26]

Table 2
Differential diagnosis of nausea and vomiting in serious illness

Central Nervous System	Gastrointestinal	Toxic/Metabolic
Increased intracranial pressure • Malignancy • Hemorrhage • Radiation	Inflammation • Medication • Infection	Medications • Chemotherapy • Nonsteroidal anti-inflammatory drugs • Opioids • Selective serotonin reuptake inhibitor • Amiodarone • Many others
Vestibular • Medication effects • Labyrinthitis • Motion sickness	Decreased motility • Gastroparesis • Constipation • Ascites • Carcinomatosis	Organ failure • Renal failure • Liver failure • Adrenal insufficiency
Anxiety, that is, anticipatory nausea and vomiting	Visceral obstruction • Gastric outlet • Small bowel • Ductal	Electrolyte abnormalities • Hypercalcemia • Hyponatremia

Ongoing symptoms of nausea and vomiting, despite the above approaches, warrant pharmacologic management using either a guideline or empiric approach. The guideline approach selects antiemetic therapy through identification of the predominantly involved pathway with accompanying receptor and neurotransmitters, where the antiemetic chosen blocks transmission of implicated neurotransmitters at the receptor level.[27] In contrast, the empiric approach leverages a D2 antagonist as the treatment for all patients.[28] A recent study comparing the 2 methods demonstrated that a guideline-directed approach improved symptoms more quickly, but no differences in outcomes were evident at 72 hours.[29]

CINV is the most widely studied and categorized as acute, delayed, and/or anticipatory. Acute CINV occurs in the first 24 hours after treatment primarily as a result of serotonin release from enterochromaffin cells. Serotonin antagonists generally are effective at decreasing or eliminating symptoms that fall into this category. Delayed CINV occurs more than 24 hours after treatment and involves a distinct mechanism. In fact, development of the 5HT3 antagonist medications has greatly reduced the incidence of acute CINV, whereas the incidence of delayed CINV has actually risen.[30] Anticipatory CINV occurs before treatment with accompanied anxiety and results from the conditioning of a variety of triggers, including sights, smells, and thoughts.

Guidelines for supportive care in cancer chemotherapy include evidenced-based recommendations for prophylactic management of CINV. These regimens are based on the level of emetogenicity of the chemotherapy regimen.[31,32] Emetogenicity refers to the percentage of patients who would be expected to vomit as a result of a treatment in the absence of antiemetic therapy. Low-emetogenicity agents have an incidence of less than 30%, whereas highly emetic chemotherapy has an incidence of more than 90%. It is thought that effective prophylactic treatment of acute CINV is the best means to prevent both delayed CINV and development of anticipatory nausea and vomiting. If symptoms remain refractory to antiemetic treatment, the chemotherapy dose can be adjusted as per the guidelines.[31,32]

Table 3 displays common medications used for the management of nausea and vomiting in serious illness along with their associated receptor activity and usual dosing regimens. Select classes of medications are described in more detail below:

- Dopamine D2 antagonists act on the chemoreceptor trigger zone to block emetogenic stimuli, such as medications, electrolyte disturbances, and bacterial toxins. Metoclopramide works via D2 receptor antagonism (and selective 5-HT3 receptor antagonism at higher doses) along with gastric motility stimulant effects via 5-HT4 receptor agonism. Olanzapine blocks many neurotransmitters with D_2, 5-HT$_{2c}$, and ACHm (acetylcholine muscarinic) antagonism likely mediating its efficacy in nausea and vomiting with moderate evidence for CINV.[33]
- Serotonin 5-HT3 antagonists work centrally at 5-HT3 receptors in the chemoreceptor trigger zone and peripherally at 5-HT3 receptors on spinal afferent and intestinal vagal nerves. The most robust evidence exists for acute CINV with some evidence available for radiation and postoperative nausea and vomiting.[34]
- Antihistamines and anticholinergic medications are useful for motion sickness and labyrinthitis. Antihistamines act at central anticholinergic (M1) and

Table 3
Select antiemetic treatments for nausea and vomiting

Antiemetic	Usual Oral Dose	Receptor Antagonized	Notes
Haloperidol	0.5–1.5 mg/dose, every 6–12 h	D2	Extrapyramidal symptoms, cardiovascular, and cerebrovascular risks
Metoclopramide	5–10 mg before meals and at bedtime, maximum 60 mg/d	D2, 5HT3	Prokinetic effects due to 5HT4 activation
Olanzapine	2.5–10 mg qd	D2, 5HT2, ACHm	5 times more potent binding at 5HT2 over D2
Prochlorperazine	5–10 mg po q 6–8 h 25 mg PR	D2	
Promethazine	12.5–25 mg po q 4–6 h	H1, ACHm, D2	Can cause dystonia, drowsiness, and sedation
Diphenhydramine	25–50 mg po q 4–6 h	H1	Delirium risk in older adults
Hyoscyamine	0.125–0.25 mg po/sl q 6 h	ACHm	Useful adjuvant for gastrointestinal colic
Scopolamine	1.25 mg q 72 h transdermal patch	ACHm,	Dry mouth Urinary retention
Ondansetron	8 mg po/odt q 8 h	5HT3	Headache Constipation
Granisetron	2 mg po daily or 1 mg po q 12 h	5HT3	Available in extended release patch
Aprepitant	125 mg 1 h before chemotherapy, then 80 mg daily for the following 2–3 d	NK-1	Receptor for substance P
Dexamethasone	4 mg po q 6 h	N/A	Give with food
Dronabinol	5 mg po q 6–8 h	CB-1	Sedation, delirium risk in older adults

antihistamine (H1) receptors to decrease vestibular and labyrinthine stimulation. Anticholinergic medications act at central muscarinic receptors and work to block the pathway from the inner ear to the brainstem and vomiting center.

- Benzodiazepines serve as antiemetics when anticipatory anxiety is contributing to symptom burden, particularly with antitumor therapy through their sedative, anxiolytic, and amnestic properties.
- Cannabinoids work primarily at CB1 in the vomiting center and possibly effect 5HT3 receptors and substance P release contributing to additional antiemetic activity.[35] Dronabinol and nabilone demonstrate efficacy and are FDA approved in refractory CINV. Medical cannabis, however, lacks similar evidence and can be associated with cannabis hyperemesis syndrome, which can occur with chronic cannabis use.[36]

Taken together, nausea and vomiting are common symptoms in patients with serious illness. Although additional evidence to guide management is needed, a range of pharmacologic and nonpharmacologic management options exist, with both guideline and empiric treatment approaches proven effective.

CONSTIPATION

Constipation is an extremely common condition that increases in frequency with serious illness with a prevalence reported as high as 87%.[37] The high rates reported in the literature result from progressive medical conditions and disease-related complications, as well as features that commonly occur in persons with serious illness. Such features may include the development of anorexia, decreased oral intake, low dietary fiber intake, dehydration, medications with anticholinergic effects along with opioid use, decreased activity, and psychosocial factors related to changes in the environment.[38] The impact of constipation can be substantial with accompanying anorexia, bloating, nausea and vomiting, urinary retention, abdominal and rectal pain, and agitation and/or confusion, each resulting in a poorer quality of life.[39]

Pathophysiology

The normal physiology of the colon benefits from peristalsis, including mass movements that occur on awakening and after meals, which move content through the colon and ultimately to the rectum for defecation.[40] Peristalsis and associated motility is highly dependent on serotonin or 5-HT. Another function of the colon is to regulate intestinal fluid and electrolytes, where sodium is actively reabsorbed, and chloride channel activation, resulting in secretion where net reabsorption of fluid occurs daily. Constipation occurs when conditions affect motility, the urge to defecate, or dysfunction of the anal sphincter.

Assessment

A comprehensive assessment incorporates a detailed history and physical examination, including a rectal examination to assess for rectal tone and to rule out an impaction. A consideration of laboratory tests, imaging, and other diagnostics depends on the afore-mentioned findings and with the goals of medical care. As part of the assessment, clinicians need to evaluate the natural history of constipation to determine if the changes in bowel habits are more acute or chronic, as this may influence the approach to care. General history questions may include asking about stool frequency and consistency, straining, inadequate evacuation, abdominal pain, bloating, and hard stool. In addition, clinicians should inquire about weight loss and any blood in the stool or rectal bleeding. Another key component of the assessment of constipation is with regard to the patient's perception of the symptoms in relation to their well-being.

More formal assessment measures of constipation may also be useful depending on the setting.[41] Commonly cited scales include the Victoria Bowel Performance Scale and The Bristol Stool Form Scale, which rank stool consistency based on visual appearance and offers insights into colonic transit time, particularly at the extremes of the scales. The constipation intensity numeric rating scale, Constipation Assessment Scale, and the Constipation Visual Analogue Scale are other standardized measures to appreciate the patient's subjective experience. The ROME IV criteria can be leveraged when determining whether a functional bowel disorder is present, including functional constipation and irritable bowel syndrome.[42] A new functional bowel disorder, opioid-induced constipation (OIC), has particular relevance to patients with serious illness.

Management

In treatment of serious illness, development of constipation should be considered with any treatment that is recommended with the intent to incorporate proactive measures to prevent its development. Once constipation occurs, clinicians focus effort on developing a treatment tailored to the individual patient's needs. That is, the patient helps define "acceptable bowel function," which means habits that are acceptable to the patient along with a decrease or cessation of previously described associated symptoms.

Nonpharmacologic approaches to the management of constipation remain commonly overlooked in patients with serious illness and include adequate hydration, sufficient dietary fiber, and increased physical activity as tolerated.[43] Each of these approaches needs to be considered within the context of the patient's underlying medical conditions, prognosis, and goals of care. In addition to lifestyle modification, medications that slow transit time should be discontinued if possible or switched to alternatives that have less impact on it. Abdominal massage is another nonpharmacologic treatment that has shown efficacy in patients with serious illness and neurologic bowel dysfunction.[44]

Laxative management of constipation seeks to either increase water content of stool or decrease transit time, which decreases water reabsorption and increases substance. The mechanism of action of laxatives is a pragmatic classification approach that includes bulking agents, surfactants, osmotic agents, stimulants, prokinetics, secretory agents, and suppositories and enemas (**Table 4**). Evidence is not available to support the use of one laxative over another, so that use is driven by patient choice, which includes tolerability, availability, and cost. A large number of laxatives are relatively inexpensive, available over the counter, and considered first-line treatment. Newer intestinal secretogog and serotonin receptor agonist prescription laxatives demonstrate efficacy but are extremely costly without a discernible benefit compared with over-the-counter preparations.[45]

Over-the-Counter Laxatives

Over-the-counter agents include bulking agents, surfactants, osmotic agents, stimulants, and suppositories and enemas. Bulking agents are generally not recommended in seriously ill populations because additional fiber can contribute to bloating and gaseousness along with the need to consume sufficient hydration, which can lead to volume overload. Moreover, inadequate hydration can potentially result in an impaction. Thus, soluble fiber in nonseriously ill populations has been found to improve symptoms.[46]

Table 4
Select laxative treatments for constipation

Generic Name	Drug Category	Adult Dose	Onset of Action (h)	Adverse Events
Psyllium	Bulking agent	Up to 30 g in 1–3 doses per day	12–72	Gas, bloating, volume overload, and impaction
Docusate sodium	Surfactant	50–500 mg/d	24–72	Rash and bitter taste
Polyethylene glycol	Osmotic agent	8.5–34 g daily	24–72	Gas, nausea, and diarrhea
Lactulose	Osmotic agent	10 g per 15 mL, max 60 mL/d	48–72	Gas, abdominal discomfort, and distention
Senna	Stimulant	2 tabs (8.6 mg sennosides/tab) at night, up to 4 tabs bid	8–12	Nausea, abdominal cramps, and diarrhea
Bisacodyl	Stimulant	5–30 mg/d	6–12	Nausea, abdominal cramps, and diarrhea
Prucalopride	Prokinetic	1–2 mg/d	2–3	Headache, abdominal pain, nausea, and diarrhea
Lubiprostone	Secretory	24 µg bid	24	Nausea and diarrhea

Surfactants, such as docusate sodium (docusate) increase fluid into the intestine and stool facilitating decreased transit time and softer stool. Docusate has had mixed results in randomized controlled trials with the most recent demonstrating no additional benefit in constipation symptoms when comparing docusate plus senna to placebo plus senna in a hospice setting.[47] In addition, the docusate arm had significantly more stools noted to be "mushy." Therefore, docusate has fallen out of favor in general for patients with serious illness, but may serve a role in select patients.

Osmotic agents contain poorly absorbed/nonabsorbable particles that draw water into the intestinal lumen thereby decreasing transit time and increasing water content of stools. More commonly used osmotic agents include polyethylene glycol (PEG) and lactulose, with the former reported to being more efficacious than the latter with improved stool frequency, stool consistency, and abdominal pain.[48] Lactulose contributes to bloating and distention through bacterial metabolism of carbohydrates and resultant gas production, which can be problematic, particularly for seriously ill patients. PEG with electrolytes is not more efficacious than PEG without electrolytes and is now available over the counter. PEG can be slowly titrated to symptomatic relief with soft but not liquid stool. Other osmotic agents are used less often, such as magnesium- and phosphate-based products, because each can contribute to electrolyte abnormalities, which can be fatal, particularly in patients with underlying renal disease.

Over-the-counter stimulants include senna and bisacodyl, which decrease water absorption, induce colonic contractions, and decrease colonic transit time. A JAMA review on constipation debunks 2 common concerns related to colonic damage and developing dependency with the use of stimulant laxatives.[40] The review noted that evidence, particularly for bisacodyl, does not support that stimulants are harmful to the colon/enteric nervous system or that they are addictive. Stimulant laxatives can produce nausea and vomiting, cramping with abdominal pain, and diarrhea. Bisacodyl is available in oral and suppository preparations, with the suppository often being administered before breakfast to benefit from the gastrocolonic effect.

Suppositories and enemas help increase water content and stimulate peristalsis, resulting in a relatively quick onset of action compared with oral laxatives to produce a bowel movement. Patients and families often report feeling uncomfortable with administering treatments via the rectum and may also be perceived as invasive, which limits use. Generally, suppositories and enemas are leveraged for short-term use because patients with severe symptoms are initiated on an oral bowel regimen. Contraindications to rectal administration include recent rectal surgery or trauma, intestinal obstruction, toxic megacolon, neutropenia, and/or thrombocytopenia. Most commonly used suppositories include bisacodyl, which has previously been mentioned, and glycerin.

Small-volume and large-volume enema preparations exist, with large-volume products requiring experienced clinicians to administer to decrease risk of complications, such as bowel perforation, traumatic injury, and hematomas, particularly if the patient is on any anticoagulation. Hypertonic sodium phosphate enema is a small-volume enema that is easy to use and generally well accepted by patients, but requires caution in persons with end-stage renal disease due to the phosphate load.[49] Normal saline and soap suds enemas distend the rectum and soften stool but the soap suds can be irritating to mucosa limiting its use. Several other enema preparations are available but beyond the scope of this review.

Prescription Laxatives

Prescription laxatives discussed in this review include prokinetic and secretory agents, with the former class recently obtaining FDA approval.[40] Prucalopride stimulates peristalsis as a 5-HT_4 agonist, where 5-HT_4 is widely distributed in the enteric nervous system leading to the release of acetylcholine and subsequent increase in gastrointestinal motility. It is a highly selective agonist and lacks affinity to the potassium channels in the heart that are responsible for cardiac arrhythmias that occurred with cisapride, which led to it being taken off the market. A comparative study did not find prucalopride to be more efficacious than PEG and thus is considered a second- or third-line treatment.[45] No reported increase in cardiovascular events has been reported, but headache, abdominal pain, nausea, and diarrhea are common adverse effects. A causal link has not been established between suicidal ideation and attempts, but these have been reported in clinical trials. The dosage of prucalopride should be reduced for renal impairment.

Intestinal secretory agents lubiprostone, linaclotide, and plecanatide are approved for the management of chronic constipation and work by increasing the release of chloride and water into the intestinal lumen.[50,51] Lubiprostone is a fatty acid derivative of prostaglandin E1 and activates type 2 chloride channels, whereas linaclotide, and plecanatide activate cystic fibrosis transmembrane conductance regulator in the intestinal epithelium through guanylate cyclase-c. In a meta-analysis, these agents increased the number of compete spontaneous bowel movements per week compared with placebo. Lubiprostone has associated nausea, whereas linaclotide and plecanatide increase likelihood of diarrhea, which seems to be dose dependent. Linaclotide and plecanatide contain black box warnings and are contraindicated in patients less than 6 years secondary to death in juvenile mice related to dehydration, and avoidance of use is recommended in patients 6 to 18 years due to lack of safety and effectiveness data.

Opioid-Induced Constipation

OIC is commonplace, with prevalence rates ranging from 40% to 60% without the development of tolerance, dictating a prophylactic approach to management. Opioid receptors are located throughout the gastrointestinal tract, so that opioid agonists result in 3 main contributors to OIC—gastrointestinal motility, secreto-absorption, and gastrointestinal sphincters.[52] Opioids increase transit time by stimulating nonpropulsive activity, intestinal segmentation, and increased tone thereby decreasing normal peristalsis activity. Opioids decrease secretion of chloride and water into the intestinal lumen, while also increasing water reabsorption through increased transit time contributing to hard and dry stools. Finally, increased contraction of the internal anal sphincter secondary to opioids contributes to opioid-induced anorectal dysfunction clinically manifested as straining and a sensation of incomplete evacuation.

The management of OIC incorporates the nonpharmacologic/lifestyle measures previously discussed along with over-the-counter laxatives, specifically osmotic agents (PEG) and stimulants (senna and bisacodyl). If patients continue to have constipation symptoms that would benefit from additional management, peripherally acting μ-opioid receptor antagonists (PAMORAs) are generally the next recommended management approach. PAMORAs include alvimopan (FDA approved for postoperative ileus, with restricted use secondary to increased cardiovascular risk), methylnaltrexone (FDA approved for noncancer pain and in adults with advanced illness receiving palliative care), naldemedine (FDA approved for noncancer pain), and naloxegol (FDA approved for noncancer pain). The drug class blocks μ receptors peripherally but not centrally, thus helping relieve constipation without loss of analgesia. A published systematic review and meta-analysis, included 31 randomized controlled trials with almost 8000 patients, found PAMORA therapy significantly improved spontaneous bowel movements, responder rate, and quality of life compared with the placebo group.[52]

Lubiprostone has been approved by the FDA for the treatment of OIC. Treatment has not been demonstrated to affect opioid analgesia but is associated with nausea, vomiting, abdominal pain, and diarrhea. Methadone does not appear to respond to lubiprostone therapy compared with other opioids, which may be dose dependent.[52]

SUMMARY

Anorexia and cachexia, nausea and vomiting, and constipation frequently accompany serious illness and adversely impact patient well-being, including a reduction in quality of life. Symptom control is generally achievable when a comprehensive assessment is conducted in conjunction with the incorporation of knowledge of underlying pathophysiology to drive relevant and targeted treatment selection.

DISCLOSURE

The authors have nothing to disclose.

REFERENCES

1. Peery AF, Crockett SD, Murphy CG, et al. Burden and cost of gastrointestinal, liver, and pancreatic diseases in the United States: update 2018. Gastroenterology 2019;156:254–72.

2. Kelly AS, Morrison RS. Palliative care for the seriously ill. N Engl J Med 2015;373: 747–55.

3. Muscaritoli M, Anker SD, Argilé J, et al. Consensus definition of sarcopenia, cachexia and pre-cachexia: joint document elaborated by special interest groups (SIG) "cachexia-anorexia in chronic wasting diseases" and "nutrition in geriatrics." Clin Nutr 2010;29:154–9.
4. Peterson SJ, Mozer M. Differentiating sarcopenia and cachexia among patients with cancer. Nutr Clin Pract 2017;32(1):30–9.
5. von Haehling S, Markus S, Anker A, et al. Prevalence and clinical impact of cachexia in chronic illness in Europe, USA, and Japan: facts and numbers update 2016. J Cachexia Sarcopenia Muscle 2016;7:507–9.
6. Baracos VE, Martin L, Korc M, et al. Cancer-associated cachexia. Nat Rev Dis Primers 2018;18(4):17105.
7. Fearon K, Strasser F, Anker SD, et al. Definition and classification of cancer cachexia: an international consensus. Lancet Oncol 2011;12(5):489–95.
8. Evans WJ, Morley JE, Argiles, et al. Cachexia: A new definition. Clin Nutr 2008; 27(6):793–9.
9. Blum D, Stene GB, Solheim TS, et al. Validation of the consensus-definition for cancer cachexia and evaluation of a classification model - a study based on data from an international multicenter project (EPCRC-CSA). Ann Oncol 2014; 25:1635–42.
10. Argilés JM, López-Soriano FJ, Toledo M, et al. The cachexia score (CASCO): a new tool for staging cachectic cancer patients. J Cachexia Sarcopenia Muscle 2011;2:87–93.
11. Carbone F, Van den Houte K, Clevers E, et al. Prucalopride in gastroparesis: a randomized placebo-controlled crossover study. Am J Gastroenterol 2019; 114(8):1265–74.
12. Yennurajalingam S, Williams JL, Chisholm G, et al. Effects of dexamethasone and placebo on symptom clusters in advanced cancer patients: a preliminary report. Oncologist 2016;21:384–90.
13. Fabbro ED. Combination therapy in cachexia. Ann Palliat Med 2019;8(1):59–66.
14. Hall CC, Cook J, Maddocks M, et al. Combined exercise and nutritional rehabilitation in outpatients with incurable cancer: a systematic review. Support Care Cancer 2019;27:2371–84.
15. van de bool C, Rutten EPA, van Helvoort A, et al. A randomized clinical trial investigating the efficacy of targeted nutrition as an adjunct to exercise training in COPD. J Cachexia Sarcopenia Muscle 2017;8(5):748–58.
16. Prommer E. Oncology update: anamorelin. Palliat Care 2017;10. 1178224217726336.
17. Greaves J, Glare P, Kristjanson LJ, et al. Undertreatment of nausea and other symptoms in hospitalized cancer patients. Support Care Cancer 2009;17(4): 461–4.
18. Solano JP, Gomes B, Higginson IJ. A comparison of symptom prevalence in far advanced cancer, AIDS, heart disease, chronic obstructive pulmonary disease and renal disease. J Pain Symptom Manage 2006;31(1):58–69.
19. Gordon P, LeGrand S, Walsh D. Nausea and vomiting in advanced cancer. Eur J Pharmacol 2014;722:187–91.
20. Singh P, Yoon SS, Kuo B. Nausea: a review of pathophysiology and therapeutics. Therap Adv Gastroenterol 2016;9(1):98–112.
21. Koch KL. Gastric dysrhythmias: a potential objective measure of nausea. Exp Brain Res 2014;232:2553–61.
22. Stern RM, Koch KL, Andrews PL. Nausea: mechanism and treatment. New York: Oxford Press; 2011.

23. Deltala AP, Fanciulli G, Maioli M, et al. Primary symptomatic adrenal insufficiency induced by megestrol acetate. Neth J Med 2013;71(1):17–21.
24. Sznol M, Postow MA, Davies MJ, et al. Endocrine-related adverse events associated with immune checkpoint blockade and expert insights on their management. Cancer Treat Rev 2017;58:70–6.
25. Richardson J, Smith JE, McCall G, et al. Hypnosis for nausea and vomiting in cancer chemotherapy: a systematic review of the research evidence. Eur J Cancer Care 2007;16(5):402–12.
26. Ezzo J, Streitberger K, Schneider A. Cochrane systematic reviews examine P6 acupuncture-point stimulation for nausea and vomiting. J Altern Complement Med 2006;12(5):489–95.
27. Stephenson J, Davies A. An assessment of aetiology-based guidelines for the management of nausea and vomiting in patients with advanced cancer. Support Care Cancer 2006;14:348–53.
28. Gupta M, Davis MP, LeGrand S, et al. Nausea and vomiting in advanced cancer: the Cleveland Clinic protocol. J Support Oncol 2013;11:8–13.
29. Hardy J, Skerman H, Glare p, et al. A randomized open-label study of guideline driven antiemetic therapy versus single agent antiemetic therapy in patients with advanced cancer and nausea not related to cancer treatment. BMC Cancer 2018;18:510.
30. Rapoport BL. Delayed chemotherapy-induced nausea and vomiting: pathogenesis, incidence and current management. Front Pharmacol 2017;8:19.
31. Rolla F, Molassiotis A, Herrstedt J, et al. 2016 MASCC and ESMO guideline update for the prevention of chemotherapy and radiotherapy-induced nausea and vomiting and of nausea and vomiting in advanced cancer patients. Ann Oncol 2016;27(Supplement 5):v119–33.
32. Berger MJ, Ettinger DS, Aston J, et al. NCCN guidelines insights: antiemesis, version 2.2017. J Natl Compr Canc Netw 2017;15(7):883–93.
33. Sutherlands A, Naessens K, Plugge E, et al. Olanzapine for the prevention and treatment of cancer-related nausea and vomiting in adults. Cochrane Database Syst Rev 2018;(9):CD012555.
34. Schwartzberg L. Getting it right the first time: recent progress in optimizing antiemetic usage. Support Care Cancer 2018;26(Suppl 1):519–27.
35. Cangemi DJ, Kuo B. Practical perspectives in the treatment of nausea and vomiting. J Clin Gastroenterol 2019;53(3):170–8.
36. Smith LA, Azariah F, Lavender VT, et al. Cannabinoids for nausea and vomiting in adults with cancer receiving chemotherapy. Cochrane Database Syst Rev 2015;(11):CD009464.
37. Larkin PJ, Skyes NP, Centeno C, et al. The management of constipation in palliative care: clinical practice recommendations. Palliat Med 2008;22(7):796–807.
38. Larkin PJ, Cherny NI, La Carpia D, et al. Diagnosis, assessment and management of constipation in advanced cancer: ESMO Clinical Practice Guidelines. Ann Oncol 2018;29(Sup 4):iv111–25.
39. Bellini M, Usai-Satta P, Bove A, et al. Chronic constipation diagnosis and treatment evaluation: the "CHRO.CO.DI.T.E." study. BMC Gastroenterol 2017;17:11.
40. Wald A. Constipation advances in diagnosis and treatment. JAMA 2016;315(2):185–91.
41. Muldrew DHL, Hasson F, Cardruff E, et al. Assessment and management of constipation for patients receiving palliative care in specialist palliative care setting: a systematic review of the literature. Palliat Med 2018;32(5):930–8.

42. Lacy BE, Mearin F, Chang L, et al. Bowel disorders. Gastroenterology 2016; 150(6):1393–407.
43. McIlfatrick S, Muldrew DHL, Beck E, et al. Examining constipation assessment and management of patients with advanced cancer receiving specialist palliative care: a multi-site retrospective case note review of clinical practice. BMC Palliat Care 2019;18:57.
44. McClurg D, Hagen S, Dickinson JK, et al. Abdominal massage for the alleviation of the symptoms of constipation in people with Parkinson's: a randomised controlled pilot study. Age Ageing 2016;45:299–303.
45. Cinca R, Chera D, Gruss HJ, et al. Randomiser clinical trial: macrogel\PEG 3350 + electrolyte versus prucalopride in the treatment of chronic constipation—a comparison in a controlled environment. Aliment Pharmacol Ther 2013; 37(9):876–86.
46. Suares NC, Ford AC. Systematic review: the effects of fibre in the management of chronic idiopathic constipation. Aliment Pharmacol Ther 2011;33(8):895–901.
47. Tarumi Y, Wilson MP, Szafran O, et al. Randomized, double-blind, placebo-controlled trial of oral docusate in the management of constipation in hospice patients. J Pain Symptom Manage 2013;45(1):2–13.
48. Lee-Robichaud H, Thomas K, Morgan J, et al. Lactulose versus polyethylene glycol for chronic constipation. Cochrane Database Syst Rev 2010;(7):CD007570.
49. Available at: https://www.geripal.org/2012/02/dangers-of-fleet-enemas.html. Accessed October 6, 2019.
50. Lasa JS, Altamirano MJ, Bracho LF, et al. Efficacy and safety of intentinal secretagogues for chronic constipation: a systemic review and meta-analysis. Gastroenterol 2018;55(Suppl 1):2–12.
51. Farmer AD, Drewes AM, Chiarioni G, et al. Pathophysiology and management of opioid-induced constipation: European expert consensus statement. United European Gastroenterol J 2019;7(1):7–20.
52. Nishie K, Yamamoto S, Yamaga T, et al. Peripherally acting μ-opioid antagonists for the treatment of opioid-induced constipation: systematic review and meta-analysis. J Gastroenterol Hepatol 2019;34(5):818–29.

Management of Respiratory Symptoms in Those with Serious Illness

Cynthia X. Pan, MD, AGSF[a,b],*, Brigit C. Palathra, MD[b,c],
Wing Fun Leo-To, PharmD, BCPS[d,e]

KEYWORDS

- Palliative • Dyspnea • Breathlessness • Cough • Malignant pleural effusions
- Hemoptysis • Airway secretions

KEY POINTS

- Dyspnea is a highly prevalent, subjective symptom. Clinicians should recognize the concept of "total dyspnea"—and consider physical, psychological, social, and spiritual factors when assessing a patient's dyspnea.
- Cough contributes to significant physical and emotional complications and poor quality of life (QOL). Clinicians should not discount patients' cough-related concerns.
- Treatment of dyspnea and cough is multimodal, and opioids are effective for treating both, in conjunction with disease-directed therapies.
- Malignant pleural effusions carry a poor prognosis. Management is guided by expert consensus guidelines.

INTRODUCTION

The clinical manifestation of respiratory symptoms is common in cancer and nonmalignant conditions, such as congestive heart failure (CHF), chronic obstructive pulmonary disease (COPD), and interstitial lung disease (ILD). The most common presenting symptom is dyspnea (breathlessness). Because of their presentation in multiple

---

[a] Division of Palliative Medicine and Geriatrics, Designated Institution Official of Graduate Medical Education, NewYork-Presbyterian Queens, 56-45 Main Street, Flushing, NY 11355, USA; [b] Weill Cornell Medical College, New York, NY, USA; [c] Hospice and Palliative Medicine Fellowship, Division of Palliative Medicine and Geriatrics, NewYork-Presbyterian Queens, 56-45 Main Street, Flushing, NY 11355, USA; [d] NewYork-Presbyterian Queens, 56-45 Main Street, Flushing, NY 11355, USA; [e] Affiliate Clinical Faculty, College of Pharmacy and Health Science, St John's University, Jamaica, NY, USA
* Corresponding author. Division of Palliative Medicine and Geriatrics, Designated Institution Official of Graduate Medical Education, NewYork-Presbyterian Queens, 56-45 Main Street, Flushing, NY 11355.
E-mail address: cxp9001@nyp.org
Twitter: @Cxpan5X (C.X.P.); @bpalathra (B.C.P.)

Med Clin N Am 104 (2020) 455–470
https://doi.org/10.1016/j.mcna.2019.12.004
medical.theclinics.com

venues of care, we as a medical community have shared accountability to address dyspnea[1] and related respiratory symptoms. Basic management of respiratory symptoms is within the scope of primary palliative care. This article aims to familiarize clinicians on how to approach these burdensome symptoms.

DYSPNEA/BREATHLESSNESS

Breathing is a continuous cycle that we unconsciously perform during a lifetime. The presence and quality of breath is assessed at birth; its absence is noted at death. Dyspnea or breathlessness is when breathing is perceived as difficult or burdensome. These terms are used interchangeably here.

Breathlessness is a prevalent symptom in patients with serious illness, cancer and noncancer alike.[2–4] Often disabling, breathlessness is accompanied by psychosocial, existential components in addition to the physical expression. There is variation in how patients often describe dyspnea (**Fig. 1**).

Definitions

Defining acute and chronic aspects of dyspnea is important, because management approach is different. Experts are advocating for better definition of dyspnea as not just an acute 1-dimensional symptom, because as a disease progresses, breathlessness becomes a complex syndrome.[5]

New onset dyspnea presents abruptly with a new diagnosis and often resolves with disease-directed management. Examples include acute asthma exacerbations and bacterial pneumonia.[6]

Chronic breathlessness syndrome occurs with a known chronic disease contributing to "the experience of breathlessness that persists despite optimal treatment of underlying pathophysiology and results in disability for the patient."[1]

Dyspnea crisis is often seen in the later phase of disease trajectory. It is best described by Mularski and colleagues[7] as "sustained and severe resting breathing discomfort that occurs in patients with advanced, often life-limiting illness and overwhelms the patient and caregivers' ability to achieve symptom relief."

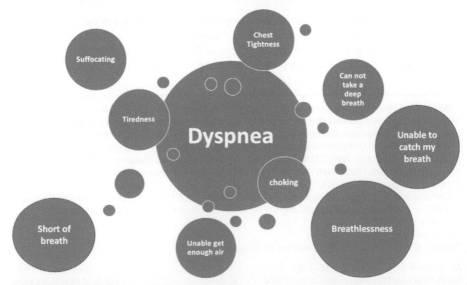

Fig. 1. Various expressions of dyspnea by patients.

Total dyspnea is a concept aligned with the "total pain" view coined by Dame Cicely Saunders. Abernethy and Wheeler[8] illustrate the synergistic effects of physical, psychological, social, and spiritual factors on a patient's breathlessness experience. The patient's subjective perception of dyspnea is complex, influenced by direct physiologic effects as well as accompanying anxiety. Likewise, when patients report poor dyspnea control, this can distress both caregivers and clinicians. The patient's own existential crisis regarding their advanced illness further complicates the breathlessness response.

Etiology

Often patients with serious illness will have multimorbidities that make dyspnea management more challenging (**Fig. 2**). Identifying the causes helps direct disease management. Risks and benefits of any intervention must be balanced with the ongoing clinical picture and overall prognosis. In advanced or end-stage illness, disease-altering therapies are likely not beneficial and could incur burden and harm.

Pathophysiology

Breathlessness can be characterized into 3 distinct qualities that are associated with specific neural mechanisms: work of breathing, air hunger, chest tightness.

Work of breathing or increased effort of respiration is often projected by respiratory muscle afferent signals to the cerebral cortex. Factors contributing to this corollary discharge to the brain include:

1. Increased resistance due to airway obstruction or external restriction (ie, COPD, tumor).
2. Muscle weakness (ie, neuromuscular disorder, cachexia, deconditioning, fatigue).
3. Increased exercise effort.[6,9–11]

Air hunger, also described as unsatisfied inspiration, often results from chemoreceptor activation. Carbon dioxide tensions play a more significant role in eliciting this response. Hypercapnia influences the medullary chemoreceptors whereas

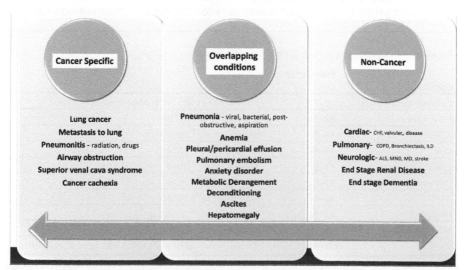

Fig. 2. Disease-specific causes of dyspnea in patients with serious illness. ALS, amyotrophic lateral sclerosis; CHF, congestive heart failure; COPD, chronic obstructive pulmonary disease; ILD, interstitial lung disease; MD, muscular dystrophy; MND, motor neuron disease.

hypoxemia affects carotid and aortic ones. The efferent-afferent mismatch occurs when the cortex receives corollary signals from the respiratory center demanding increased ventilatory drive but the respiratory response does not meet this request.[6,9–11]

Chest tightness is frequently associated with bronchoconstriction. Airway receptors are stimulated, triggering pulmonary afferents to the brain. This neuromechanical dissociation is distinct from the work of breathing and stimulation of chemoreceptors.[6,9–11]

Prevalence

Breathlessness is frequently seen in palliative care patients across a spectrum of diseases and is well described in the literature (**Table 1**).[2,12–15]

Evaluation and Assessment

History, physical examination, and appropriate diagnostic testing should be performed to assess dyspnea. Various scales are used in assessing severity of breathlessness in the palliative care population.[6,16] The modified Borg scale is easy to administer and practical to implement. Edmonton Symptom Assessment System is a more global scale that assesses for concurrent symptoms, such as pain, nausea, depression, anxiety, drowsiness, appetite, and sensation of well-being. To guide diagnosis and treatment, it is useful to clarify if this is a new symptom (acute dyspnea), ongoing process (chronic breathlessness), or an acute on chronic process (dyspnea crisis).

Assessment begins with the initial encounter and is ongoing and repeated throughout the disease course. Management may need ongoing titration or modification as disease progresses.[6,16–18] Evaluation should include the "total dyspnea" perspective of patients, families, and caregivers, as breathlessness is distressing for both reporters and observers.

Management

If a new disease process, change in chronic illness, or hypoxemia is identified, specific treatment targeting the underlying cause is recommended. Concurrent consultation

Table 1
Prevalence of dyspnea in serious illness patients based on disease

Condition	Prevalence (%)	References
Cancer—unspecified	16–77	Ripamonti et al,[2] 1998; Moens et al,[12] 2014
Lung cancer	62–95	Currow et al,[13] 2010
COPD	56–98	Moens et al,[12] 2014
CHF	18–88	Moens et al,[12] 2014
ESRD	11–82	Moens et al,[12] 2014
Dementia	12–52	Moens et al,[12] 2014
AIDS	43–62	Moens et al,[12] 2014
MND/ALS	81–88	Moens et al,[12] 2014
MS	26	Moens et al,[12] 2014
Stroke	37–44	Addington-Hall et al,[14] 1995; Menezes et al,[15] 2018

Abbreviations: ALS, amyotrophic lateral sclerosis; CHF, congestive heart failure; COPD, chronic obstructive pulmonary disease; ESRD, end-stage renal disease; MND, motor neuron disease; MS, multiple sclerosis.
Data from Refs.[2,12–15]

with a specialist (ie, pulmonary, cardiology, oncology) may be required.[1,7,18,19] Particularly in patients with serious illness, clinicians must weigh the risks and benefits of any diagnostic or therapeutic intervention. This is to assure care is concordant with patient values and preferences regarding medical care and what they perceive as an acceptable quality of life (QOL). This shared decision-making approach is important at any point of the disease trajectory.

Often disease-directed therapy alone may not have an impact on the sensation of dyspnea in advanced illness. Clinicians can offer changing focus of care to more symptomatic management that is, described below.

Nonpharmacologic

1. *Positioning:* Positioning can help mitigate dyspnea. In patients with COPD, a forward leaning position with pursed lip breathing is helpful. In patients with malignant pleural effusions (MPEs) or effusions, laying with the effusion side down is helpful to aerate the less affected lung.[20]
2. *Fan therapy:* A systematic review showed limited direct evidence from randomized controlled trials of patients with nonmalignant and malignant diseases. However, there is evidence that hand-fan therapy may effectively alleviate dyspnea.[21] The most common nonmalignant disease was COPD and most common duration of fan therapy was 5 minutes. Fans are inexpensive, low risk, and patients may benefit from a trial.
3. *Pulmonary rehabilitation:* In patients with COPD who can undergo pulmonary rehabilitation, it has been shown to improve dyspnea and fatigue, as well as QOL and exercise tolerance. Hospital-based programs had better QOL improvement scores versus community-based ones.[22] In patients with a life expectancy of months or less, the benefit is not known.[18]
4. *Oxygen:* Oxygen therapy is recommended for hypoxic patients or those with exertional hypoxemia.[6,10,11,17,23,24] An international double-blind randomized controlled trial examined response of oxygen versus medical (room) air to relieve breathlessness in patients with life-limiting illness, refractory dyspnea, and Pao_2 greater than 55 mm Hg. The intensity of dyspnea improved comparably in both arms. The authors hypothesized that air stimulating the nasal passages reduced sensation of breathlessness,[25] but there were subgroup differences. Subsequent systematic reviews found that use of oxygen in nonhypoxemic patients with COPD[26] improved dyspnea whereas nonhypoxemic patients with cancer did not have the same relief.[27] Thus, we recommend that patients with cancer who are nonhypoxemic should be assessed for opioids or fan therapy before consideration of O_2.
5. *Other interventions:* Cochrane Systematic Review found breathing training, walking aids, neuroelectrical muscle stimulation, and chest wall vibration to help relieve dyspnea in advanced disease. There is some evidence that acupuncture or acupressure may be helpful.[28,29]
6. *Use of noninvasive ventilation in end of life:* Noninvasive ventilation (NIV) is used frequently for dyspnea management in end of life but time limited trials are highly recommended. When using NIV, there must be appropriate, achievable, patient-centered, short-term goals.[30] In a prospective study, NIV did not affect QOL and did not provide significant dyspnea relief of symptoms in over half the patients.[31]

Pharmacologic

1. Systemic opioids:
   - *Overview:* Existing evidence and expert societies support using oral and parenteral opioids for dyspnea in advanced illness patients with chronic

breathlessness and acute dyspnea crisis, when disease-directed therapy is limited.[6,17,24,32–34] When appropriately used, opioids can be beneficial earlier in the trajectory of serious illness by improving QOL and functional goals.[18,35]

- *Mechanism of action:* Dyspnea relief is theorized by: (1) central opioid receptor actions—direct (cortical opioid receptors) and indirect (corollary discharge from respiratory center to sensory cortex), (2) peripheral receptor actions in the respiratory tract, and (3) alleviating anxiety.[36]
- *Safety profile:* Current evidence supports the use of opioids in advanced cancer, COPD, and ILD without concern of induced mortality or respiratory side effects, if managed responsibly.[9,11,18,32,33,35–40] Long-acting morphine was beneficial and safe in treating chronic dyspnea.[39] There is anecdotal support in amyotrophic lateral sclerosis (ALS)[11] and benefit is unclear in CHF.[11,18] Initiation and maintenance of opioid therapy for dyspnea requires informed decision making and ongoing counseling. Patients and families must be informed about common side effects and advised to monitor for them (constipation, nausea, somnolence, and hallucinations).
- *Starting doses:* **Fig. 3** shows dosing recommendations.[17,23,37,39,41–44] It is reasonable to start low and go slow, especially in the serious illness population. When initiating opioids, clinicians should consider frailty, body habitus, renal and hepatic clearance, comorbidities, and current medications when picking both the opioid and the dose.[11]
- *Episodic versus chronic breathlessness:* As needed, low-dose morphine can be used to treat episodic breathlessness, whereas sustained release formulations are reserved for chronic breathlessness.
- *Current opioid epidemic climate inhibits opioid use due to recent Centers for Disease Control (CDC) guidelines:* In 2016, the CDC released their guidelines for prescribing opioids for chronic pain *outside of* active cancer treatment, palliative care, and end-of-life care.[45]

These CDC guidelines refer to chronic pain and do not apply to patients being managed for palliative needs, end of life, and hospice settings. It is still important to risk-stratify patients with potential for substance use disorder, addiction, and diversion, and monitor for misuse. We recommend clinicians to follow local state laws and national guidelines.

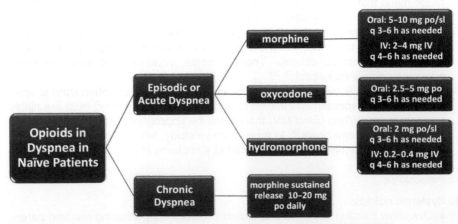

Fig. 3. Starting doses for opioid naive patients. (*Data from* Refs.[23,37,39,41,42,44])

2. Nebulized medications:
   - There is not strong evidence to support the use of nebulized opioids in improving dyspnea or exercise tolerance.[11,32,33,46,47]
   - Current evidence weakly suggests that aerosolized furosemide may reduce dyspnea in patients with advanced cancer and COPD.[46,47]
   - Aerosolized saline may have some therapeutic effect on breathlessness, but this has not been fully defined.[46]
3. Benzodiazepines and anxiolytics:
   - *Benzodiazepines*: According to a 2016 Cochrane Review, there is no conclusive evidence for using or avoiding benzodiazepines for breathlessness in patients with advanced cancer and COPD. Benzodiazepines were more sedating compared with morphine. No statistically significant differences found with benzodiazepine type, dose, administration route, frequency, or treatment duration. If opioids fail to alleviate symptoms, benzodiazepines may be considered as an alternate treatment, but further research is needed.[48]
   - *Buspirone:* In patients with cancer, buspirone failed to show a benefit for dyspnea or anxiety relief, and there is no definitive evidence for use in COPD.[46,49]
4. Corticosteroids:
   - The role of steroids in nonmalignant conditions, such as COPD and ILD is clearly defined.
   - Although steroids are used in various cancer-related conditions that cause breathlessness, such as treatment-induced pneumonitis (radiation or drug) or superior vena caval syndrome, evidence is lacking to support or avoid use in cancer-related dyspnea as a primary agent.[50] A recent prospective observation study suggested that lymphangitis carcinomatosis did not appear to be steroid responsive.[51]
   - Multiple traditional and novel antineoplastic agents are linked to drug-induced pneumonitis that is, treated with high doses of steroids.[52]
   - When initiating corticosteroids in patients with advanced cancer with dyspnea, clinicians should monitor patients for the development of delirium, as many patients are at risk from poor functional status.[53] Concerns exist regarding steroids side effects at high doses, including psychomotor agitation, hyperglycemia, fluid retention.
5. Other medications:
   - Current evidence is inconclusive regarding the role of antidepressants, herbal medications, and cannabinoids for treatment of dyspnea.[46]
6. Palliative sedation:
   - In rare instances, the above measures do not improve dyspnea symptoms. Palliative sedation can be a last resort option and to be performed only by clinicians who are trained and experienced. We would recommend specialist palliative care consultation.

Prognosis

The presence of dyspnea is a risk factor for overall mortality, independent of age, smoking history, lung function.[54] Dyspnea is associated with shortened survival in multiple conditions, such as advanced cancer,[55] COPD,[56] ILD,[57] and cardiac disease.[58]

Palliative extubation

The decision to forego life sustaining treatment occurs in 75% of deaths in US hospitals.[59,60] For patients with terminal illnesses and respiratory failure, palliative extubation is the withdrawal of ventilator support when congruent with patients' treatment goals and preferences. There are different approaches to withdrawing ventilator support and managing dyspnea and air hunger.[61] Expert opinions agree that neuromuscular blockers are not indicated during withdrawal of life support.[62] Both opioids and benzodiazepine are used to control symptoms. Clinicians must individualize symptom management for different patients, to avoid underdoing or overdosing. Clinicians may request specialty palliative care consultation to help with symptom optimization and anticipatory counseling of patients/families.[63]

COUGH
Background

Cough is inherently protective as it expels aspirates and secretions from the respiratory tract.[11] It is common in patients with cancer and COPD. Although cathartic when isolated, it can be a distressing symptom when persistent that causes physical problems, including musculoskeletal pain, rib fractures, urinary incontinence, fatigue, and insomnia. Physical sequelae in turn contribute to negative psychosocial impact and isolation.[64] Chronic cough contributes to other physical and emotional complications and poor QOL. Therefore, patients' concerns should not be minimized.[65]

Cough is caused by stimulation of afferent vagal receptors—the physiologic response, and by upregulation of these afferents-cough hypersensitivity.[11,66]

Evaluation and Assessment

Assessment mirrors what was discussed for breathlessness. Clinicians should clarify patient-centered needs and goals, and their prognosis, when determining whether extensive workup and treatment is warranted or offered.

The American College of Chest Physicians recently updated guidelines on the initial evaluation of cough. Clinical approach begins with determining acuity of cough: acute (<3 weeks), subacute (3–8 weeks), or chronic (>8 weeks).[67]

Management

If clinically appropriate, clinicians should investigate and treat the primary cause of cough. In the seriously ill, cough management is symptom based. Often extensive workup is forgone if patient is at end of life.

Management strategies may include: (1) a medication review to remove offending agents (ie, angiotensin-converting enzyme inhibitors)[66–72] and (2) exploring atypical causes of cough. Association of gastrointestinal symptoms, such as reflux (acid and nonacid) and nausea seem to have a strong presence in the palliative care population, suggesting management of cough may involve acid suppression and promotility agents.[66,70,72]

For mild cough, linctus (honey, syrup), inhaled sodium cromoglycate and peripherally acting agents, such as benzonatate and levodropropizine are potential options.[11,66,72] Guaifenesin, a commonly used expectorant and mucolytic agent, works by loosening mucus in the airway to make cough more productive. Dextromethorphan can be effective in suppressing acute cough but has weak evidence in palliative care settings; advantages include low toxicity and wide availability.[72] For moderate to severe cough or failure of mild cough interventions, centrally acting agents are indicated.

Opioids offer effective cough suppression. Most experts recommend morphine and hydrocodone. Codeine should be avoided because of adverse effects, minimal effectiveness, unpredictable bioavailability due to genetic variability metabolism.[73]

Gabapentin and pregabalin have been described as potential agents to reduce cough by muting cough hypersensitivity.

From a nonpharmacological approach, specialized speech pathology therapy may be helpful.[74–76]

MALIGNANT PLEURAL EFFUSIONS
Overview

MPEs are common causes of exudative effusions and contribute to hospitalizations and associated yearly hospital expenditure exceeding $5 billion.[77] Common cancers causing MPEs are lung (38%), breast (15.2%), hematologic (11.2%), gynecologic (9%), and gastrointestinal (11%).[77,78]

Effusions can be caused by indirect effects of malignancy also known as paramalignant effusions: reactive pleuritis due to underlying lung cancer, airway obstruction, atelectasis, radiation-induced pleuritis.[79] Paramalignant effusions do not have consensus treatment guidelines.

Prognosis

MPEs confer a poor prognosis. In primary lung cancer, the expected survival ranges from 4 to 7 months.[80] Thus, palliation of symptoms is goal of management. Clive and colleagues[81] validated the LENT prognostic score, which uses pleural lactate dehydrogenase, Eastern Cooperative Oncology Group score, neutrophil-lymphocyte ratio and type of cancer. This last factor is significant as there is variation in median survival based on tumor morphology (Lung cancer 74d versus Mesothelioma 339d). Median survivals for LENT scores: low risk, 319 days; medium risk, 130 days; and high risk, 44 days.[81]

Management

There is lack of high-grade evidence to support a specified therapeutic approach. In 2018, American Thoracic Society (ATS), Society of Thoracic Surgeons, and Society of Thoracic Radiology published guidelines based on best available evidence and expert opinion to provide clinically applicable and patient-centered recommendations.[82,83] Ost and colleagues[84] retrospectively reviewed Medicare patients and found fewer repeat pleural interventions procedures and complications when using guideline-consistent care.[85]

Diagnostic thoracentesis should be used in asymptomatic patients as tumor type and stage greatly influence antineoplastic therapy options and responses to treatment. Therapeutic large volume fluid removal should be reserved for symptomatic patients.

2018 ATS guidelines[82,83] support: (1) using ultrasound guidance for thoracentesis to avoid complications and (2) using indwelling pleural catheter (IPC) when there is loculated effusion, lung has not reinflated after large volume thoracentesis, or failed chemical pleurodesis. In symptomatic patients where lung is thought to be re-expandable, IPC or talc pleurodesis can be pursued.

Advantages to IPC include insertion as outpatient, can be managed at home, less hospital days, and reduced pleural procedures. Potential risk of IPCs include localized soft tissue infections, which experts recommend treating with attempts to salvage IPC if possible.[82,83,86,87]

AIRWAY SECRETIONS

In ALS and COPD, manually assisted cough and mechanical insufflation-exsufflation probably assists with airway secretion management, because cough efficiency is weak.[88]

Death rattle or noisy breathing is a common symptom in the dying process. Prevalence rates of death rattle range from 12% to 92%.[89] It distresses families and clinicians alike, often compelling one to intervene. Although a Cochrane Review failed to identify a superior intervention to address this system,[90] use of antimuscarinic is common in practice. These medications can cause anticholinergic side effects. Scopolamine, atropine, hyoscyamine cross the blood-brain barrier and are likely to cause delirium and sedation whereas glycopyrrolate (quaternary amine) will not.[91]

HEMOPTYSIS

Hemoptysis is the expectoration of blood from a pulmonary origin. When defining massive hemoptysis, there is no recognized universal volume (100 mL to ≥ 1 L/24 hours).[11] Increased mortality has been associated with alcoholism, cancer, aspergillosis, pulmonary artery involvement, infiltrates involving ≥ 2 quadrants on chest film, and ventilatory support.[92] In the palliative care patient, hemoptysis may occur with malignancy, anticoagulation, coagulopathy, lung infections and abscess, cystic fibrosis, bronchiectasis, and iatrogenic from either medication or interventional treatment.[11] Massive hemoptysis is seen with tuberculosis, bronchiectasis, lung abscesses, and rarely patients with lung cancer.

Management should be tailored to the patient's diagnosis and previous history, prognosis, functional status, likelihood of an intervention being successful (including risks and benefits associated with said intervention), individual preferences and what patient deems acceptable to endure.

Bronchoscopy with direct endobronchial treatment, interventional radiologic procedure, such as embolization or surgery may be appropriate depending on cause and location of bleeding and if such interventions align with treatment goals.[11]

There are no extensive studies to support pharmacologic treatments. Some treatments used in massive hemoptysis described in the literature include systemic or inhaled tranexamic acid[11,93,94] as well as aerosolized vasopressin.[95] Although rare, massive hemoptysis may directly cause death. Important strategies include:

1. Psychologically preparing families and clinicians caring for the patient.
2. Clarifying resuscitation preferences.
3. Having a plan in place to ensure physical comfort for the patient and emotional support to the family when the event occurs.

Patient comfort is addressed with anxiolysis and dyspnea control, best positioning to avoid accumulation of blood in the pharynx or well-functioning airways. Families should be supported, position the family so that hemorrhage is not in direct view, and use dark bedding and towels to obscure the sight of blood.[11]

SUMMARY

Respiratory symptoms are common in patients living with serious illness, both in cancer and nonmalignant conditions. Common symptoms include dyspnea (breathlessness), cough, MPEs, airway secretions and hemoptysis. Beyond physical effects, these symptoms exert significant psychological, social, existential, and spiritual impact on the patients' experience. Basic management of respiratory symptoms is within the scope of primary palliative care, with escalation to specialty palliative care consultations as appropriate. Treating respiratory symptoms requires pharmacologic and nonpharmacologic approaches. Opioids play an important role in relieving dyspnea and cough in patients with advanced illnesses, and should be considered alongside disease-directed therapies. There is need for robust research regarding palliative management of respiratory symptoms to inform practice guidelines of various respiratory conditions.

DISCLOSURE

The authors have nothing to disclose.

REFERENCES

1. Johnson MJ, Yorke J, Hansen-Flaschen J, et al. Towards an expert consensus to delineate a clinical syndrome of chronic breathlessness. Eur Respir J 2017;49(5) [pii:1602277].
2. Ripamonti C, Fulfaro F, Bruera E. Dyspnoea in patients with advanced cancer: incidence, causes and treatments. Cancer Treat Rev 1998;24(1):69–80.
3. Blinderman CD, Homel P, Billings JA, et al. Symptom distress and quality of life in patients with advanced congestive heart failure. J Pain Symptom Manage 2008; 35(6):594–603.
4. Blinderman CD, Homel P, Billings JA, et al. Symptom distress and quality of life in patients with advanced chronic obstructive pulmonary disease. J Pain Symptom Manage 2009;38(1):115–23.
5. Mularski RA. Advancing a common understanding and approach to dyspnea management. consensus proposal for the chronic breathlessness syndrome. Ann Am Thorac Soc 2017;14(7):1108–10.
6. Parshall MB, Schwartzstein RM, Adams L, et al. An official American Thoracic Society statement: update on the mechanisms, assessment, and management of dyspnea. Am J Respir Crit Care Med 2012;185(4):435–52.
7. Mularski RA, Reinke LF, Carrieri-Kohlman V, et al. An official American Thoracic Society workshop report: assessment and palliative management of dyspnea crisis. Ann Am Thorac Soc 2013;10(5):S98–106.
8. Abernethy AP, Wheeler JL. Total dyspnoea. Curr Opin Support Palliat Care 2008; 2:110–3.
9. Thomas JR, von Gunten CF. Clinical management of dyspnoea. Lancet Oncol 2002;3(4):223–8.
10. Lansing RW, Gracely RH, Banzett RB. The multiple dimensions of dyspnea: review and hypotheses. Respir Physiol Neurobiol 2009;167(1):53–60.
11. Chan K, Tse D, Sham M. Dyspnoea and other respiratory symptoms in palliative care. In: Cherny NI, editor. Oxford textbook of palliative medicine - 5th ed. Oxford: Oxford University Press; 2015. p. 421–34.
12. Moens K, Higginson IJ, Harding R, EURO IMPACT. Are there differences in the prevalence of palliative care-related problems in people living with advanced cancer and eight non-cancer conditions? A systematic review. J Pain Symptom Manage 2014;48(4):660–77.
13. Currow DC, Smith J, Davidson PM, et al. Do the trajectories of dyspnea differ in prevalence and intensity by diagnosis at the end of life? A consecutive cohort study. J Pain Symptom Manage 2010;39(4):680–90.
14. Addington-Hall J, Lay M, Altmann D, et al. Symptom control, communication with health professionals, and hospital care of stroke patients in the last year of life as reported by surviving family, friends, and officials. Stroke 1995;26(12):2242–8.
15. Menezes KKP, Nascimento LR, Alvarenga MTM, et al. Prevalence of dyspnea after stroke: a telephone-based survey. Braz J Phys Ther 2019;23(4):311–6.

16. Kamal AH, Maguire JM, Wheeler JL, et al. Dyspnea review for the palliative care professional: assessment, burdens, and etiologies. J Palliat Med 2011;14(10): 1167–72.
17. Mahler DA, Selecky PA, Harrod CG, et al. American College of Chest Physicians consensus statement on the management of dyspnea in patients with advanced lung or heart disease. Chest 2010;137(3):674–91.
18. Weinberg R, Ketterer B. Management of chronic dyspnea #376. J Palliat Med 2019;22(7):858–60.
19. Kamal AH, Maguire JM, Wheeler JL, et al. Dyspnea review for the palliative care professional: treatment goals and therapeutic options. J Palliat Med 2012;15(1): 106–14.
20. Puntillo K, Nelson JE, Weissman D. Palliative care in the ICU: relief of pain, dyspnea, and thirst–a report from the IPAL-ICU Advisory Board. Intensive Care Med 2014;40(2):235–48.
21. Qian Y, Wu Y, Rozman de Moraes A, et al. Fan therapy for the treatment of dyspnea in adults: a systematic review. J Pain Symptom Manage 2019;58(3):481–6.
22. McCarthy B, Casey D, Devane D, et al. Pulmonary rehabilitation for chronic obstructive pulmonary disease. Cochrane Database Syst Rev 2015;(2):CD003793.
23. Lanken PN, Terry PB, Delisser HM, et al, ATS End-of-Life Care Task Force. An official American Thoracic Society clinical policy statement: palliative care for patients with respiratory diseases and critical illnesses. Am J Respir Crit Care Med 2008;177(8):912–27.
24. Vogelmeier CF, Criner GJ, Martinez FJ, et al. Global strategy for the diagnosis, management, and prevention of chronic obstructive lung disease 2017 report. GOLD executive summary. Am J Respir Crit Care Med 2017;195(5):557–82.
25. Abernethy AP, McDonald CF, Frith PA, et al. Effect of palliative oxygen versus room air in relief of breathlessness in patients with refractory dyspnoea: a double-blind, randomised controlled trial. Lancet 2010;376(9743):784–93.
26. Ekström M, Ahmadi Z, Bornefalk-Hermansson A, et al. Oxygen for breathlessness in patients with chronic obstructive pulmonary disease who do not qualify for home oxygen therapy. Cochrane Database Syst Rev 2016;(11):CD006429.
27. Uronis HE, Currow DC, McCrory DC, et al. Oxygen for relief of dyspnoea in mildly- or non-hypoxaemic patients with cancer: a systematic review and meta-analysis. Br J Cancer 2008;98(2):294–9.
28. Bausewein C, Booth S, Gysels M, et al. Non-pharmacological interventions for breathlessness in advanced stages of malignant and non-malignant diseases. Cochrane Database Syst Rev 2008;(2):CD005623.
29. Jobst K, Chen JH, McPherson K, et al. Controlled trial of acupuncture for disabling breathlessness. Lancet 1986;2(8521–22):1416–9.
30. Quill CM, Quill TE. Palliative use of noninvasive ventilation: navigating murky waters. J Palliat Med 2014;17(6):657–61.
31. Vilaça M, Aragão I, Cardoso T, et al. The role of noninvasive ventilation in patients with "Do Not Intubate" order in the emergency setting. PLoS One 2016;11(2): e0149649.
32. Barnes H, McDonald J, Smallwood N, et al. Opioids for the palliation of refractory breathlessness in adults with advanced disease and terminal illness. Cochrane Database Syst Rev 2016;3(3):CD011008.
33. Jennings AL, Deavies AN, Higgins JP, et al. A systematic review of the use of opioids in the management of dyspnoea. Thorax 2002;57(11):939–44.

34. Vargas-Bermudez A, Cardenal F, Porta-Sales J. Opioids for the management of dyspnea in cancer patients: evidence of the last 15 years - a systematic review. J Pain Palliat Care Pharmacother 2015;29(4):341–52.

35. Davis MP, Behm B, Balachandran D. Looking both ways before crossing the street: assessing the benefits and risk of opioids in treating patients at risk of sleep -disorderedbreathing for pain and dyspnea. J Opioid Manag 2017;13: 183–96.

36. Mahler DA. Opioids for refractory dyspnea. Expert Rev Respir Med 2013;7(2): 123–34.

37. Abernethy AP, Currow DC, Frith P, et al. Randomised, double blind, placebo controlled crossover trial of sustained release morphine for the management of refractory dyspnoea. BMJ 2003;327(7414):523–8.

38. Ben-Aharon I, Gafter-Gvili A, Paul M, et al. Interventions for alleviating cancer-related dyspnea: a systematic review. J Clin Oncol 2008;26(14):2396–404.

39. Currow DC, McDonald C, Oaten S, et al. Once-daily opioids for chronic dyspnea: a dose increment and pharmacovigilance study. J Pain Symptom Manage 2011; 42:388–99.

40. Hallenbeck J. Pathophysiologies of dyspnea explained: why might opioids relieve dyspnea and not hasten death? J Palliat Med 2012;15:848.

41. Yamaguchi T, Matsuda Y, Matsuoka H, et al. Efficacy of immediate-release oxyco-done for dyspnoea in cancer patient: cancer dyspnoea relief (CDR) trial. Jpn J Clin Oncol 2018;48(12):1070–5.

42. Gallagher R. The use of opioids for dyspnea in advanced disease. CMAJ 2011; 183(10):1170.

43. Clemens KE, Klaschik E. Effect of hydromorphone on ventilation in palliative care patients with dyspnea. Support Care Cancer 2008;16:93–9.

44. Clemens KE, Quednau I, Klaschik E. Is there a higher risk of respiratory depres-sion in opioid-naïve palliative care patients during symptomatic therapy of dys-pnea with strong opioids? J Palliat Med 2008;11(2):204–16.

45. Dowell D, Haegerich TM, Chou R. CDC guideline for prescribing opioids for chronic pain–United States, 2016. JAMA 2016;315(15):1624–45.

46. Barbetta C, Currow DC, Johnson MJ. Non-opioid medications for the relief of chronic breathlessness: current evidence. Expert Rev Respir Med 2017;11(4): 333–41.

47. Kallet RH. The role of inhaled opioids and furosemide for the treatment of dys-pnea. Respir Care 2007;52(7):900–10.

48. Simon ST, Higginson IJ, Booth S, et al. Benzodiazepines for the relief of breath-lessness in advanced malignant and non-malignant diseases in adults. Cochrane Database Syst Rev 2016;(10):CD007354.

49. Peoples AR, Bushunow PW, Garland SN, et al. Buspirone for management of dys-pnea in cancer patients receiving chemotherapy: a randomised placebo-controlled URCC CCOP study. Support Care Cancer 2016;24(3):1339–47.

50. Haywood A, Duc J, Good P, et al. Systemic corticosteroids for the management of cancer-related breathlessness (dyspnoea) in adults. Cochrane Database Syst Rev 2019;(2):CD012704.

51. Mori M, Shirado AN, Morita T, et al. Predictors of response to corticosteroids for dyspnea in advanced cancer patients: a preliminary multicenter prospective observational study. Support Care Cancer 2017;25(4):1169–81.

52. Vahid B, Marik Pe. Pulmonary complications of novel antineoplastic agents for solid tumors. Chest 2008;133:528–38.

53. Morita T, Tei Y, Inoue S. Impaired communication capacity and agitated delirium in the final week of terminally ill cancer patients: prevalence and identification of research focus. J Pain Symptom Manage 2003;26(3):827–34.

54. Pesola GR, Ahsan H. Dyspnea as an independent predictor of mortality. Clin Respir J 2016;10(2):142–52.

55. Maltoni M, Pirovano M, Scarpi E, et al. Prediction of survival of patients terminally ill with cancer. Results of an Italian prospective multicentric study. Cancer 1995; 75(10):2613–22.

56. Nishimura K, Izumi T, Tsukino M, et al. Dyspnea is a better predictor of 5-year survival than airway obstruction in patients with COPD. Chest 2002;121(5):1434–40.

57. Nishiyama O, Taniguchi H, Kondoh Y, et al. A simple assessment of dyspnoea as a prognostic indicator in idiopathic pulmonary fibrosis. Eur Respir J 2010;36(5): 1067–72.

58. Abidov A, Rozanski A, Hachamovitch R, et al. Prognostic significance of dyspnea in patients referred for cardiac stress testing. N Engl J Med 2005;353(18): 1889–98.

59. Prendergast TJ, Claessens MT, Luce JM. A national survey of end-of-life care for critically ill patients. Am J Respir Crit Care Med 1998;158(4):1163–7.

60. AMA Council on Ethical and Judicial Affairs. AMA code of medical ethics' opinions on care at the end of life opinion 2.20 - withholding or withdrawing life-sustaining medical treatment. Virtual Mentor 2013;12(12):1038–40.

61. von Gunten C, Weissman DE. Ventilator withdrawal protocol. J Palliat Med 2003; 6(5):773–4.

62. Campbell ML. How to withdraw mechanical ventilation: a systematic review of the literature. AACN Adv Crit Care 2007;18(4):397–403 [quiz: 344–5].

63. Pan CX, Platis D, Maw MM, et al. How long does (S)he have? Retrospective analysis of outcomes after palliative extubation in elderly, chronically critically ill patients. Crit Care Med 2016;44(6):1138–44.

64. Molassiotis A, Lowe M, Ellis J, et al. The experience of cough in patients diagnosed with lung cancer. Support Care Cancer 2011;19(12):1997–2004.

65. Irwin RS. Complications of cough: ACCP evidence-based clinical practice guidelines. Chest 2006;129(1 Suppl):54S–8S.

66. Morice AH, Shanks G. Pharmacology of cough in palliative care. Curr Opin Support Palliat Care 2017;11(3):147–51.

67. Irwin R, French C, Change A, et al. Classification of cough as a symptom in adults and management algorithms. CHEST 2018;153(1):196–209.

68. Jiang M, Guan WJ, Fang ZF, et al. A critical review of the quality of cough clinical practice guidelines. Chest 2016;150(4):777–88.

69. Molassiotis A, Bailey C, Caress A, et al. Interventions for cough in cancer. Cochrane Database Syst Rev 2015;(5):CD007881.

70. Harle ASM, Blackhall FH, Molassiotis A, et al. Cough in patients with lung cancer: a longitudinal observational study of characterization and clinical associations. Chest 2019;155(1):103–13.

71. Molassiotis A, Smith JA, Mazzone P, et al, CHEST Expert Cough Panel. Symptomatic treatment of cough among adult patients with lung cancer: CHEST guideline and expert panel report. Chest 2017;151(4):861–74 [Erratum appears in: Chest. 2017 Nov;152(5):1095].

72. Wee B, Browning J, Adams A, et al. Management of chronic cough in patients receiving palliative care: review of evidence and recommendations by a task group of the Association for Palliative Medicine of Great Britain and Ireland. Palliat Med 2012;26(6):780–7.

73. Smith HS. Opioid metabolism. Mayo Clin Proc 2009;84(7):613–24.
74. Ryan NM, Birring SS, Gibson PG, et al. Gabapentin for refractory chronic cough: a randomised, double-blind, placebo-controlled trial. Lancet 2012;380(9853): 1583–9.
75. Vertigan AE, Theodoros DG, Gibson PG, et al. Efficacy of speech pathology management for chronic cough: a randomised placebo controlled trial of treatment efficacy. Thorax 2006;61:1065–9.
76. Vertigan AE, Kapela SL, Ryan NM, et al. Pregabalin and speech pathology combination therapy for refractory chronic cough: a randomized controlled trial. Chest 2016;149:639–48.
77. Taghizadeh N, Fortin M, Tremblay A. US hospitalizations for malignant pleural effusions: data from the 2012 National Inpatient Sample. Chest 2017;151(4): 845–54.
78. Roberts ME, Neville E, Berrisford RG, et al, BTS Pleural Disease Guideline Group. Management of a malignant pleural effusion: British Thoracic Society Pleural Disease Guideline 2010. Thorax 2010;65(Suppl 2):ii32–40.
79. Feller-Kopman D, Light R. Pleural disease. N Engl J Med 2018;378(8):740–51.
80. Porcel JM, Gasol A, Bielsa S, et al. Clinical features and survival of lung cancer patients with pleural effusions. Respirology 2015;20:654–9.
81. Clive AO, Kahan BC, Hooper CE, et al. Predicting survival in malignant pleural effusion: development and validation of the LENT prognostic score. Thorax 2014;69:1098–104.
82. Feller-Kopman DJ, Reddy CB, DeCamp MM, et al. Management of malignant pleural effusions. An official ATS/STS/STR clinical practice guideline. Am J Respir Crit Care Med 2018;198(7):839.
83. Reddy CB, DeCamp MM, Diekemper RL, et al. Summary for clinicians: clinical practice guideline for management of malignant pleural effusions. Ann Am Thorac Soc 2019;16(1):17–21.
84. Ost DE, Niu J, Zhao H, et al. Quality gaps and comparative effectiveness of management strategies for recurrent malignant pleural effusions. Chest 2018;153: 438–52.
85. Shieh B, Beaudoin S, Gonzalez AV. The pathway to definitive palliation of malignant pleural effusions. Ann Am Thorac Soc 2019;16(5):639–41.
86. Tremblay A, Michaud G. Single-center experience with 250 tunnelled pleural catheter insertions for malignant pleural effusion. Chest 2006;129:362–8.
87. Kheir F, Shawwa K, Alokla K, et al. Tunneled pleural catheter for the treatment of malignant pleural effusion: a systematic review and meta-analysis. Am J Ther 2016;23(6):e1300–6.
88. Arcuri JF, Abarshi E, Preston NJ, et al. Benefits of interventions for respiratory secretion management in adult palliative care patients - a systematic review. BMC Palliat Care 2016;15:74.
89. Lokker ME, van Zuylen L, van der Rijt CC, et al. Prevalence, impact, and treatment of death rattle: a systematic review. J Pain Symptom Manage 2014;47(1): 105–22.
90. Wee B, Hillier R. Interventions for noisy breathing in patients near to death. Cochrane Database Syst Rev 2008;(1):CD005177.
91. Bickel K, Arnold RM. Death rattle and oral secretions–second edition #109. J Palliat Med 2008;11(7):1040–1.
92. Fartoukh M, Khoshnood B, Parrot A, et al. Early prediction of in-hospital mortality of patients with hemoptysis: an approach to defining severe hemoptysis. Respiration 2012;83(2):106–14.

93. Komura S, Rodriguez RM, Peabody CR. Hemoptysis? Try inhaled tranexamic acid. J Emerg Med 2018;54(5):e97–9.
94. Segrelles Calvo G, De Granda-Orive I, López Padilla D. Inhaled tranexamic acid as an alternative for hemoptysis treatment. Chest 2016;149(2):604.
95. Anwar D, Schaad N, Mazzocato C. Aerosolized vasopressin is a safe and effective treatment for mild to moderate recurrent hemoptysis in palliative care patients. J Pain Symptom Manage 2005;29(5):427–9.

Cannabis for Symptom Management in Older Adults

Cari Levy, MD, PhD[a,b], Emily Galenbeck, BA[a,*], Kate Magid, MPH[a]

KEYWORDS

- Medical marijuana • Cannabinoids • Cannabis • Palliative care
- Symptom management • Older adults

KEY POINTS

- Few randomized controlled trials (RCTs) have focused on medical cannabis for the older adult population. Existing studies have small sample sizes (N <100) and indicate a lack of high-quality evidence for the efficacy and safety of medical cannabis for older adults. In total, fewer than 250 older adults have been included in these studies.
- Mixed evidence suggests no strong indication that medical cannabis effectively reduces neuropsychiatric symptoms associated with dementia or cancer-related pain and its side effects.
- Low to moderate evidence suggests medical cannabis effectively reduces pain, particularly at the 30% level relative to pre-intervention pain.
- Studies assessing tolerability and safety report higher rates of mild adverse events and study withdrawal due to treatment-related side effects in participants receiving cannabinoids.
- There is no clear recommendation of use of medical cannabis for most indications relevant to palliative care.

INTRODUCTION

As of June 2019, 33 states and the District of Columbia have legalized medical cannabis use, and 11 states and the District of Columbia have legalized recreational marijuana use among adults (**Fig. 1**).[1] The federal government, however, classifies marijuana as a Schedule I controlled substance.[2] Substances classified as Schedule I are considered illegal to possess under federal regulations, regardless of state regulations. Additionally, there are extensive restrictions on conducting research with

[a] Research, Rocky Mountain Regional Veterans Affairs Medical Center, Denver-Seattle Center of Innovation, 1700 North Wheeling Street, Aurora, CO 80045, USA; [b] Division of Health Care Policy and Research, School of Medicine, University of Colorado, 1700 North Wheeling Street, Aurora, CO 80045, USA
* Corresponding author.
E-mail address: Emily.galenbeck@va.gov
Twitter: @cari_levy (C.L.); @EGalenbeck (E.G.); @Katie_Magid (K.M.)

Med Clin N Am 104 (2020) 471–489
https://doi.org/10.1016/j.mcna.2020.01.004
0025-7125/20/© 2020 Elsevier Inc. All rights reserved.

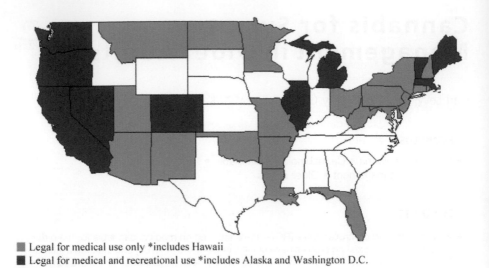

■ Legal for medical use only *includes Hawaii
■ Legal for medical and recreational use *includes Alaska and Washington D.C.
☐ Not legal

Fig. 1. Map of state laws related to medical and recreational marijuana. (*Adapted from* National Conference of State Legislatures (NCSL). State Medical Marijuana Laws. Available at: www.ncsl.org/research/health/state-medical-marijuana-laws.aspx. Accessed July 29 2019; with permission.)

Schedule I drugs. Due to these restrictions and the relatively recent legalization of marijuana in certain states, there is limited medical cannabis research, especially for symptom management in serious illness and advanced age. Existing studies vary widely in sample size, duration, and types of cannabis used.

As a Schedule I drug, federal regulations create a barrier to research on marijuana use by older adults, particularly among residents in nursing facilities. Nursing facilities receiving Medicare or Medicaid funding are required to abide by all federal, state, and local laws. The discontinuity between legalization within the state and the federal regulations creates a tension for nursing facilities between following federal regulations and striving to respect the rights of residents who may desire to use cannabis through a state-authorized program. One nursing facility, Hebrew Home at Riverdale, located in the Bronx, New York, has developed an innovative program to afford residents the ability to legally obtain and utilize medical cannabis for symptom management within the skilled nursing facility, while staying in compliance with state regulations.[3] To mitigate violation of federal laws, Hebrew Home has written a policy for the use of medical cannabis in the facility. The policy directs that only residents with qualifying conditions may use medical cannabis, that residents are required to buy their own cannabis product from a state-certified dispensary, and that the resident and their family are responsible for self-administering so that facility staff are not involved. Given that use of medical cannabis among older adults continues to increase, research on clinical efficacy in this demographic group is paramount.[4–6] Data from the 2016 National Survey on Drug Use and Health indicate that 9% of adults ages 50 years to 64 years and 2.9% of adults ages greater than or equal to 65 years used cannabis either medically or recreationally within the past year.[7]

Currently, physicians lack clear, evidence-based guidelines for the clinical use of medical cannabis; yet, many believe there are potential benefits. As a result, knowledge about the efficacy of medical cannabis and comfort in discussing this treatment with patients vary among providers.[8] For example, a survey of providers in Washington State found that although 74% believed medical cannabis could be useful for chronic conditions, knowledge on the topic was low and served as a barrier to issuing authorizations.[9] Among those surveyed who were legally permitted to write medical cannabis authorizations, only 21% had ever issued an authorization. A recent survey by Costantino and colleagues[10] of 310 hospice staff found that 91% support using medical cannabis for hospice patients. Of the 36 physicians surveyed, only half reported certifying for medical cannabis, and, among those who did, the majority recommended medical cannabis to patients less than once a month. Survey respondents cited discordance between state and federal legal status and a general lack of knowledge on how to handle medical cannabis due to the dearth of guidelines as barriers to use of medical cannabis in hospice care. As with respondents to the 2019 survey, a 2011 study of hospice providers found overwhelming (86%) support for the belief in the benefits of medical cannabis.[11] Additionally, approximately half of respondents reported receiving questions about medical cannabis from patients.

The purpose of this article is to present evidence on the efficacy and safety of medical cannabis as a therapy for symptom management in palliative care, while recognizing that no strong recommendations can be made based on the available evidence. This article is not an exhaustive review of the literature, but rather a summary of the best available evidence for conditions typically encountered in the treatment of patients receiving palliative care. First, this article summarizes recent research on the use of medical cannabis for symptom management in older adults. Next, this article provides an overview of the evidence on the risks and benefits of using medical cannabis for the indications of chronic pain, cancer-related pain, cancer cachexia, dementia, and Alzheimer's disease. Finally, this article identifies gaps in the medical cannabis research and provides suggestions for future studies. Each section provides a summary of key findings prior to a more detailed description of relevant data.

LITERATURE SEARCH METHODOLOGY

The initial objective of this article was to describe the available literature on use of medical cannabis among older adult populations. To accomplish this objective, a structured search in PubMed initially identified studies on the use, efficacy, and safety of medical cannabis for older adults. Potential studies met all the following criteria:

1. Participant population included older adults ($\geq$65 years) or mean age of participant population was $\geq$65 years
2. Sample size $\geq$10 participants
3. Data reported separately for older adults
4. Treatment arm of study included medical cannabis
5. The design was a randomized, quasi-randomized, or non-randomized clinical trial
6. The study published between January 1, 2009, and July 20, 2019

The search strategy included a combination of terms related to older adults (eg, aged or elder), medical cannabis, and study design (**Table 1** lists search queries). The search identified 888 records. After screening abstracts and full text articles, the authors identified 8 studies that met all inclusion criteria. **Fig. 2** provides a summary of the review process and reasons for record exclusion.

MEDICAL MARIJUANA RESEARCH AMONG OLDER ADULT POPULATIONS

- Few randomized controlled trials (RCTs) have focused on medical cannabis for the older adult population.

Table 1		
Search strategy for patients who are older adults		
ID	**Search**	**Results**
1	Search quasi-experiment* or quasiexperiment* or quasi-random* or quasirandom* or non-random* or nonrandom* or compar* or randomized controlled trial [pt] OR controlled clinical trial [pt] OR randomized controlled trials [mh] OR random allocation [mh] OR double-blind method [mh] OR single-blind method [mh] OR clinical trial [pt] OR clinical trials [mh] OR ("clinical trial" [tw]) OR ((singl* [tw] OR doubl* [tw] OR trebl* [tw] OR tripl* [tw]) AND (mask* [tw] OR blind* [tw])) OR (placebos [mh] OR placebo* [tw] OR random* [tw] OR research design [mh:noexp] OR comparative study [pt] OR evaluation studies [mh] OR follow-up studies [mh] OR prospective studies [mh] OR control* [tw] OR prospectiv* [tw] OR volunteer* [tw]) NOT (animals [mh] NOT human [mh])	8469736
2	Search cannabis[mh] OR cannabis[tiab] OR hemp[tiab] OR marijuana[tiab] OR ganja[tiab] OR hashish[tiab] OR marihuana[tiab] OR bhang[tiab] OR cannabinoids[mh] OR cannibinoids[tiab] OR cannibinoid[tiab] OR marinol [tiab] OR dronabinol[tiab] OR nabilone[tiab] OR cesamet[tiab] OR dexanabinol[tiab] OR sativex[tiab] OR tetrahydrocannabinol[tiab]	37650
3	Search ((("Aged"[Mesh]) OR "Aged, 80 and over"[Mesh] OR elder OR geriatric)))	3003853
4	Search #1 and #2 and #3	888

- Existing studies have small sample sizes (N <100) and lack high-quality (due to short follow-up periods and insufficient sample size to generalize to clinical populations) evidence for the efficacy and safety of medical cannabis for older adults.

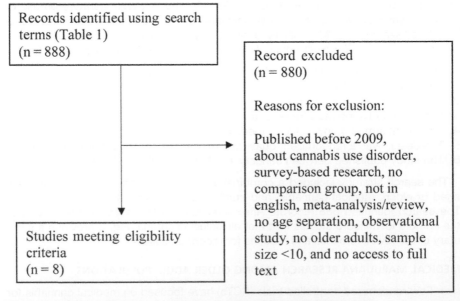

Fig. 2. Search flow diagram of medical cannabis studies with older adults.

The search identified 8 RCTs on the efficacy of medical cannabis for older adults (**Table 2**).[12-19] These studies examined the efficacy of medical cannabis in 4 indications: dementia and Alzheimer's disease, appetite and chemosensory perception in cancer patients, Parkinson disease, and chronic obstructive pulmonary disease (COPD). There are more than 100 cannabinoid compounds in the cannabis plant, including tetrahydrocannabinol (THC) and cannabidiol (CBD). CBD can be extracted from hemp or marijuana. Hemp plants contain less than 0.3% THC whereas marijuana plants contain higher concentrations of THC, which is the main psychoactive compound in marijuana responsible for the high sensation. The studies used various cannabinoids, including THC, CBD, THC:CBD oromucosal spray, and nabilone (**Table 3**). Sample sizes in the studies were small, ranging from 10 to 50 participants, and intervention durations were all shorter than 12 weeks. Given the small sample sizes and short intervention durations across studies, the evidence from the 8 studies is low quality.

Although literature on the efficacy and safety of medical cannabis has increased in general populations, RCTs focusing on older adults are lacking (See **Table 2**). A recent review of medical cannabis for older adults underscored the paucity of evidence for the efficacy of medical cannabis for symptoms frequently experienced by older adults, such as pain, neurologic symptoms, and mood disorders.[20] The current lack of research indicates the pressing need for high-quality research studies that examine the risks and benefits of medical cannabis for physical, emotional, and quality-of-life outcomes in older adults. Additionally, future research is warranted because older adults are likely to experience side effects from cannabis use that may differ from those experienced by younger populations.[20] Until further studies are conducted, physicians are unlikely to have sufficient evidence on the efficacy of medical cannabis in older adults to make informed recommendations and clinical decisions.

EXPANDED SYNTHESIS OF MEDICAL MARIJUANA LITERATURE FOR SYMPTOM RELIEF

Due to the limited RCT evidence on the efficacy of medical cannabis, specifically in older adults, the rest of this article summarizes evidence on the efficacy and safety of medical cannabis for conditions that are approved indications by the majority of states and are relevant to older adults and palliative care patients. These include chronic pain, cancer-related pain, dementia and Alzheimer's disease, and cachexia. To identify the highest-quality studies on these indications, the authors conducted a PubMed search of systematic reviews and meta-analyses published in the past 10 years and report the summary of the data in this article.

CANCER AND CANCER-ASSOCIATED SYMPTOMS

- Medical cannabis has been studied for several cancer-related indications, including pain, cachexia, nausea, vomiting, and reduced appetite.
- Evidence is mixed for the benefit of cannabis for cancer-related indications, and studies suggesting a positive impact often are low quality and published before 2009.

Persons with cancer often experience cachexia and symptoms of pain, nausea, vomiting, and anorexia.[21,22] New treatments to address and mediate these symptoms are in high demand. Several states have approved cannabinoids for cancer-related pain and cancer-related nausea, cachexia, vomiting, and anorexia.[1]

Table 2
Randomized controlled trials of medical cannabis for older adults

Study	Study Design	Medical Indication	N	Mean Age ± SD (Years)	Type of Cannabis, (Dose)	Primary and Secondary Outcomes	Conclusion
Pickering et al,[16] 2011	RCT	Breathlessness in COPD patients	11	67 (66–68) (THC:CBD) 58 (51–67) (placebo)	THC:CBD extract Sublingual spray (2.7-2.5 mg 1–4 times per day on 2 separate days at least a week apart)	Breathlessness, respiratory measurements	Provides low-quality evidence of no significant difference in breathlessness and respiratory measurements between MC and placebo
Brisbois et al,[13] 2011	RCT	Chemosensory outcomes and appetite in cancer patients	46	67.0 ± 10.9 (dronabinol) 65.5 ± 8.0 (placebo)	Dronabinol Oral capsule (2.5 mg once daily for the first 3 d and then 2 times per day from day 4 to day 21	Sensory perception, appetite, caloric intake, quality of life	Provides low-quality evidence of significant enhancement in chemosensory perception and appetite with MC relative to placebo. Found no significant changes in total caloric intake or quality of life between MC compared with placebo
Chagas et al,[14] 2014	RCT	PD	21	65.9 ± 10.6 (CBD 75 mg) 63.4 (± 6.5) (CBD 300 mg) 67.3 (± 7.2) (placebo)	CBD Oral capsule (75 mg or 300 mg per day for 6 wk)	PD symptoms and functioning	Provides low-quality evidence of no significant difference in PD symptoms but significant improvement in overall functioning and well-being scores

Study	Design	Population	N	Age	Intervention	Outcomes	Results
Ahmed et al,[12] 2015	RCT	Dementia	10	77.3 ± 5.6	THC Oral tablet (0.75 mg twice daily for 3 d per week during weeks 1–6 and 1.5 mg twice daily for 3 d during weeks 7–12)	Safety of THC, side effects	Provides low-quality evidence of no significant difference in incidence of serious side effects and significant changes in heart rate, blood pressure, body sway, and internal perception with MC relative to placebo
Herrmann et al,[15] 2019	RCT	Agitation in Alzheimer's disease	39	87 ± 10	Nabilone Oral capsule (1–2 mg per day for 6 wk)	Agitation, NPSs, caregiver distress, side effects	Provided low-quality evidence of significant improvements in agitation, NPSs, and caregiver distress with MC relative to placebo. Also reported significantly higher incidence rate of side effects with MC relative to placebo
van den Elsen et al,[17] 2015	RCT	Neuropsychiatric dementia symptoms	50	78.4 ± 7.4	THC, oral tablet (1.5 mg 3 times per day for 3 wk)	NPSs, agitation, quality of life, activities of daily living, side effects	Provides low-quality evidence of no significant difference in NPSs, agitation, quality of life, activities or daily

(continued on next page)

Table 2
(continued)

Study	Study Design	Medical Indication	N	Mean Age ± SD (Years)	Type of Cannabis, (Dose)	Primary and Secondary Outcomes	Conclusion
							living, or incidence of side effects between MC and placebo
van den Elsen et al,[18] 2017	RCT	Balance and gait in dementia patients	18	77 ± 6	THC, Oral tablet (1.5 mg twice a day for 3 d for 1 wk	Gait, balance, side effects	Provides mixed low-quality evidence of differences of balance and gait between MC and placebo. No significant difference in incidence of side effects
van den Elsen et al,[19] 2015	RCT	Dementia behaviors	22	76.4 ± 5.3	THC Oral tablet (0.75 mg twice daily for 3 d during weeks 1–3 and 1.5 mg twice a day for 3 d during weeks 4–6)	NPSs, behavior, agitation, caregiver burden, and side effects	Provides low-quality evidence of no significant difference in NPSs or incidence of side effects between MC and placebo

Abbreviations: CBD, cannabidiol; MC, medical cannabis; NPS, neuropsychiatric symptoms; PD, Parkinson disease.

Table 3
Common terminology, formulations, and routes of delivery

Terminology	Definition	Formulations	Synthetic Formulations	Routes of Delivery
Cannabinoid	Compound from	Cannabis	Dronabinol	Oral
CBD	cannabis plant	extract	Nabilone	Smoking
THC	or synthetic	Herbal	NIB, oral nitrogen	Vaporizing
Oral	equivalent	cannabis	analog of THC	Topical
cannabis	Cannabinoid	Oromucosal	Nabiximols spray	Mucous membrane
extract	compound	spray	Levonantradol	absorption
Oromucosal	Cannabinoid	THC:CBD	Ajulemic acid	
spray	compound	spray	capsules/ CT-3	
Cannabis	Typically, a pill	THC:CBD	Benzopyranoperidine	
sativa	or capsule	extract	CT-3	
	made by	THC		
	extracting	extract		
	cannabinoids	THC		
	from whole-	sublingual		
	plant cannabis	spray		
	Sublingual form			
	of oral cannabis			
	extract			
	containing THC			
	and CBD			
	Cannabis species			
	used for			
	medical cannabis			

Data from Maslach C, Schaufeli WB, Leiter MP. Job Burnout. Annu Rev Psychol 2001;52:397-422.

Recent meta-analyses and systematic reviews present different conclusions on the efficacy and safety of medical cannabis for cancer-related pain, cachexia, nausea/vomiting, and anorexia (**Table 4**). Both Hauser and colleagues[23] and Mucke and colleagues[24] reported no differences in pain relief from medical cannabis compared with placebo. In contrast, another systematic review concluded that cannabinoids produced greater cancer pain relief and analgesic effects relative to placebo or comparison drug.[25] Several studies included nabiximols, which are oromucosal sprays of a formulated extract of the cannabis sativa plant that contains THC and CBD in a 1:1 ratio along with other minor cannabinoids and noncannabinoid compounds. Two RCTs comparing nabiximols oromucosal spray to placebo found that medical cannabis was no better than the placebo at reducing self-reported pain in cancer patients.[26] Conversely, an RCT published in 2012 suggested that low doses of oromucosal spray are beneficial for reducing cancer pain and superior to placebo.[27] Overall, level of evidence for cancer pain management is inconclusive, formulations and dosing across studies vary widely, and existing studies offer low-quality evidence.

Medical cannabis frequently has been studied for cancer-related cachexia. A systematic review and meta-analysis of 3 RCTs testing the use of medical cannabis for cancer cachexia suggested that there is no evidence of a therapeutic benefit.[28] Two of the studies in the review reported no significant differences between treatment groups for appetite and/or nausea, whereas the third study observed that THC was superior to placebo for increasing appetite in cancer patients.[13,29,30]

In terms of nausea and vomiting, meta-analyses provide mixed evidence. For example, Mucke and colleagues[24] reported pooled data indicating no significant difference in nausea and vomiting whereas Whiting and colleagues[31] found that cancer

Table 4
Evidence for medical cannabis in cancer and cancer-associated symptoms

Study (Condition)	Study Details	Type of Cannabis	Primary Outcomes	Side Effects	Conclusion
Hauser et al,[23] 2019	Study design: SR Indication: cancer pain Number of RCTs: 5 Pooled sample size: 1534	• Nabiximols oromucosal spray • Oromucosal THC spray	• No significant differences in 30% pain reduction, 50% pain reduction, or opioid use compared with placebo	• Mild/moderate: significantly higher compared with placebo • Serious: no difference	No difference Provides low-quality evidence of no difference in cancer-related pain reduction between MC and placebo
Wang et al,[28] 2019[b]	Study design: SR/MA Indication: cancer cachexia Number of RCTs: 3 Pooled sample size: 592	• Oral THC capsule • THC:CBD extract • THC extract • Cannabis extract	• No significant difference in increased appetite compared with placebo	[b]	No difference Provides low-quality evidence of no difference in increased appetite between MC and placebo
Mucke et al,[24] 2018	Study design: SR/MA Indication: cancer pain; cancer-related anorexia Number of RCTs: 5 Pooled sample size: 758	• Dronabinol oral • Oromucosal spray THC extract • THC:CBD oromucosal spray • THC:CBD oral	• No significant differences in pain reduction, weight, caloric intake, appetite, or nausea/vomiting compared with placebo	• Tolerability: no difference • Mild/moderate: no difference • Serious: no difference	No difference Provides low-quality evidence of no difference in caloric intake, appetite, nausea/vomiting, or pain reduction, between MC and placebo

Tateo et al,[25] 2017[a]	Study design: SR Indication: cancer pain Number of RCTs: 8 pooled sample size: 683	• Oral THC • Nabiximols oromucosal spray • Oral NIB • Oral benzopyra-noperidine	• Mixed evidence in pain reduction compared with placebo and/or comparison drug [a]	Mixed evidence Provides low-quality, mixed evidence for cancer-related pain reduction
Whiting et al,[31] 2015[c]	Study design: SR/MA Indication: chemotherapy induced nausea/vomiting Number of RCTs: 28 Pooled sample size: 1772	• Nabilone • Dronabinol • Nabiximols oromucosal spray • Levonantradol • THC	• Significant evidence of greater odds of achieving complete nausea and vomiting response with MC relative to placebo and/or comparison drug [c]	Significant benefit Provides low-quality evidence for improvements in chemotherapy-induced nausea and vomiting with MC compared with placebo and/or comparison drug

Abbreviations: MA, meta-analysis; MC, medical cannabis; SR, systematic review.
a Side effects are broadly reported without specifics on severity, tolerability, or comparison between study arms.
b Side effects are examined and compared between study arms without reporting of statistical significance.
c Side effects not separated for studies on the specific indication.

patients treated with cannabinoids had greater odds of improvements in nausea and vomiting relative to the placebo or active comparison. Evidence on improved cachexia-relevant outcomes in cancer patients is limited, with a lack of data on the effect of medical cannabis on weight, and a paucity of high-quality, recently published studies.

CHRONIC PAIN

- Medical cannabis is approved in almost all states with medical marijuana programs for chronic, noncancer pain, including neuropathic pain.
- Low-quality to moderate-quality evidence suggests that, compared with placebo or active control, medical cannabis increases the number of participants reporting pain relief of 30% or greater relative to pre-intervention pain.

Chronic pain, most often defined as pain lasting longer than 6 months, is a medical cannabis indication approved in almost all states. Current Centers for Disease Control and Prevention recommendations suggest using nonpharmacologic therapy and nonopioid pharmacologic therapy for treatment of chronic pain.[32] Medical cannabis for pain management could be a safer option than opioid medications, given the differences in overdose potential between opioids and medical cannabis. More than 165,000 people between 1999 and 2014 died from an opioid-related overdose.[32] Although marijuana can have side effects, overdose is unlikely.[33] Legalizing medical cannabis also may reduce Medicare costs. For example, when examining Medicare Part D claims for prescription drugs from 17 states where medical marijuana was legal in 2013, opioid use fell, and the investigators estimated that Part D would save $165 million per year from this reduction in opioid use.[34] Importantly, the evidence for the use of medical cannabis to treat chronic pain varies, as is discussed later.

Five recent systematic reviews and meta-analyses on chronic pain categorize pain into 2 categories: chronic noncancer pain and chronic neuropathic pain (**Table 5**). One meta-analysis of medical cannabis for treatment of chronic noncancer pain reported that the proportion of participants achieving at least 30% pain reduction compared with baseline levels was significantly higher with medical cannabis relative to placebo; however, there was no significant difference in the proportion achieving a 50% reduction in their pain.[35] Aviram and colleagues[36] also found that medical cannabis resulted in a significant decrease in pain relative to placebo when data was pooled from 43 RCTs. In contrast, a meta-analysis conducted by Whiting and colleagues[31] found no significant difference in pain reduction between medical cannabis and placebo treatments in the majority of standard pain measures, excluding 1 numeric pain scale that favored medical cannabis. There is some evidence to support medical cannabis having an analgesic effect; however, the evidence is low quality to moderate quality and is variable.

Two meta-analyses examined chronic neuropathic pain and reported significant evidence for the benefits of medical cannabis in the reduction of pain.[37,38] Mucke and colleagues[37] found that significantly more participants achieved a 30% and 50% reduction in pain relative to baseline pain with medical cannabis compared with placebo or active control. Nugent and colleagues[38] also found that medical cannabis was preferred to placebo for achieving a 30% reduction in pain scores post-intervention but did not find a significant difference for the outcome of 50% pain reduction. In an RCT done with participants experiencing neuropathic pain, there was a significant decrease in pain intensity with vaporized THC compared with placebo.[39] Both high and low THC doses showed significant decreases in pain for 2 hours after inhalation.

Table 5
Evidence for medical cannabis in chronic pain

Study	Method	Type of Cannabis	Primary Outcomes	Side Effects	Conclusion
Stockings et al,[35] 2018	Study design: SR/MA Indication: chronic noncancer pain Number of RCTs: 17 Pooled sample size: 2535	• THC:CBD oral • THC extract oromucosal spray • THC extract oral • THC:CBD extract oral • Dronabinol oral • Nabilone oral • Nabiximols oromucosal spray • Cannabis sativa (vaporized or smoked) • CT-3	• Significant differences in proportion of participants achieving 30% reduction in pain, no significant difference in proportion of participants achieving 50% reduction in pain compared with placebo	• Mild/moderate: no significant difference • Serious: no significant difference	Significant benefits Provides moderate-quality evidence for 30% pain reduction with MC compared with placebo
Aviram et al,[36] 2017	Study design: SR/MA Indication: chronic pain Number of RCTs: 43 Pooled sample size: 2437	• THC oral capsules • CT-3 oral capsules • THC:CBD extract oromucosal spray • THC oromucosal spray • CBD oromucosal spray • Sativex oromucosal spray • Dronabinol oral • Ajulemic acid oral • Nabilone oral • Cannabis (smoked) • THC (smoked, vaporized)	• Significant decrease in pain compared with placebo	• Significant increase in central nervous system, gastrointestinal, psychological, vision, and hearing-related side effects • No significant effect on cardiac or musculoskeletal side effects	Mixed evidence Provides moderate-quality evidence for pain reduction and greater incidence of side effects with MC compared with placebo

(continued on next page)

Table 5
(continued)

Study	Method	Type of Cannabis	Primary Outcomes	Side Effects	Conclusion
Mucke et al,[37] 2018	Study design: SR/MA Indication: chronic pain Number of RCTs: 16 Pooled sample size: 1750	• THC:CBD oromucosal spray • Inhaled herbal cannabis • Nabilone oral • Dronabinol	• Significant difference in proportion of participants reporting at least a 30% reduction in pain, 50% reduction in pain, and difference in mean pain intensity compared with placebo or active control	• Tolerability: significant difference • Mild/moderate: significant difference • Serious: no difference	Significant benefits Provides low-quality evidence for pain reduction and higher incidence of mild/moderate side effects with MC compared with placebo or active control
Nugent et al,[38] 2017[a]	Study design: SR/MA Indication: neuropathic pain Number of RCTs: 13 Pooled sample size: 748	• Smoked THC • Nabiximols oromucosal spray • THC Sublingual spray • Vaporized THC	• Significant difference in proportion of participants reporting at least 30% reduction in pain compared with placebo or no treatment	[a]	Significant Provides low-quality evidence for pain reduction with MC compared with placebo or no treatment
Whiting et al,[31] 2015[b]	Study design: SR Indication: chronic neuropathic pain Number of RCTs: 28 Pooled sample size: 2454	• Nabiximols oromucosal spray • Smoked THC • THC oromucosal spray • Nabilone • Dronabinol • Vaporized cannabis • Ajulemic acid capsules • Oral THC	• No significant difference on most standardized pain measures compared with placebo • Significant reduction in pain using a 10-point numeric rating scale compared with placebo or active control	[b]	Mixed evidence Provides minimal, low-quality evidence for MC to treat chronic pain when data pooled for select measures, compared with placebo or active control

Abbreviations: MA, meta-analysis; MC, medical cannabis; SR, systematic review.
[a] Side effects are examined and compared between study arms without reporting of statistical significance.
[b] Side effects not separated for studies on the specific indication.

Although side effects did occur, incidence was lower with the low dose. Serpell and colleagues[40] also found that a greater number of participants achieved at least 30% reduction in peripheral neuropathic pain relative to pre-intervention pain after receiving a high dose or low dose of THC/CBD oromucosal spray, when compared with placebo. Observed therapeutic benefit was similar between doses, suggesting that a lower dose may be superior when considering potential side effects.

DEMENTIA

- Few RCTs have focused on medical cannabis for dementia-related neuropsychiatric symptoms (NPSs); only 117 participants total across RCTs have been studied to date.
- Evidence is mixed, with no strong indication that medical cannabis effectively reduces NPSs.

Dementia is used as an overarching term to describe a variety of neurodegenerative illnesses, including Alzheimer's disease. Research on medical cannabis to alleviate NPS associated with dementia is limited. In a recent systematic review, 6 RCTs related to dementia and NPS were evaluated (**Table 6**).[41] Significant improvements were reported in only 1 of these studies, in which the sample size was 2 participants. In 2 of the RCTs with the largest sample sizes, no significant reductions were found in NPS based on the Neuropsychiatric Inventory when using oral THC compared with placebo.[17,19] There is not enough quality evidence to suggest any impact on NPS when using medical cannabis.

SIDE EFFECTS

- Cannabis-based medicines are associated with various nonserious side effects.
- Studies assessing tolerability and safety report higher rates mild side effects and study withdrawal due to treatment-related side effects in participants receiving cannabinoids.

Evidence on the efficacy of medical cannabis should be weighed with safety and tolerability considerations. Although medical cannabis offers potential benefits for

Table 6
Evidence for medical cannabis in dementia

Study	Method	Type of Cannabis	Primary Outcomes	Side Effects	Conclusion
Hillen et al,[41] 2019[a]	Study design: systematic review Indication: dementia Number of RCTs: 6 Pooled sample size: 117	• Oral THC • Dronabinol	• No significant difference in NPS compared with placebo • Significant improvement in 1 RCT (n = 2) compared with placebo	[a]	No difference Provides low-quality evidence of no difference in NPS between medical cannabis and placebo

[a] Side effects are broadly reported without specifics on severity, tolerability, or comparison between study arms.

various indications, there are several risks associated with use of medical cannabis that may reduce the potential clinical benefit. As **Tables 4–6** indicate, studies on the efficacy of medical cannabis for cancer and related symptoms, chronic pain, and dementia report myriad side effects. Across studies, investigators categorize the majority of these treatment-related events as mild or moderate. The most common side effects include dizziness, nausea, fatigue, dry mouth, somnolence, disorientation, drowsiness, confusion, balance issues, euphoria, and hallucinations.[31] Several systematic reviews and meta-analyses report suggest that rates of participant withdrawal are significantly higher among participants using cannabinoids compared with those taking placebo.[23,31,37] Available evidence indicates that the frequency of mild side effects is higher in cannabis treatment groups compared with control groups.[23,31,37] For example, a systematic review of the side effects of medical cannabinoids found that the rate of mild side effect was 1.86-times higher in participants receiving medical cannabis than controls.[42] Studies also indicate rate of study withdrawal because of side effects occurrence was significantly higher among those taking nabiximols and THC compared with those taking placebo. Overall, existing evidence suggest that there is no significant difference in rates of serious side effects, defined as side effects that result in hospitalization or disability or are life-threatening, between patients taking medical cannabis relative to placebo.[23,24,37,42] Based on existing evidence, it is unclear whether the potential benefits of cannabinoids outweigh the harms.

DISCUSSION

The authors are unable to recommend the use of medical cannabis in the majority of indications relevant to common symptoms experienced by older adults and patients receiving palliative care. The possible exception is for chronic pain based on the available evidence. Currently, there is insufficient evidence to determine the effectiveness and safety of medical cannabis for cancer-related pain, cancer cachexia, dementia, and Alzheimer's disease. Overall, the literature investigating the benefits and risks of medical cannabis is primarily composed of low-quality studies with small sample sizes, variation in formulations and dosing, and short intervention durations. Due to the paucity of high-quality studies, the authors are not able to establish the efficacy of medical cannabis for most indications explored in this article.

Future research is required before palliative care clinicians can make evidence-based decisions on the integration of medical cannabis as adjunct therapies. Moreover, as the older adult population and number of patients receiving palliative care grows, demand for alternative medications to manage symptoms, such as pain, reduced appetite, nausea, and vomiting, likely will increase. There is a pressing need for high-quality studies that address existing gaps in the literature. First, the ideal dosage, ratio of THC to CBD, administration route, and medical cannabis type for different indications has yet to be established. Second, more studies that compare medical cannabis to available treatments rather than placebo are warranted. Third, future research should assess the clinical significance of medical cannabis using standardized outcomes, assess minor and serious side effects, and examine long-term effects of medical cannabis use. The authors recognize that the feasibility of conducting these studies will be shaped by the legislative environment and the classification of cannabis. The regulatory environment almost certainly will continue to shift as states introduce laws to allow the use of medical marijuana.

DISCLOSURE

The authors have nothing to disclose.

REFERENCES

1. National Conference of State Legislatures. State medical marijuana laws. Available at: www.ncsl.org/research/health/state-medical-marijuana-laws.aspx. Accessed July 29, 2019.
2. United States Drug Enforcement Administration. Drug scheduling. Available at: https://www.dea.gov/drug-scheduling. Accessed July 2, 2019.
3. Palace ZJ, Reingold DA. Medical cannabis in the skilled nursing facility: a novel approach to improving symptom management and quality of life. J Am Med Dir Assoc 2019;20(1):94–8.
4. Substance Abuse and Mental Health Services Administration. National survey on drug use and health: summary of national findings, 2014(NSDUH Series H-48, HHS Publication No. (SMA) 14-4863). Rockville (MD): Author; 2013.
5. Lloyd SL, Striley CW. Marijuana use among adults 50 years or older in the 21st century. Gerontol Geriatr Med 2018;4. 2333721418781668.
6. Salas-Wright CP, Vaughn MG, Cummings-Vaughn LA, et al. Trends and correlates of marijuana use among late middle-aged and older adults in the United States, 2002-2014. Drug Alcohol Depend 2017;171:97–106.
7. Han BH, Palamar JJ. Marijuana use by middle-aged and older adults in the United States, 2015-2016. Drug Alcohol Depend 2018;191:374–81.
8. Morris NP. Educating physicians about marijuana. JAMA Intern Med 2019;179(8): 1017–8. [Epub ahead of print].
9. Carlini BH, Garrett SB, Carter GT. Medicinal Cannabis: a survey among health care providers in Washington State. Am J Hosp Palliat Care 2017;34(1):85–91.
10. Costantino RC, Felten N, Todd M, et al. A survey of hospice professionals regarding medical cannabis practices. J Palliat Med 2019;22(10):1208–12.
11. Uritsky TJ, McPherson ML, Pradel F. Assessment of hospice health professionals' knowledge, views, and experience with medical marijuana. J Palliat Med 2011; 14(12):1291–5.
12. Ahmed AI, van den Elsen GA, Colbers A, et al. Safety, pharmacodynamics, and pharmacokinetics of multiple oral doses of delta-9-tetrahydrocannabinol in older persons with dementia. Psychopharmacology 2015;232(14):2587–95.
13. Brisbois TD, de Kock IH, Watanabe SM, et al. Delta-9-tetrahydrocannabinol may palliate altered chemosensory perception in cancer patients: results of a randomized, double-blind, placebo-controlled pilot trial. Ann Oncol 2011;22(9):2086–93.
14. Chagas MH, Zuardi AW, Tumas V, et al. Effects of cannabidiol in the treatment of patients with Parkinson's disease: an exploratory double-blind trial. J Psychopharmacol 2014;28(11):1088–98.
15. Herrmann N, Ruthirakuhan M, Gallagher D, et al. Randomized placebo-controlled trial of Nabilone for agitation in Alzheimer's disease. Am J Geriatr Psychiatry 2019;27(11):1161–73.
16. Pickering EE, Semple SJ, Nazir MS, et al. Cannabinoid effects on ventilation and breathlessness: a pilot study of efficacy and safety. Chron Respir Dis 2011;8(2): 109–18.
17. van den Elsen GA, Ahmed AI, Verkes RJ, et al. Tetrahydrocannabinol for neuropsychiatric symptoms in dementia: a randomized controlled trial. Neurology 2015;84(23):2338–46.
18. van den Elsen GA, Tobben L, Ahmed AI, et al. Effects of tetrahydrocannabinol on balance and gait in patients with dementia: a randomised controlled crossover trial. J Psychopharmacol 2017;31(2):184–91.

19. van den Elsen GAH, Ahmed AIA, Verkes RJ, et al. Tetrahydrocannabinol in behavioral disturbances in dementia: a crossover randomized controlled trial. Am J Geriatr Psychiatry 2015;23(12):1214–24.

20. Minerbi A, Hauser W, Fitzcharles MA. Medical cannabis for older patients. Drugs Aging 2019;36(1):39–51.

21. Argiles JM, Busquets S, Stemmler B, et al. Cancer cachexia: understanding the molecular basis. Nat Rev Cancer 2014;14(11):754–62.

22. Van Lancker A, Velghe A, Van Hecke A, et al. Prevalence of symptoms in older cancer patients receiving palliative care: a systematic review and meta-analysis. J Pain Symptom Manage 2014;47(1):90–104.

23. Hauser W, Welsch P, Klose P, et al. Efficacy, tolerability and safety of cannabis-based medicines for cancer pain: a systematic review with meta-analysis of randomised controlled trials. Schmerz 2019;33(5):424–36.

24. Mucke M, Weier M, Carter C, et al. Systematic review and meta-analysis of cannabinoids in palliative medicine. J Cachexia Sarcopenia Muscle 2018;9(2):220–34.

25. Tateo S. State of the evidence: Cannabinoids and cancer pain-A systematic review. J Am Assoc Nurse Pract 2017;29(2):94–103.

26. Fallon MT, Albert Lux E, McQuade R, et al. Sativex oromucosal spray as adjunctive therapy in advanced cancer patients with chronic pain unalleviated by optimized opioid therapy: two double-blind, randomized, placebo-controlled phase 3 studies. Br J Pain 2017;11(3):119–33.

27. Portenoy RK, Ganae-Motan ED, Allende S, et al. Nabiximols for opioid-treated cancer patients with poorly-controlled chronic pain: a randomized, placebo-controlled, graded-dose trial. J Pain 2012;13(5):438–49.

28. Wang J, Wang Y, Tong M, et al. Medical cannabinoids for cancer cachexia: a systematic review and meta-analysis. Biomed Res Int 2019;2019:2864384.

29. Johnson JR, Burnell-Nugent M, Lossignol D, et al. Multicenter, double-blind, randomized, placebo-controlled, parallel-group study of the efficacy, safety, and tolerability of THC:CBD extract and THC extract in patients with intractable cancer-related pain. J Pain Symptom Manage 2010;39(2):167–79.

30. Strasser F, Luftner D, Possinger K, et al. Comparison of orally administered cannabis extract and delta-9-tetrahydrocannabinol in treating patients with cancer-related anorexia-cachexia syndrome: a multicenter, phase III, randomized, double-blind, placebo-controlled clinical trial from the Cannabis-In-Cachexia-Study-Group. J Clin Oncol 2006;24(21):3394–400.

31. Whiting PF, Wolff RF, Deshpande S, et al. Cannabinoids for medical use: a systematic review and meta-analysis. JAMA 2015;313(24):2456–73.

32. Dowell D, Haegerich TM, Chou R. CDC guideline for prescribing opioids for chronic pain - United States, 2016. MMWR Recomm Rep 2016;65(1):1–49.

33. Centers for Disease Control and Prevention. Marijuana and public health. Available at: https://www.cdc.gov/marijuana/faqs/overdose-bad-reaction.html. Accessed August 14, 2019.

34. Bradford AC, Bradford WD. Medical marijuana laws reduce prescription medication use in medicare part D. Health Aff (Millwood) 2016;35(7):1230–6.

35. Stockings E, Campbell G, Hall WD, et al. Cannabis and cannabinoids for the treatment of people with chronic noncancer pain conditions: a systematic review and meta-analysis of controlled and observational studies. Pain 2018;159(10):1932–54.

36. Aviram J, Samuelly-Leichtag G. Efficacy of Cannabis-based medicines for pain management: a systematic review and meta-analysis of randomized controlled trials. Pain Physician 2017;20(6):e755–96.
37. Mucke M, Phillips T, Radbruch L, et al. Cannabis-based medicines for chronic neuropathic pain in adults. Cochrane Database Syst Rev 2018;(3):CD012182.
38. Nugent SM, Morasco BJ, O'Neil ME, et al. The effects of cannabis among adults with chronic pain and an overview of general harms: a systematic review. Ann Intern Med 2017;167(5):319–31.
39. Wilsey B, Marcotte TD, Deutsch R, et al. An exploratory human laboratory experiment evaluating vaporized cannabis in the treatment of neuropathic pain from spinal cord injury and disease. J Pain 2016;17(9):982–1000.
40. Serpell M, Ratcliffe S, Hovorka J, et al. A double-blind, randomized, placebo-controlled, parallel group study of THC/CBD spray in peripheral neuropathic pain treatment. Eur J Pain 2014;18(7):999–1012.
41. Hillen JB, Soulsby N, Alderman C, et al. Safety and effectiveness of cannabinoids for the treatment of neuropsychiatric symptoms in dementia: a systematic review. Ther Adv Drug Saf 2019;10. 2042098619846993.
42. Wang T, Collet JP, Shapiro S, et al. Adverse effects of medical cannabinoids: a systematic review. CMAJ 2008;178(13):1669–78.

Delirium at the End of Life

Meera Agar, MBBS, MPC, FRACP, FAChPM, PhD[a,*],
Shirley H. Bush, MBBS, DRCOG, DCH, MRCGP, PgDip Pall Med, FAChPM[b,c,d,e]

KEYWORDS

- Delirium • Delirium pathophysiology • Delirium screening • Delirium prevention
- Antipsychotics • Benzodiazepines • Palliative care • End of life

KEY POINTS

- Delirium is highly prevalent in palliative care and is associated with significant distress and high mortality.
- The extent of assessment for delirium depends on goals of care, disease trajectory, potential reversibility, and burdens of the diagnostic workup and treatment of delirium.
- Institute nonpharmacologic measures and strategies as a part of essential care, tailored to the individual to decrease delirium distress.
- Support for carers is essential, which should include education on delirium.
- Pharmacologic management should be reserved for severe perceptual disturbance and agitation that has not responded to nonpharmacologic approaches, considering potential for loss of meaningful interactions with the patient owing to sedation and other adverse effects.

INTRODUCTION

Delirium is a highly prevalent and serious neuropsychiatric disorder in people with progressive life-limiting illness (people receiving palliative care).[1] The prevalence of delirium in the end of life period[2] (last weeks to days of life) increases exponentially.[1] Delirium presents as a constellation of disturbances in attention and awareness, cognitive changes (eg, disorientation, memory deficit, language, visuospatial ability or perception), and altered psychomotor behavior, mood, and sleep–wake cycle.[3] These changes occur acutely, usually fluctuate, and occur in the context of acute

[a] IMPACCT (Improving Palliative, Aged and Chronic Care Through Clinical Research and Translation) Faculty of Health, University of Technology Sydney, Building 10, Level 3, 235 Jones Street, Ultimo, New South Wales 2007, Australia; [b] The Ottawa Hospital, General Campus, 501 Smyth Road, Box 206, Ottawa, ON K1H 8L6, Canada; [c] Bruyère Research Institute, 85 Primrose Ave, Ottawa, ON K1R 6M1, Canada; [d] Ottawa Hospital Research Institute, 053 Carling Ave, Ottawa, ON K1Y 4E9, Canada; [e] Palliative Care, Bruyère Continuing Care, The Ottawa Hospital, 43, Bruyère Street, Ottawa, Ontario K1N 5C8, Canada
* Corresponding author.
E-mail address: meera.agar@uts.edu.au
Twitter: @meera_agar (M.A.)

Med Clin N Am 104 (2020) 491–501
https://doi.org/10.1016/j.mcna.2020.01.006
0025-7125/20/© 2020 Elsevier Inc. All rights reserved.

medical.theclinics.com

medical precipitants, which often are multiple.[4] The symptoms of delirium cause distress for the person themselves, their family, and the health professionals who care for them. Delirium is associated with significant morbidity, and increases the risk of falls, other medical complications, and functional and cognitive decline. In people with advanced illness it is also an independent predictor of mortality, and hence can herald the transition into the end-of-life period in those with a serious illness.[5] In the patient with a serious illness, it can prolong hospitalization or precipitate a hospital admission for those being cared for in the community.

Delirium prevalence on admission to palliative care units or hospices ranges from 13.3% to 42.3%, and the incidence after admission ranges from 3% to 45%.[6] The median period prevalence before death is 75% (range, 58%–88%).[1,4,6] In the community, delirium point prevalence is reported to be between 4% and 12%.[1]

The pathophysiology of delirium is highly complex and remains poorly understood. Increasingly the view is that, rather than a singular model, there are likely many pathophysiologic pathways that account for the range of precipitants and clinical phenotype and symptoms, further influenced by the biopsychosocial factors that promote healthy cognition.[7,8] These pathways include putative mechanisms that are mediated by neurotransmitter abnormalities, impaired functional connectivity, central neuroinflammation, inadequate oxidative mechanisms, abnormal glucose metabolism, the hypothalamic–pituitary–adrenal axis, or circadian rhythm dysregulation.[8,9]

DELIRIUM ASSESSMENT
Risk Assessment

A high degree of suspicion is required to ensure early detection and prompt diagnosis of delirium in the patients in palliative care, especially those who are at higher risk. Patients in palliative care are already in a high-risk group by nature of having an advanced illness. Furthermore, other risk factors to consider include visual and hearing impairment, age greater than 65, preexisting cognitive impairment (including dementia), dehydration, immobility, multiple medications, and comorbid illness.[10] A small number of studies exploring risk factors in cancer implicate psychoactive medications, hypoalbuminemia, metabolic disturbance, and metastases to bone, liver, and brain.[11]

Delirium Screening

It is recommended that routine screening be implemented for at-risk patients, with those who screen positive then proceeding to a full assessment to establish a diagnosis of delirium.[11] Several validated instruments are available for delirium screening.[12] Those studied in palliative care populations include the Confusion Assessment Method,[13] the Nursing Delirium Screening Scale,[14] and initial work exploring the 4AT.[15] The choice of screening approach should consider psychometrics of the tool, the training required to maintain its optimal use, degree of patient burden, and also take into account the local policy recommendations so that the one's approach to delirium screening is aligned with the broader health service where possible.

A collateral history from family members or carers is also a critical part of the assessment, because they often notice the changes in cognition and attention more promptly. A reported disturbance in cognition or awareness from a family member or carer should prompt a detailed assessment for delirium from the clinical team.

Delirium Diagnosis

The gold standard for the diagnosis of delirium is a clinician assessment utilizing standard diagnostic criteria. These criteria are either the *Diagnostic and Statistical Manual of Mental Disorders* (DSM), fifth edition (DSM-5), or alternatively, the *International Classification of Diseases*, 11th edition, of the World Health Organization.[3,16] The DSM-5 classification requires disturbance of attention and awareness (representing a change from baseline), a change in cognition, short and fluctuating chronology, and the presence of an underlying medical condition; these changes cannot occur in the context of a severely decreased level of arousal, such as a coma. The recent *International Classification of Disease*, 11th edition, classification requires disturbed attention and awareness that develop over a short period of time and tend to fluctuate, associated with other cognitive impairments, and with disturbance of sleep–wake cycle in some cases. Clinicians can use delirium assessment scales to assist in operationalizing these criteria and monitoring severity, for example, the Memorial Delirium Assessment Scale[17] and the Delirium Rating Scale—Revised 98,[18,19] both of which have been validated in people with advanced illness and cancer.

It is also important to assess the presence of other symptoms; although not required for diagnosis, it contributes to the person's experience of delirium and will assist in determining an individualized management plan to relieve distress. These symptoms include:

- Perceptual disturbance (misperceptions, illusions, hallucinations commonly visual, delusions),
- Thought disorder,
- Language difficulties (word finding difficulty, dysgraphia, dysnomia, paraphasia),
- Altered affect (anger, irritability, depression, apathy, lability, fear, and anxiety), and
- Sleep–wake disturbance (reversal of the normal sleep–wake cycle, dreams and nightmares, fragmented sleep).

Although not included in the DSM-5 diagnostic criteria, 3 subtypes of delirium assist in identifying some common presentations based on the psychomotor features and arousal levels. Subsyndromal presentations also occur, which fall on the continuum from single symptoms to full delirium.[20,21] Patients with hypoactive delirium seem to be lethargic and drowsy, respond slowly to questions, do not initiate movement, and have reduced awareness of surroundings; this presentation is common in patients approaching the end of life.[22] Hypoactive delirium can be easily misdiagnosed as fatigue or depression.[23] In contrast, patients with the hyperactive delirium subtype have restlessness, agitation, and psychomotor overactivity, as well as a higher rate of perceptual disturbance and delusions, mimicking the anxiety of psychosis.[24] In some patients, the presentation fluctuates between these 2 subtypes (mixed delirium).

It is particularly challenging to distinguish delirium from dementia, or diagnose a delirium superimposed on a preexisting dementia. Arousal is generally preserved, even in advanced dementia, and the temporal onset of symptoms in dementia are more subacute.[25] There are several approaches to assess inattention that can be used at the bedside, for example, reciting the months of the year backwards.[25] Cognitively simple tests assessing focusing and sustaining attention rather than those that require manipulating information or testing memory may be particularly useful to distinguish delirium and dementia (such as evaluating a patient's ability to follow a slowly moving simple picture in front of the patient's face when verbally prompted to look at the picture).[25] Family recognition of change in behavior from baseline is also a helpful clue.

Identifying the Precipitant(s)

A detailed history and examination should be conducted to identify the possible etiologies of delirium and determine whether they are potentially reversible. It should be expected that there will be 3 precipitants on average (range, 1–6 precipitants), with common etiologies including infection, substance withdrawal (alcohol and nicotine), metabolic abnormalities (eg, hypercalcemia), hypoxia, and psychoactive medications (corticosteroids, opioids, anticholinergics, and benzodiazepines).[4,11,19,26] Brain or leptomeningeal malignancy, cognitive effects of anticancer therapies and paraneoplastic syndromes also are possible.[11]

To confirm the diagnosis of etiologies, laboratory testing, imaging, and less commonly electroencephalogram or lumbar puncture may be required. Careful consideration of the patient's goals of care and preferences, prior function and disease trajectory, potential reversibility of the precipitant(s), and potential adverse impacts and burden of the treatment options should be undertaken before investigations are planned.[11,27] There are several reasons for why identifying the precipitant(s) can be helpful in people who have delirium at the end of life, even if this is based on bedside assessment, and regardless of whether intervention is planning to be pursued. First, it may not yet be clinically obvious that the person is imminently dying, and thus it will assist in determining if the etiology is irreversible. Second, it underpins an explanation to the person and their family about what delirium is and why it has occurred.

DELIRIUM PREVENTION

Multicomponent nonpharmacologic strategies, which include reorientation, early mobilization, therapeutic activity, optimizing oral hydration and nutrition, sleep strategies, and maximizing hearing and vision, are effective in decreasing delirium incidence in hospitalized older adults, with a decrease in delirium incidence of up to 44%.[20,29] A recent review of the participant diagnoses, illness severity, and mortality in these studies suggested that patients at the end of life were included despite palliative care patients often being a formal exclusion criteria. However, neither the ability of palliative care patients to participate in the interventions or their outcomes was formally reported.[30] It is reasonable, however, to institute nonpharmacologic measures and strategies wherever possible, as essentials in care with the knowledge they may contribute to decreasing delirium risk. A personalized approach should be used, with adaptation of these measures and strategies to the individual and setting where necessary.

DELIRIUM MANAGEMENT
General Principles

It is essential that delirium care is interdisciplinary, with care delivered in a coordinated and collaborative way (**Box 1**). Delirium can affect decision capacity, but it is important to remember that, because delirium is a fluctuating condition, there may be periods where it is possible to discuss the options for care directly with the person themselves.[11] Delirium occurrence in the palliative care patient should prompt open discussion with the person themselves and proxy decision makers including the implications for prognosis and also treatment choices.[5]

Individuals receiving palliative care with delirium will often look medically unwell and can present similarly to the person who is imminently dying, making the determination of whether delirium is refractory to treatment difficult, and it may only become clear

---

Box 1
Guiding principles of delirium care at the end of life

- Do not consider the person with delirium as a list of fragmented problems and risks
- Enable and foster choice
- Understand the person's background and context, and discover what is important to them
- Foster connectivity with staff, family, and loved ones
- Provide clear explanations about what is happening and the context
- Understand that delirium disrupts sense of continuity and is unfamiliar; acknowledge and value concerns
- Make the environment more familiar, and consider if home with support is the better location for care
- Treat the person with respect and dignity

---

over time or after lack of response to a time-limited trial of initial treatment that the person is at the end of life.[11]

The plan for delirium management should consider, and address as needed the following issues:

- The safety of the patient and those surrounding the patient (other patients, family, staff);
- The best location of care (eg, admission may be required for a more investigational approach or if family carers are exhausted, but a familiar home environment may be more conducive to minimizing symptoms);
- Information and education for the person with delirium and their family and carers;
- Correction of underlying causes if possible;
- Minimization of concurrent issues that can exacerbate symptoms (eg, urinary retention, constipation, pain, assistance with repositioning);
- Institute approaches to support delirium recovery if possible (treating underlying cause and essential nonpharmacologic care);
- Determination of the mediators of distress for the individual with delirium, remembering that it is highly individual and address symptoms accordingly;
- An assessment of the distress of carers and staff;
- Consideration of the patient priority in relation to mental awareness and periods of lucidity;
- Recognition that delirium presents as a loss of the person the family knew;
- Determination of the risk of poor prognosis and communication to family and carers of the potential for deterioration.

Nonpharmacologic Interventions

The same nonpharmacologic approaches that have been effective in preventing delirium are also useful to continue as part of delirium care. In addition to those strategies, the following also should be considered:

- Thorough medication review, reducing (for those that cannot be abruptly stopped) and ceasing unnecessary psychoactive medication and minimizing drug interactions;
- Pain assessment and management;

- Bladder and bowel care;
- Minimize use of physical restraints and other tethers (such as intravenous lines, indwelling bladder catheter).

A clear explanation in lay terms should be given about what delirium is and what has caused it.[11,31] Providing carers with information on how to communicate with the person with delirium and to care for them is also critical (**Box 2**). An example explanation[31] in lay terms could be "Delirium is common. It is a disturbance in brain function that can happen when a person is medically unwell. Common causes include medication and infections (such as chest and urine infection). Often there is more than one cause."

Pharmacologic Interventions

Internationally, there is no registered medication for delirium. There remains no definitive evidence that antipsychotics reduce delirium duration or severity in older hospitalized adults[32,33]; or reduce duration of delirium or coma, and survival, length of intensive care unit and hospital stay in patients in intensive care.[34,35]

In palliative care populations, there are few placebo-controlled trial data to inform clinical practice. One study found greater delirium symptoms (inappropriate communication, inappropriate behavior or perceptual disturbance) in participants who received oral haloperidol and risperidone in comparison to placebo after 72 hours of treatment.[36] Another study was in a population of patients with advanced cancer in the last days or weeks of life, with agitation and delirium despite scheduled haloperidol.[37] This study showed a decrease in agitation (with associated sedation) with the

---

Box 2
Recommended topics to cover in the provision of delirium information to palliative care patients and their families

Explanation of delirium, especially its fluctuating nature, and subtypes

Potential causes of the delirium episode

Signs and symptoms of delirium
- Differentiate the features of hypoactive and hyperactive delirium.
- Describe the change in sleep–wake cycle that often occurs in people with delirium.
- Describe perceptual changes, such as hallucinations and delusions.

The management of delirium

How to communicate with a person with delirium
- Explain that the person with delirium may not understand what people are saying and also feel that they are not being understood.
- Outline helpful strategies to improve communication and reassure the person with delirium.

How the family can help to care for the person with delirium
- Provide guidance on nonpharmacologic interventions that can be done by the family
  - For example, reorientation of the person with delirium
  - For example, use of eyeglasses, hearing aids, and dentures
  - For example, increase exposure to daylight during the day
  - For example, minimize light, noise, and disruptions during the night

In addition:
   Advise the person with delirium to inform the health care team if they are feeling confused, frightened, or having hallucinations.
   Advise the family to inform the health care team if the person seems more confused.
   An example of a Delirium Information Leaflet for Palliative Care patients and their families can be found here: https://www.bruyere.org/en/Delirium[32]

addition of a single dose of intravenous lorazepam to scheduled haloperidol compared with placebo after 8 hours.[37] The evidence thus points to pharmacologic strategies predominantly mediating effects through sedation, without impacting on the underlying delirium pathology. It also serves as a reminder that delirium is a constellation of symptoms, and adding a pharmacologic agent may make not improve the overall symptom burden, for example, by changing a hyperactive presentation to a hypoactive one, which can be equally distressing for the patient.

Before the institution of any pharmacologic strategy, the clinician should have a thorough understanding of the causes and degree of distress, the patient's and/or family's interpretation of the symptoms and signs, and have made an assessment of whether the agitation is more distressing than the possible distress caused by the potential sedation and loss of meaningful communication which could occur from a pharmacologic approach. Pharmacologic approaches should never be the sole approach, with concurrent nonpharmacologic approaches and information and support crucial.[11] As with any medication therapy, net clinical benefit needs to be considered, with clear target symptom and consideration of unintended side effects that could contribute further to the constellation of cognitive symptoms that makes delirium distressing (**Fig. 1**).

The potential risks associated with antipsychotic drug treatment should be considered including extrapyramidal adverse effects, sedation, anticholinergic side effects, cardiac arrhythmias, and possible drug–drug interactions. A US Food and Drug Administration warning exists for the increased risk of mortality associated with antipsychotics in elderly patients with dementia-related behavioral disturbances.[38]

Until further evidence emerges, clinicians should be guided by principles outlined in the guidelines developed by the National Institute for Health and Clinical Excellence[10] and the European Society for Medical Oncology[11]; that is, antipsychotics should be limited to situations in which nonpharmacologic strategies have been ineffective and the delirious patient is distressed or considered a risk to themselves or others (**Box 3**). The pharmacologic management of delirium should not be viewed as a quick

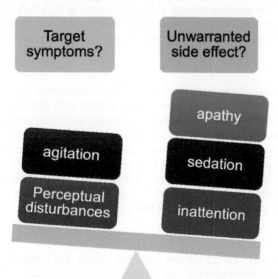

Fig. 1. Pharmacologic therapy for delirium management should consider the target symptom, balanced with their potential for adverse effects.

Box 3
Prescribing practice points

- Reflect carefully on whose distress you are aiming to treat—be cautious of treating the patient solely to relieve the distress of family and staff.
- Articulate clearly what is the symptom(s) you are aiming to treat and the rationale for your medication choice and the intent (treating perceptual disturbance, sedation, pharmacologic restraint).
- Consider if all other aspects of care have been put in place and if it expected that these will improve situation soon. Consider if watchful waiting is an option.
- Remember prescribing is off label—this practice requires informed consent and shared decision making with the person or their proxy decision maker.
- Delirium is a medical emergency requiring senior clinician input
- Reassess regularly

---

fix solution for a complex medical emergency, delegated to the preordered as-needed chart. Senior clinician input should guide prescribing, even if this occurs after hours. This process will ensure that the required discussion with the patient or proxy decision maker occurs and a shared decision is made to proceed with a pharmacologic approach to decrease the risk of inappropriate prescribing and dosing. It has been identified that families often have ambivalence about the intent of prescribing in this situation,[39] which can be mitigated by appropriate discussion, shared decision-making and informed consent.

If the decision is to proceed with prescribing medications to manage delirium symptoms, then the short-term, low-dose use of an antipsychotic agent is recommended, and only for specific symptoms of perceptual disturbance or severe agitation where distress has been identified or if there are safety concerns.[40] Patients should be monitored for the effectiveness of administered antipsychotics in ameliorating delirium symptoms, as well as adverse effects. A benzodiazepine may be indicated for benzodiazepine or alcohol withdrawal, as a crisis medication for severe agitation from delirium and distress, or when the agreed therapeutic goal is sedation.[11,40]

SUMMARY

A systematic approach to early detection of delirium supported by collaborative interdisciplinary care will allow optimal care for the person with delirium at the end of life. Thorough bedside assessment, in conjunction with communication with the patient and his or her family, is essential to identify the etiology, symptoms experienced, and cause of distress. To make informed decisions about the treatment approach the person if able and their family need to understand what delirium is, and the treatment options available to them and their relative risks and benefits. Taking into account this assessment and the person's preferences will foster an individualized management plan to optimize quality of life and minimize distress.

DISCLOSURE

M. Agar has received funding from the National Health and Medical Council, National Breast Cancer Foundation and Cancer Australia for Delirium Clinical Trials. S.H. Bush has received research funding from the Bruyère Academic Medical Organization, National Breast Cancer Foundation and Cancer Australia for Delirium Clinical Trials. M. Agar and S.H. Bush did not receive any funding for this article.

REFERENCES

1. Watt CL, Momoli F, Ansari MT, et al. The incidence and prevalence of delirium across palliative care settings: a systematic review. Palliat Med 2019;33(8):865–77.
2. Hui D, Nooruddin Z, Didwaniya N, et al. Concepts and definitions for "actively dying," "end of life," "terminally ill," "terminal care," and "transition of care": a systematic review. J Pain Symptom Manage 2014;47(1):77–89.
3. American Psychiatric Association. Delirium, Neurocognitive disorders. In: Diagnostic and statistical manual of mental disorders. 5th edition. Washington, DC: DSM-5; 2013. p. 596.
4. Lawlor PG, Gagnon B, Mancini IL, et al. Occurrence, causes, and outcome of delirium in patients with advanced cancer: a prospective study. Arch Intern Med 2000;160(6):786–94.
5. Agar MR, Quinn SJ, Crawford GB, et al. Predictors of mortality for delirium in palliative care. J Palliat Med 2016;19(11):1205–9.
6. Hosie A, Davidson PM, Agar M, et al. Delirium prevalence, incidence, and implications for screening in specialist palliative care inpatient settings: a systematic review. Palliat Med 2013;27(6):486–98.
7. Oldham MA, Flaherty JH, Maldonado JR. Refining delirium: a transtheoretical model of delirium disorder with preliminary neurophysiologic subtypes. Am J Geriatr Psychiatry 2018;26(9):913–24.
8. Maldonado JR. Delirium pathophysiology: an updated hypothesis of the etiology of acute brain failure. Int J Geriatr Psychiatry 2018;33(11):1428–57.
9. MacLullich AMJ, Ferguson KJ, Miller T, et al. Unravelling the pathophysiology of delirium: a focus on the role of aberrant stress responses. J Psychosom Res 2008;65(3):229–38.
10. National Institute for Health and Clinical Excellence (NICE) National Clinical Guideline centre. Delirium: diagnosis, prevention and management London. London: National Institute for Health and Clinical Excellence; 2010. Available at: https://www.nice.org.uk/guidance/cg103. Accessed August 23, 2019.
11. Bush SH, Lawlor PG, Ryan K, et al. Delirium in adult cancer patients: ESMO clinical practice guidelines. Ann Oncol 2018;29(Suppl 4):iv143–65. available online.
12. De J, Wand AP. Delirium screening: a systematic review of delirium screening tools in hospitalized patients. Gerontologist 2015;55(6):1079–99.
13. Ryan K, Leonard M, Guerin S, et al. Validation of the confusion assessment method in the palliative care setting. Palliat Med 2009;23(1):40–5.
14. Barnes CJ, Webber C, Bush SH, et al. Rating delirium severity using the nursing delirium screening scale: a validation study in patients in palliative care. J Pain Symptom Manage 2019. https://doi.org/10.1016/j.jpainsymman.2019.06.027.
15. Baird L, Spiller JA. A quality improvement approach to cognitive assessment on hospice admission: could we use the 4AT or Short CAM? BMJ Open Qual 2017; 6(2):e000153.
16. World Health Organisation. 6D70 Delirium 2018. Available at: https://icd.who.int/browse11/l-m/en#/http://id.who.int/icd/entity/897917531. Accessed August 25, 2019.
17. Breitbart W. The memorial delirium assessment scale. J Pain Symptom Manage 1997;13(3):128–37.
18. Trzepacz PT, Mittal D, Torres R, et al. Validation of the Delirium Rating Scale-revised-98: comparison with the delirium rating scale and the cognitive test for delirium. J Neuropsychiatry Clin Neurosci 2001;13(2):229–42.

19. Leonard M, Raju B, Conroy M, et al. Reversibility of delirium in terminally ill patients and predictors of mortality. Palliat Med 2008;22(7):848–54.
20. Cole MG. Subsyndromal delirium in old age: conceptual and methodological issues. Int Psychogeriatr 2013;25(6):863–6.
21. Leonard MM, Agar M, Spiller JA, et al. Delirium diagnostic and classification challenges in palliative care: subsyndromal delirium, comorbid delirium-dementia, and psychomotor subtypes. J Pain Symptom Manage 2014;48(2):199–214.
22. Breitbart W, Alici Y. Evidence-based treatment of delirium in patients with cancer. J Clin Oncol 2012;30(11):1206–14.
23. Meagher DJ, Trzepacz PT. Motoric subtypes of delirium. Semin Clin Neuropsychiatry 2000;5(2):75–85.
24. Boettger S, Passik S, Breitbart W. Treatment characteristics of delirium superimposed on dementia. Int Psychogeriatr 2011;23(10):1671–6.
25. Morandi A, Davis D, Bellelli G, et al. The diagnosis of delirium superimposed on dementia: an emerging challenge. J Am Med Dir Assoc 2017;18(1):12–8.
26. Breitbart W, Alici Y. Agitation and delirium at the end of life: "We couldn't manage him". JAMA 2008;300(24):2898–910.
27. Leonard M, Agar M, Mason C, et al. Delirium issues in palliative care settings. J Psychosom Res 2008;65(3):289–98.
28. Hshieh TT, Yue J, Oh E, et al. Effectiveness of multicomponent nonpharmacological delirium interventions: a meta-analysis. JAMA Intern Med 2015;175(4): 512–20.
29. Siddiqi N, Harrison JK, Clegg A, et al. Interventions for preventing delirium in hospitalised non-ICU patients. Cochrane Database Syst Rev 2016;(3):CD005563.
30. Hosie A, Siddiqi N, Featherstone I, et al. Inclusion, characteristics and outcomes of people requiring palliative care in studies of non-pharmacological interventions for delirium: a systematic review. Palliat Med 2019;33(8):878–99.
31. Bush SH. Élisabeth Bruyère palliative care delirium clinical practice guidelines development team. Information for palliative care patients and their families about delirium. 2017. Available at: https://www.bruyere.org/en/Delirium. Accessed August 25, 2019.
32. Burry L, Mehta S, Perreault MM, et al. Antipsychotics for treatment of delirium in hospitalised non-ICU patients. Cochrane Database Syst Rev 2018;(6):CD005594.
33. Neufeld KJ, Yue J, Robinson TN, et al. Antipsychotic medication for prevention and treatment of delirium in hospitalized adults: a systematic review and meta-analysis. J Am Geriatr Soc 2016. https://doi.org/10.1111/jgs.14076.
34. Girard TD, Pandharipande PP, Carson SS, et al. Feasibility, efficacy, and safety of antipsychotics for intensive care unit delirium: the MIND randomized, placebo-controlled trial. Crit Care Med 2010;38(2):428–37.
35. Girard TD, Exline MC, Carson SS, et al. Haloperidol and ziprasidone for treatment of delirium in critical illness. N Engl J Med 2018;379(26):2506–16.
36. Agar MR, Lawlor PG, Quinn S, et al. Efficacy of oral risperidone, haloperidol, or placebo for symptoms of delirium among patients in palliative care: a randomized clinical trial. JAMA Intern Med 2017;177(1):34–42. Accessed August 25, 2019.
37. Hui D, Frisbee-Hume S, Wilson A, et al. Effect of lorazepam with haloperidol vs haloperidol alone on agitated delirium in patients with advanced cancer receiving palliative care: a randomized clinical trial. JAMA 2017;318(11): 1047–56.

38. Schneider LS, Dagerman KS, Insel P. Risk of death with atypical antipsychotic drug treatment for dementia: meta-analysis of randomized placebo-controlled trials. JAMA 2005;294(15):1934–43.
39. Wright DK, Brajtman S, Macdonald ME. A relational ethical approach to end-of-life delirium. J Pain Symptom Manage 2014;48(2):191–8.
40. Bush SH, Tierney S, Lawlor PG. Clinical assessment and management of delirium in the palliative care setting. Drugs 2017;77(15):1623–43.

Management of Grief, Depression, and Suicidal Thoughts in Serious Illness

Kanako Y. McKee, MD[a,b,*], Anne Kelly, LCSW[c]

KEYWORDS

- Serious illness • Grief • Prolonged grief • Depression • Death contemplation
- Suicidal ideation • Antidepressants • Psychotherapy

KEY POINTS

- Psychological distress is a common cause of suffering in patients and families facing serious illness.
- Grief is an adaptive and individualized process that may occur in response to any form of loss.
- Prolonged grief and major depressive disorder (MDD) are discrete conditions that warrant individualized assessment and treatment.
- Differentiating between grief, prolonged grief, MDD, and other conditions marked by depressive symptoms is important to provide appropriate support and treatment.
- Although thoughts about death may be normative in patients nearing the end of life, they must be differentiated from active suicidal ideation in which a patient actively seeks to take one's own life.

INTRODUCTION

Serious illness causes a cascade of life changes for patients and their families. The varied physical, social, and psychological stressors that accompany advanced disease can be burdensome and cause intense emotional suffering, hindering the ability of patients to cope in day-to-day life and affecting their ability to endure or adhere to recommended treatments. Clinicians may find it challenging to distinguish normative symptoms of grief from other conditions that may have overlapping symptoms but require further clinical attention, such as prolonged grief and major depression.

[a] Division of Geriatrics, Department of Medicine, University of California San Francisco San Francisco, San Francisco, CA, USA; [b] San Francisco Veterans Affairs Health Care System, 4150 Clement Street, Box 181G, San Francisco, CA 94121, USA; [c] San Francisco Veterans Affairs Health Care System, 4150 Clement Street (NH 181), San Francisco, CA 94121, USA
* Corresponding author.
E-mail address: kanako.mckee@ucsf.edu

Med Clin N Am 104 (2020) 503–524
https://doi.org/10.1016/j.mcna.2020.01.003
0025-7125/20/Published by Elsevier Inc.

medical.theclinics.com

Suicide assessments in this population are complicated by the reality that seriously ill patients and their caregivers may frequently contemplate or talk about death without having active suicidal thoughts. This article addresses key concepts for the assessment and management of commonly encountered types of psychological distress among patients and families living with serious illness.

GRIEF AND LOSS IN SERIOUS ILLNESS
Grief

Grief is a natural, albeit painful, response to a loss. Patients and families facing serious health conditions are likely to experience many types of loss over the course of illness, including physical functioning, cognitive functioning, meaningful social roles, and financial resources. They may also include loss of control, certainty, or hopes and expectations for the future. Bereavement is a term used to describe the event of losing of a loved one through death, which is considered to be among life's most stressful events and a time often marked by considerable grief.

Assessment and Diagnosis

Grief is a highly individualized process, although there are common traits that clinicians can identify or anticipate. Symptoms fluctuate and may manifest across multiple domains:

- Emotional—numbness, guilt, sadness, yearning, relief, anger
- Physical—decreased energy, tension in the body
- Cognitive—difficulty concentrating, thoughts focused on the loss
- Behavioral—changes in sleep and appetite, crying, social withdrawal
- Spiritual—questions of meaning, relationship to one's faith may be strengthened or challenged

Although grief is a dynamic process without prescribed stages, the difficulties experienced in grief dissipate with time. In the context of bereavement, surviving loved ones may initially feel an acute form of grief marked by strong waves of sadness, disbelief, and persistent yearning. Sleep disturbances and social withdrawal can occur, and some individuals report seeing, hearing, or feeling the presence of the deceased.[1,2] However, the intensity of grief subsides as the griever comes to grasp the reality of the loss and adapts to a changed life and future. As the loss is integrated into daily life, bereaved individuals regain the desire and ability to engage in pleasurable activity and meaningful relationships while maintaining a sense of connection to the deceased. Acute symptoms of grief commonly subside within 6 months to a year after the death has occurred.[3] However, important reminders of the loss, such as holidays, birthdays, and anniversaries may trigger strong feelings of grief to re-emerge.

Although grief is difficult and may cause temporary or intermittent changes in functioning, distress is largely attributed to the loss itself and does not preclude individuals from also experiencing pleasure, joy, and hope. A normative grief process is not characterized by problems with self-worth or sustained impairments in social or occupational functioning. The intensity, duration, and expression of grief is influenced by a variety of factors including the type of loss, how the loss occurred, gender, cultural and spiritual norms, age, health, and the griever's support system.[4]

Treatment

On its own, grief does not require formal medical or psychiatric intervention for distress levels to improve.[5] For many, the empathy and reassurance received from family, friends, or a spiritual community are enough to foster healthy coping. Clinicians can actively support grieving patients by offering empathic listening and normalizing their experience in the context of the loss. Educating patients and families about what to expect while grieving can help them navigate an unfamiliar and difficult process while also dispelling myths that grief adheres to prescribed traits or stages. In situations where an informal support system feels inadequate to the griever, a referral to a peer support group, chaplain, or mental health provider should be considered. For bereaved individuals seeking grief support, local hospice agencies may be an apt resource. Bereaved families of hospice may receive counseling services for up to a year after the death of a loved one and many hospices make their bereavement programs available to the wider public regardless of hospice enrollment.

The risk of developing distinct mood, anxiety, and substance use disorders is heightened during bereavement.[2,4] Because the symptoms that frequently characterize grief may also appear in other health conditions, a careful and culturally sensitive assessment is warranted to avoid either pathologizing a natural grief response or neglecting to identify and address a co-occurring illness. In circumstances where sleep disturbances are affecting daily functioning, it may be appropriate to consider targeted treatment of insomnia.

PROLONGED GRIEF

Prolonged grief is a severe and debilitating grief reaction that is estimated to occur in 10% of bereaved adults,[6] possibly affecting more than 1 million Americans annually.[7] Associated with reduced quality of life, poor health, and high-risk behaviors,[8,9] prolonged grief is a discrete mental health condition that can lead to substantial and long-lasting consequences.

The concept of prolonged grief in bereavement has been explored using different definitions and names, including complicated grief and traumatic grief. The World Health Organization included a new diagnosis of Prolonged Grief Disorder (PGD) in their release of the *International Classification of Diseases, 11th Revision*. The American Psychological Association's *Diagnostic and Statistical Manual, Fifth Edition (DSM-5)*[10] included a variant of this diagnosis, Persistent Complex Bereavement Disorder (PCBD), in section III, "Conditions for Further Study." The Yale Bereavement Study found no significant difference between the patient populations identified by PGD and PCBD.[11] For consistency, the term "prolonged grief" will be used throughout this article.

Assessment and Diagnosis

Prolonged grief is characterized not simply by the presence of grief symptoms over time but rather by the protracted duration of intense grief that causes impairments in daily functioning. In prolonged grief, acute cognitive, emotional, and behavioral grief symptoms remain unremitting for most of the time at least 6 months to a year after the death of a loved one and are inconsistent with cultural, spiritual, or social norms.[1,12–14]

Fundamental to this condition is the persistent yearning for or preoccupation with the deceased person. This is often accompanied by unrelenting feelings of anger, guilt, or shock. The griever may have difficulty accepting the reality of the death, feel they have lost a part of themselves, and/or actively avoid people, places, or things that trigger memories of the loss. Feelings of guilt may be centered around regrets related to the deceased or blaming themselves/others for their inability to prevent the death from happening. For the griever, the process may feel never-ending and worrisome or, alternatively, it may feel that grief is what maintains their connection to the deceased. Disturbed sleep and suicidal thinking can occur in prolonged grief independent of a comorbid mood or anxiety disorder.[8,15] Suicidal thoughts may particularly stem from the griever's longing to be with the deceased.

Prolonged grief is associated with other health problems including cardiac disease, hypertension, cancer, and substance use.[9] Bereaved people with a history of trauma, previous losses, mood and anxiety disorders, substance use disorders, inadequate social support, and women are among those more vulnerable to developing prolonged grief; losing a loved one in sudden or violent circumstances also raises the risk.[1,13,16]

Clinicians are cautioned not to screen for or diagnose PGD within the first 6 months of bereavement to avoid pathologizing a normative grief process, and guidelines proposed for PCBD do not allow a diagnosis to be made for at least 12 months into bereavement. If severe grief symptoms are persistent and causing impairments within important areas of functioning 6 months to a year after the death of a loved one, patients should be screened for prolonged grief. Because the presenting symptoms may initially appear similar to or exist alongside a mood or anxiety disorder (**Table 1**), clinicians should identify all presenting conditions to inform an appropriate treatment plan.

There are multiple assessment tools that have been shown to reliably distinguish normative grief from prolonged grief. Examples include:

- The Inventory of Complicated Grief: consists of 19 self-rated items; scores greater than 25 warrant further clinical assessment.[17]
- The Brief Grief Questionnaire: consists of 5 self-rated items; scores greater than 5 warrant further clinical assessment.[18,19]
- Prolonged Grief Disorder-13: consists of 12 self-rated items; diagnostic criteria warranting further clinical assessment are specified.[14]

Table 1
Differences between prolonged grief and major depression

Symptom	Prolonged Grief	Major Depression
Negative thoughts & emotions	Centered around the deceased and persistent longing	Generalized and pervasive, feelings of hopelessness
Feelings of pleasure	Able to experience positive emotions alongside preoccupation with the deceased	Inability to enjoy daily activities
Feelings of guilt	Centered around regrets in relation to the deceased	Global feelings of guilt, worthlessness, and being a burden on others
Avoidant behaviors	Avoidance of places, objects, and people that remind them of the reality of the loss	General avoidance and social withdrawal
Physical symptoms	Sleep disturbance	Sleep disturbance, changes in appetite/weight, psychomotor agitation/retardation, fatigue/loss of energy
Suicidal thoughts	Commonly associated with a wish to be with the deceased	Rooted in feelings of hopelessness and worthlessness, intolerable suffering, and feeling a burden to others

Treatment

When prolonged grief is suspected, patients should be referred to a mental health provider for specialized assessment and treatment. Psychotherapeutic interventions designed to treat prolonged grief seem to be more effective than standard interventions used in the treatment of depression.[7,20] Many targeted treatments have been studied with promising results.[21–24] One such intervention is Complicated Grief Treatment (CGT), which has demonstrated positive outcomes across 3 randomized control trials.[7,20,25] The treatment is a manualized, 16-session cognitive behavioral therapy which incorporates strategies used in interpersonal therapy and motivational interviewing.[26] The role of pharmacotherapy in treating prolonged grief remains unclear. Some studies have examined the concurrent use of antidepressants in patients receiving CGT, but the results are mixed and the evidence base remains limited.[27]

All clinicians caring for individuals with prolonged grief can offer added support through empathic listening and gentle reassurance around their attempts to resume daily activities. Educating the griever about prolonged grief may offer a framework for their distress and foster hope for improvement. They should be encouraged to use support available through their family, friends, and spiritual community. Clinicians should also remain vigilant to suicidal thinking or behaviors and assess a griever's risk for self-harm.

DEPRESSION IN SERIOUS ILLNESS

Depressive symptoms are common among patients with serious illness and take a major toll on quality of life. Depression can exacerbate the physical burdens of advanced disease including pain, fatigue, poor appetite, and sleep disturbance.[28] It has been associated with decreased treatment adherence,[29,30] increased disability,[31,32] increased health service costs,[33] increased caregiver burden,[34] poor prognosis,[35] and—in some diseases—higher mortality.[36–39] In addition, major depression is a well-established risk factor for suicide.[40] Although estimates of depression prevalence among the seriously ill vary widely due to differences in definitions used and populations studied, available studies consistently show that patients with serious illness experience depression at higher rates than the general population. Compared with a 4% 1-year pooled prevalence of major depressive disorder (MDD) in the general population,[41] a 2011 meta-analysis found prevalence ranges of 5% to 30% for depression among patients with cancer in palliative care settings, with a pooled prevalence of 15% for MDD and about 10% for minor depression.[42] Rates of depressive symptoms are also high at the very end of life: 1 study found that 43% of all home hospice patients experienced moderate-to-severe symptoms of depression, as rated by caregivers using the Edmonton Symptom Assessment Scale.[43] Unfortunately, clinical depression remains underdiagnosed and undertreated in palliative care.

Assessment and Diagnosis

The DSM-5 defines a major depressive episode as greater than 2 weeks of pervasive and functionally debilitating depressed mood or anhedonia, accompanied by at least 4 of the following additional symptoms of depression:

1. Changes in weight or appetite
2. Insomnia or hypersomnia
3. Psychomotor agitation or retardation
4. Fatigue or loss of energy
5. Feelings of worthlessness or excessive guilt

6. Poor concentration or indecisiveness
7. Recurrent thoughts of death, suicidal ideation, or suicidal behavior[10]

Many screening instruments are used in clinical practice. The simplest of these is a 2-question screen, which is considered positive if a patient answers "Yes" to both of the following questions: "Are you depressed?" and "Have you experienced loss of interest in things or activities that you would normally enjoy?"[44] In a meta-analysis of 5 studies of patients with cancer and patients receiving palliative care, this 2-question screen had a pooled sensitivity of 91% and a specificity of 86%.[45] Other depression screening tools used in palliative care include the 4-question Brief Case Find for Depression,[46] Patient Health Questionnaire-9,[47] and the Hospital Anxiety and Depression Scale.[48]

In-Depth Assessment

For patients who screen positive for depression, clinicians should conduct a more detailed assessment starting with the history of present illness. The history is essential to establishing the presence of depressive symptoms and their chronology, their impact on functioning, any alleviating or aggravating factors, and comorbid medical and psychiatric conditions. Special attention should be paid to the patient's underlying serious illness—including disease and symptom burden, current and past treatment history, and medication review. Because the somatic symptoms of depression are often caused by the patient's underlying illness, assessments of depression in the seriously ill often give greater weight to psychological symptoms and require clinicians to carefully consider the time course of symptoms, changes from baseline, and proportionality or intensity of symptoms in relation to the situation.[49,50] Finally, clinicians should assess patients for suicidal ideation/risk, obtain a social history, and perform focused physical and mental status examinations.[51]

The differential diagnosis for MDD includes adjustment disorder with depressed mood, demoralization syndrome, and prolonged grief—all of which can present with symptoms of distress. Adjustment disorder with depressed mood occurs in response to an identifiable stressor, with patients experiencing distress out of proportion to the stressor itself; the distress resolves within 6 months of resolution of the identified stressor.[10] Demoralization syndrome, although not currently recognized as a distinct psychiatric syndrome, is marked by existential despair, hopelessness, and a profound sense of helplessness and incompetence. The distress arising from demoralization can be profound—even leading to a desire for hastened death—and studies suggest that it is clinically significant in 13% to 18% of patients with progressive disease or cancer.[52] Prolonged grief has been discussed in detail above. For cases in which making a diagnosis is particularly challenging, consultation with a specialist is recommended.

Treatment

Whenever possible, management of major depression in patients with serious illness should combine patient and family education/support, supportive psychotherapy, and antidepressant pharmacotherapy.

Nonpharmacologic Therapy

All health care providers can take an active role in providing psychosocial support for patients and families. Evidence from randomized controlled trials (RCTs) in patients with cancer shows that:

- Interactions that convey empathy and active listening promotes psychological adjustment

- Providing anticipatory guidance about what to expect in the future promotes psychological well-being
- Opportunities to discuss feelings with a health professional reduce psychological distress[53]

Offering compassion, listening deeply, clarifying and validating patient concerns, encouraging adaptive coping mechanisms, engaging existing social supports, reframing cognitive distortions, and helping patients with meaning-making are all interventions that can decrease psychological suffering.[49,54,55]

For more formal psychotherapy, patients should be referred to a mental health provider. Multiple RCTs have demonstrated that psychotherapy is an efficacious treatment of unipolar major depression in healthy adults, comparable with treatment with antidepressants.[56,57] A meta-analysis of psychotherapy for depression treatment in patients with advanced cancer found a statistically significant decrease in depression scores indicating a moderate clinical effect.[58] Cognitive behavioral therapy,[57,58] supportive-expressive therapy,[59] dignity therapy,[55,60] and meaning-centered psychotherapy[61] are examples of psychotherapies used in treatment of depression for patients with serious illness.

Pharmacotherapy

Antidepressants are prescribed at lower rates for depressed patients with concurrent physical illness compared with their physically healthy counterparts,[62] perhaps due to clinicians' uncertainty about the appropriateness and efficacy of pharmacotherapy.[62,63] A 2010 Cochrane systematic review and meta-analysis found antidepressants to be effective and appropriate for the treatment of depression in patients with physical illness,[64] and a follow-up study in 2011 reached a similar conclusion for depressed patients with life-threatening illness.[65] Specifically, the latter found antidepressants to be superior to placebo at every time point starting at 4 to 5 weeks after initiation, with effect size increasing over time up to 9 to 18 weeks. Interestingly, this meta-analysis also suggested that, in the palliative care population, antidepressants may be effective in reducing depressive symptoms not only in MDD, but also in milder mood disorders, such as adjustment disorder with depressed mood and dysthymia (now classified under persistent depressive disorder in the *DSM-5*).[65] As noted by a 2018 Cochrane review and meta-analysis of antidepressant use in patients with cancer, however, the evidence base remains limited and better trials are needed.[66]

Numerous studies on standard antidepressant pharmacotherapy in physically healthy patients demonstrate similar efficacy across and within antidepressant classes.[56] The choice of antidepressant in palliative care thus depends on factors such as the patient's symptoms, preferences, and prognosis; the medication's side effect profile and other distinguishing features; and drug-drug interactions (DDIs). **Table 2** summarizes commonly used antidepressants, recommended dosing ranges, and notable characteristics. Selective serotonin reuptake inhibitors (SSRIs), widely used as first-line therapy for depression, have a positive safety profile for patients with serious illness and have fewer autonomic and anticholinergic side effects than tricyclic antidepressants (TCAs).[56,65] Common side effects of SSRIs include transient nausea, gastrointestinal upset, headache, and sexual dysfunction; some (especially citalopram) can cause dose-dependent QTc prolongation.[56] Serotonin/norepinephrine reuptake inhibitors (SNRIs) have a similar antidepressant efficacy and side effect profile as SSRIs. In addition, SNRIs may be more effective than SSRIs in treating concomitant anxiety and are effective for the treatment of neuropathic pain—very useful in palliative care.[67] Two other first-line antidepressants with atypical mechanisms of action deserve mention for their distinguishing

Table 2
Antidepressants commonly used in palliative care

Medication	Typical Starting Dosage	Typical Dosage Range	Notes on Titration & Available Formulations	Clinical Considerations
SSRIs				• Positive safety profile in patients with serious illness; generally well tolerated • Common side effects: transient nausea, gastrointestinal upset, headache, sexual dysfunction
Citalopram (Celexa)	10–20 mg/d	20–40 mg/d	• Start at 20 mg/d; may increase dose after >1 wk • Available as tabs, liquid	• Well tolerated • Few DDIs • Max dose 20 mg/d older patients • Significant risk of QTc prolongation at doses >40 mg/d
Escitalopram (Lexapro)	5–10 mg/d	10–20 mg/d	• Start at 5–10 mg/d; may increase dose after >1 wk • Available as tabs, liquid	• Well tolerated • Few DDIs • Max dose 10 mg/d in older patients • Dose-dependent QTc prolongation • Taper to DC when possible • Some evidence suggests that escitalopram and sertraline provide best combination of efficacy and acceptability among SSRIs
Fluoxetine (Prozac)	10–20 mg/d	20–60 mg/d	• Start at 10–20 mg/d; may increase dose after >1 wk • Available as tabs, capsules, liquid	• Many DDIs (potent CYP2D6 inhibition) • Associated with weight loss (most other SSRIs associated with weight gain) • May be activating in some patients • Wide dose range: up to 80 mg/d • Very long $t^{1/2} \rightarrow$ tapering to DC less important

Paroxetine (Paxil)	10–20 mg/d	20–40 mg/d	• Start at 10–20 mg/d; may increase dose after >1 wk
			• Available as tabs, liquid
				• Many DDIs (potent CYP2D6 inhibition)
				• Very short $t^{1/2}$
				  ○ Taper to DC to avoid significant discontinuation syndrome
				  ○ Caution if oral route unreliable

Sertraline (Zoloft)	25–50 mg/d	50–200 mg/d	• Start at 25–50 mg/d; may increase dose by 50 mg weekly up to 200 mg/d • Available as tabs, liquid	• Well tolerated • Few DDIs • Taper to DC when possible • Some evidence suggests that escitalopram and sertraline provide best combination of efficacy and acceptability among SSRIs
SNRIs				• Similar antidepressant efficacy and side effect profile as SSRIs • May be more effective than SSRIs for concomitant anxiety • Effective treatment of neuropathic pain

Venlafaxine (Effexor)	37.5–75 mg/d	75–225 mg/d	• Start at 37.5–75 mg/d; may increase by 75 mg every 4 d up to 225 mg/d
			• Available as tabs, capsules
			• Capsule granules are difficult to administer through feeding tubes
			• Extended-release formulation can be given qd. Otherwise, divide the total daily dose bid–tid
				• Effective treatment of neuropathic pain (higher doses)
				• Very short $t^{1/2}$
				  ○ Taper to DC to avoid significant discontinuation syndrome
				  ○ Caution if oral route unreliable
				• Common side effects: insomnia, headache, hypertension
				• Decrease dose by 25%–50% in renal impairment and by 50% in mild-mod hepatic impairment.

(continued on next page)

Table 2
(continued)

Medication	Typical Starting Dosage	Typical Dosage Range	Notes on Titration & Available Formulations	Clinical Considerations

Duloxetine (Cymbalta)	30–60 mg/d	60–120 mg/d	• Start at 30–60 mg/d; may increase by 30 mg weekly
			• Available as capsules
			• Capsule granules are difficult to administer through feeding tubes
				• Effective treatment of neuropathic pain (higher doses)
				• Doses >60 mg/d are rarely more effective for depression, although ok to increase up to 120 mg/d for neuropathic pain.
				• Short t½
				  ○ Taper to DC to avoid significant discontinuation syndrome (although less severe than venlafaxine)
				  ○ Caution if oral route unreliable
				• Contraindicated in renal impairment (CrCl < 30) and hepatic impairment/ cirrhosis.

Atypical agents			• Buproprion, mirtazapine, and methylphenidate may be used as single agents or in combination with SSRIs/SNRIs • Esketamine is currently available on a restricted basis only for treatment-resistant depression; it must be given with an oral antidepressant	
Bupropion (Wellbutrin)	150 mg/d	300–450 mg/d	• Start at 150 mg/d; may increase to 300 mg/d after 3 d and then to 450 mg/ d after 2 wk • Available as tabs • Multiple formulations (IR, SR, XL); XL allows for once daily dosing	• Weak norepinephrine and dopamine reuptake inhibitor • Useful in patients working on smoking cessation • Lowers seizure threshold → contraindicated in seizure disorder and eating disorder • Mild stimulant effect → useful in fatigue, but may worsen anxiety or insomnia • May improve concentration • Minimal sexual side effects

| Mirtazapine (Remeron) | 7.5–15 mg/d | 15–45 mg/d | • Increase dose by 15 mg every 1–2 wk | • Exact mechanism of action unknown. Increases central serotonergic and noradrenergic activity
• Side effects include sedation and appetite gain
  ○ Useful in patients with insomnia, anorexia, weight loss
  ○ Dose at bedtime
• May help with nausea
• Common side effect: orthostatic hypotension
• Antidepressant effect may peak at 30 mg/d, then decrease at higher doses
• A few studies suggest slightly faster onset of action compared with standard antidepressants |
| Methylphenidate (Ritalin) | 2.5–5 mg/d | 10–30 mg/d | • Start at 2.5 mg once daily or 2.5 mg bid. Increase by 5 mg/d (or 2.5 mg/dose) every 5 d, up to 15 mg bid | • Psychostimulant medication
• Rapid antidepressant effect (within 1–3 d)
  ○ Consider choosing as first-line therapy for patients with short prognoses (days to <2 mo)
• Well tolerated in most patients
• Most have good response at lower dosages
• Dose qam or bid. If dosing bid, administer 2nd dose no later than 2 PM to avoid insomnia
• May also help with fatigue, opioid-induced sedation, and appetite
• Side effects: anxiety, restlessness, insomnia
• Caution/avoid in patients with history of tachyarrhythmias |

(continued on next page)

Table 2
(continued)

Medication	Typical Starting Dosage	Typical Dosage Range	Notes on Titration & Available Formulations	Clinical Considerations
Ketamine	?	?		• *N*-methyl-ᴅ-aspartate antagonist traditionally used as an anesthetic • Various dosing regimens studied (iv/po), but studies are small • Rapid onset of antidepressant effect (within minutes to hours) observed in studies
Esketamine (Spravato)	56 mg intranasally on day 1		56–84 mg intranasally twice weekly during 4-wk induction phase, then 56–84 mg q 1–2 wk during maintenance phase	• Esketamine: intranasal formulation Food and Drug Administration approved for treatment-resistant depression in conjunction with an oral antidepressant • Restricted distribution (Risk Evaluation and Mitigation Strategy) in the US: must be administered under observation • Side effects: dissociation, dizziness, nausea, sedation
TCAs				• Not a first-line medication class in palliative care due to side effect profile (anticholinergic/autonomic side effects are common), DDIs, and narrow therapeutic window with potential for overdose • Helps with neuropathic pain as well as depression

| Nortriptyline (Pamelor) | 10–25 mg/d | 50–150 mg/d | • Start at 10–25 mg/d; may increase by 25–50 mg/d every 2–3 d (10–25 mg/d every 2–3 d in older adults).
 • Available as tabs | • Side effects: sedation, delirium, urinary retention, orthostatic hypotension
 ○ Administer at bedtime
 ○ Nortriptyline has fewer anticholinergic adverse effects than amitriptyline
 • Many DDIs
 • Narrow therapeutic window; cardiotoxicity, risk of fatal overdose
 • Effective for neuropathic pain, but generally not used as first-line (SNRIs preferred) |

Abbreviation: DC, discontinuation

features. Bupropion causes less sexual dysfunction than SSRIs, is useful in patients who want treatment of comorbid tobacco dependence, and has mild stimulant properties—which may be helpful to patients with significant fatigue, or potentially bothersome to patients with anxiety.[56] Mirtazapine is an effective antidepressant, with a few studies suggesting a faster time to onset than other antidepressants.[56] Its side effects of sedation and increased appetite are helpful to patients suffering from insomnia, anorexia, and weight loss, and data support its use in nausea management.[68] Finally, other patient factors may influence the choice of antidepressant. For patients with a history of abruptly stopping medications or for those at risk of losing the oral route in the near future, clinicians may want to avoid medications with significant discontinuation syndromes such as paroxetine or SNRIs (venlafaxine more so than duloxetine). For patients with severe depression expressing suicidal ideation, clinicians should exercise caution in prescribing TCAs, which carry the potential for fatal overdose. In fact, although TCAs are effective for depression and neuropathic pain, they are not considered first-line agents due to their side effect profile, narrow therapeutic window, and frequent DDIs.[56,67]

One challenge to treatment of MDD in palliative care is the lengthy time course to effectiveness for all of the antidepressants discussed above. Although early responders may see symptom improvement as early as 1 to 2 weeks after drug initiation, a 4- to 8-week trial at the target dose is necessary to ascertain effectiveness.[56] Patients nearing the end of life may die before standard antidepressants have had time to work. For patients with very short prognoses, alternatives should be considered. Psychostimulants such as methylphenidate can reduce depressive symptoms in the short term (up to 4 weeks),[69] and a therapeutic trial can be completed in a matter of days by initiating treatment at a low dose and titrating up daily or every few days until the clinical target or unwanted side effects are reached. Another option is ketamine: an *N*-methyl-D-aspartate receptor antagonist traditionally used as an anesthetic that has garnered attention as a promising new treatment of refractory depression. A 2019 review article examined 11 studies of ketamine used as an antidepressant in the palliative care population; all reported positive results.[70] In these studies, significant improvement in depressive symptoms occurred as early as 40 minutes to a few hours after administration, with the effect of a single dose typically lasting 6 to 7 days and daily dosing regimens showing sustained alleviation of depression for many weeks. In March 2019, the Food and Drug Administration-approved Spravato (esketamine) nasal spray, in conjunction with an oral antidepressant, for the treatment of treatment-resistant depression.[71]

SUICIDAL THOUGHTS IN SERIOUS ILLNESS

Living with a chronic or serious illness often prompts patients and their families to think about death and the way in which they might one day die. Death contemplation is increasingly common as people approach the end of life and is likely to be accompanied by a variety of emotional responses, possibly including passive suicidal ideation (SI). Passive SI is characterized by thoughts of wanting life to end and must be distinguished from active SI, which is marked by the desire and/or intent to end one's own life. In patients with advanced illness, active SI may also be expressed through the desire for a hastened death.

It is estimated that 4% of American adults report SI annually[72] with even higher rates noted among older adults,[73] the bereaved,[4] and as many as 30% of nursing home residents in a given month.[74] The palliative care patient population is at an increased risk for SI given that a number of the risk factors for suicide are inherent for many people living with serious illness. For example, having one or more physical illnesses that cause functional limitations, pain, respiratory problems, or impaired vision are associated with an increased risk for suicide.[75,76] Feeling a lack of control, a lack of meaning or purpose in one's life, and feeling a burden to others also pose greater risk for suicide and are not uncommon among people living with advanced illness.[77,78] Although a co-occurring mental illness, such as depression, is frequently present in patients who report SI, it is not requisite for suicidal thoughts and behaviors to occur.

Proactively identifying and assessing SI in seriously ill patients is an essential yet complex task for health care providers. Many professionals find it challenging to respond to psychosocial suffering and worry that discussing difficult issues could provoke strong emotions or intensify patients' psychological distress.[53] Their discomfort may lead them to avoid the topic of SI or change the subject for fear of saying the wrong thing in response. The perpetuation of common myths regarding suicide assessment is another factor that may inhibit professionals from exploring the topic with patients. Two common myths claim that asking about suicide could cause SI to occur and that there is nothing a clinician can do if a patient is determined to die by suicide. However, evidence shows that asking about suicidal thoughts does not create SI in a patient's mind, and that accurate assessment for suicide risk gives clinicians the ability to intervene with a treatment plan to decrease suicidal behaviors, attempts, and ultimately death.

Table 3
Risk factors, warning signs, and protective factors for suicide

Risk Factors: Suggest Risk Over a Longer Timeframe (1 Year ~ Lifetime)	Warning Signs: Specific to the Current State; Implies Imminent Risk	Protective Factors: Need to Be Both Available & Accessible
• Previous history of psychiatric diagnoses ◦ Comorbidity and recent onset of illness increase risk • Previous suicide attempts • Male gender • Same-sex sexual orientation • Age (y): >45, highest risk >64 • Veteran status • History of abuse • Family history of suicide • Significant loss (actual or perceived) • Physical illness, pain, insomnia • Impaired functional capacity • Isolation, limited social connectedness • Hopelessness • Perceived burdensomeness • Impulsivity or aggressive tendencies • Easy access to lethal means	• Talking about wanting to die or kill oneself • Looking for ways to kill oneself: seeking access to pills, weapons, or other means • Increasing or excessive alcohol/drug use • Hopelessness • Purposeless: no reasons for living • Talking about being a burden to others • Withdrawing from friends, family, society • Feeling trapped—like there is no way out • Being in unbearable pain • Rage, anger, seeking revenge • Acting reckless or engaging in risky activities (unthinkingly) • Anxiety, agitation, sleeping too little or too much • Displaying extreme mood swings	• Effective & active medical and mental health care • Social supports • Connectedness • Reasons for living • Meaning & purpose in life • Hopefulness • Adaptive problem-solving skills • Cultural & religious beliefs that discourage suicide • Restricted access to lethal means • Children present in the home • Fear of death or suicide

Data from Refs.[40,79,80]

Step 1: Assess for the presence of active suicidal thoughts.

Ask:

- *Have you been thinking about killing yourself?*
- *Have you thought about suicide?*

- Differentiate between suicidal thoughts (wanting to kill oneself) and death contemplation (thoughts of death, dying, or wanting to be dead but not active thoughts of killing oneself).

- Use precise, unambiguous language.

 "Yes"

Step 2: Ask an open-ended question (without providing prompts) to assess the specificity of the patient's suicidal thinking.

- *Can you tell me exactly what you've been thinking?*

Step 3: Get details

Assess specificity of thinking. Use the acronym **FIDS** (frequency, intensity, duration, and specificity - including access).

- How *often* do you have thoughts about killing yourself?
        (Once a day, more than once a day, once a week, once a month?)
- Can you tell me how *intense* or *severe* the thoughts are?
- When you have these thoughts, how *long* do they last? *(A few seconds, minutes, or longer?)*
- Have you been thinking about *how* you might do this? Do you have a plan? How would you go about killing yourself?
    - *Tip: Do NOT provide options to choose from when questioning about method.*
- Have you thought about *when* or *where* you would kill yourself?
- Do you have *access* to [method] or have you taken steps to get access?
- Have you thought about *any other method* of suicide? *[Ask this question until the patient says no.]*

"No"

- Document that the patient did not express active suicidal thoughts.

- Include a specific quote in documentation.

- It is still important to assess suicidal history.

Step 4: Assess intent, including reasons for dying and both subjective & objective markers of intent.

Greater specificity and detail in the how, when, where, and why suggest greater intent.

- *It sounds like you're going through a hard time. What led you to think of committing suicide?*
- *What are your reasons for dying? Why do you want to kill yourself?*
- *What triggers your thoughts about suicide?*
- *Do you have any intention of acting on your thoughts? Can you rate your intent on a scale of 1 to 10, with 1 being 'no intent at all' to 10 being 'certain that you'll act on them as quickly as you can'?*
- *Have you taken steps to act on your suicidal thoughts?*
- *Have you done anything in preparation for your death (e.g. will, life insurance, letters to loved ones)?*

Step 5: Assess prior history of suicidality and other risk factors / warning signs.

- *Can you tell me about the first time you ever thought about suicide?*
- *What was going on at that time?*
- *Did you make a suicide attempt?*
- *What was the outcome? Were you injured? Did you get medical care?*
- *How did you feel about surviving?*
- *How many suicide attempts have you made?*

Step 6: Assess protective factors, including reasons for living.

- *Even though you've had a very difficult time, something has kept you going. What are your reasons for living?*
- *Are you hopeful about the future?*
- *What keeps you going in difficult times like this? Who do you rely on during difficult times?*
- *Has treatment been effective for you in the past?*
- *Does your family know that you feel this way? Did you share this with anyone else?*

Fig. 1. Suggested framework for suicide assessment and risk stratification. (*Adapted from* Rudd MD. The assessment and management of suicidality. Journal of Contemporary Psychotherapy 2007;37(4):235; and Substance Abuse and Mental Health Services Administration (SAMHSA). SAFE-T: Suicide assessment five-step evaluation and triage. HHS Publication No. (SMA) 09-4432, CMHS-NSP-0193; Printed 2009; with permission.)

Assessment and Management

In responding to a patient expressing thoughts about death, it is important to be alert to one's own responses, allow for time to explore the patient's thoughts, and resist the

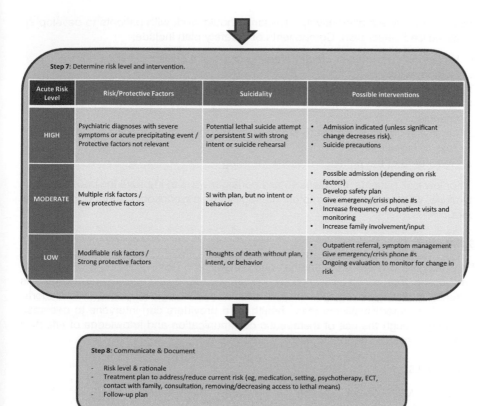

Fig. 1. (*continued*).

urge to rush to conclusions. Serious illness communication techniques continue to be valuable in this setting. Active listening skills, the appropriate use of silence, responding to emotions with empathy, and acknowledging the patient's experience can all aid clinicians in the assessment, and can be done without actively supporting that person's desire to die. Using precise, unambiguous language is particularly important in performing a suicide assessment because it lays the foundation for honesty and bluntness in the therapeutic relationship, signals to a patient that the clinician will not shy away from painful details, and provides the details needed to make an accurate risk assessment. Precision and clarity in written documentation is likewise critical in this setting.[40]

Key components of an SI assessment include:

1. Differentiating between nonsuicidal death contemplation and SI/behavior
2. Assessing the patient's suicidal thoughts, intent, and planning behaviors
3. Assessing for risk factors, warning signs, and protective factors (**Table 3**)[40,79,80]

Based on these elements, a clinician makes a clinical judgment as to the patient's risk level for suicide. One framework for suicide assessment, adapted from "The Assessment and Management of Suicidality" by M. David Rudd,[40] is outlined in **Fig. 1**.

The risk assessment informs the appropriate actions a clinician should take to mitigating a patient's suicide risk. When risk level is high, patients generally require inpatient admission and suicide precautions. For moderate risk patients, hospitalization may be considered; alternatively, clinicians should work with patients to develop an individualized safety plan. Components of a safety plan include:

1. Helping the patient self-identify warning signs of a crisis
2. Coping strategies
3. Available supports, including safe people and places
4. Specific people to contact for help, including family, friends, and professionals/agencies
5. Modifying the environment to promote safety, including removing or reducing access to lethal means
6. Reminders of the patient's reasons for living

For low-risk patients, clinicians should consider ways to improve the patient's quality of life, whether through symptom management, psychosocial support, or spiritual care.[40,80]

SUMMARY

Psychological distress is common among patients and families coping with the stress and losses that accompany serious illness. Accurate and routine assessment is essential to distinguishing between normative and pathologic responses. In collaboration with an interdisciplinary team, health care providers can intervene to decrease suffering through the use of therapeutic communication and knowledge of effective pharmacologic and nonpharmacologic treatments.

REFERENCES

1. Shear MK. Clinical practice. Complicated grief. N Engl J Med 2015;372(2): 153–60.
2. Zisook S, Iglewicz A, Avanzino J, et al. Bereavement: course, consequences, and care. Curr Psychiatry Rep 2014;16(10):482.
3. Bonanno GA, Wortman CB, Lehman DR, et al. Resilience to loss and chronic grief: a prospective study from preloss to 18-months postloss. J Pers Soc Psychol 2002;83(5):1150–64.
4. Stroebe M, Schut H, Stroebe W. Health outcomes of bereavement. Lancet 2007; 370(9603):1960–73.
5. Jordan JR, Neimeyer RA. Does grief counseling work? Death Stud 2003;27(9): 765–86.
6. Lundorff M, Holmgren H, Zachariae R, et al. Prevalence of prolonged grief disorder in adult bereavement: a systematic review and meta-analysis. J Affect Disord 2017;212:138–49.
7. Shear K, Frank E, Houck PR, et al. Treatment of complicated grief: a randomized controlled trial. JAMA 2005;293(21):2601–8.
8. Latham AE, Prigerson HG. Suicidality and bereavement: complicated grief as psychiatric disorder presenting greatest risk for suicidality. Suicide Life Threat Behav 2004;34(4):350–62.
9. Prigerson HG, Bierhals AJ, Kasl SV, et al. Traumatic grief as a risk factor for mental and physical morbidity. Am J Psychiatry 1997;154(5):616–23.
10. Association AP. Diagnostic and statistical manual of mental disorders, fifth edition: DSM-5. 5th edition. Arlington (VA): American Psychiatric Association; 2013.
11. Maciejewski PK, Maercker A, Boelen PA, et al. "Prolonged grief disorder" and "persistent complex bereavement disorder", but not "complicated grief", are

one and the same diagnostic entity: an analysis of data from the Yale Bereavement Study. World Psychiatry 2016;15(3):266–75.

12. Simon NM, Wall MM, Keshaviah A, et al. Informing the symptom profile of complicated grief. Depress Anxiety 2011;28(2):118–26.

13. Zisook S, Shear K. Grief and bereavement: what psychiatrists need to know. World Psychiatry 2009;8(2):67–74.

14. Prigerson HG, Horowitz MJ, Jacobs SC, et al. Prolonged grief disorder: psychometric validation of criteria proposed for DSM-V and ICD-11. PLoS Med 2009; 6(8):e1000121.

15. Hardison HG, Neimeyer RA, Lichstein KL. Insomnia and complicated grief symptoms in bereaved college students. Behav Sleep Med 2005;3(2):99–111.

16. Lobb EA, Kristjanson LJ, Aoun SM, et al. Predictors of complicated grief: a systematic review of empirical studies. Death Stud 2010;34(8):673–98.

17. Prigerson HG, Maciejewski PK, Reynolds CF 3rd, et al. Inventory of complicated grief: a scale to measure maladaptive symptoms of loss. Psychiatry Res 1995; 59(1–2):65–79.

18. Shear KM, Jackson CT, Essock SM, et al. Screening for complicated grief among Project Liberty service recipients 18 months after September 11, 2001. Psychiatr Serv 2006;57(9):1291–7.

19. Ito M, Nakajima S, Fujisawa D, et al. Brief measure for screening complicated grief: reliability and discriminant validity. PLoS One 2012;7(2):e31209.

20. Shear MK, Wang Y, Skritskaya N, et al. Treatment of complicated grief in elderly persons: a randomized clinical trial. JAMA Psychiatry 2014;71(11):1287–95.

21. Bryant RA, Kenny L, Joscelyne A, et al. Treating prolonged grief disorder: a randomized clinical trial. JAMA Psychiatry 2014;71(12):1332–9.

22. Kersting A, Dolemeyer R, Steinig J, et al. Brief Internet based intervention reduces posttraumatic stress and prolonged grief in parents after the loss of a child during pregnancy: a randomized controlled trial. Psychother Psychosom 2013; 82(6):372–81.

23. Eisma MC, Boelen PA, van den Bout J, et al. Internet-based exposure and behavioral activation for complicated grief and rumination: a randomized controlled trial. Behav Ther 2015;46(6):729–48.

24. Rosner R, Pfoh G, Kotoucova M, et al. Efficacy of an outpatient treatment for prolonged grief disorder: a randomized controlled clinical trial. J Affect Disord 2014; 167:56–63.

25. Shear MK, Reynolds CF 3rd, Simon NM, et al. Optimizing treatment of complicated grief: a randomized clinical trial. JAMA Psychiatry 2016;73(7):685–94.

26. The Center for Complicated Grief CUSoSW. Complicated grief. 2017. Available at: www.complicatedgrief.columbia.edu. Accessed August 05, 2019.

27. Bui E, Nadal-Vicens M, Simon NM. Pharmacological approaches to the treatment of complicated grief: rationale and a brief review of the literature. Dialogues Clin Neurosci 2012;14(2):149–57.

28. Wilson KG, Chochinov HM, Skirko MG, et al. Depression and anxiety disorders in palliative cancer care. J Pain Symptom Manage 2007;33(2):118–29.

29. DiMatteo MR, Lepper HS, Croghan TW. Depression is a risk factor for noncompliance with medical treatment: meta-analysis of the effects of anxiety and depression on patient adherence. Arch Intern Med 2000;160(14):2101–7.

30. Mathes T, Pieper D, Antoine SL, et al. Adherence influencing factors in patients taking oral anticancer agents: a systematic review. Cancer Epidemiol 2014; 38(3):214–26.

31. Hays RD, Wells KB, Sherbourne CD, et al. Functioning and well-being outcomes of patients with depression compared with chronic general medical illnesses. Arch Gen Psychiatry 1995;52(1):11–9.
32. Wells KB, Stewart A, Hays RD, et al. The functioning and well-being of depressed patients. Results from the Medical Outcomes Study. JAMA 1989;262(7):914–9.
33. Unutzer J, Schoenbaum M, Katon WJ, et al. Healthcare costs associated with depression in medically ill fee-for-service medicare participants. J Am Geriatr Soc 2009;57(3):506–10.
34. Rhondali W, Chirac A, Laurent A, et al. Family caregivers' perceptions of depression in patients with advanced cancer: a qualitative study. Palliat Support Care 2015;13(3):443–50.
35. Hata M, Yagi Y, Sezai A, et al. Risk analysis for depression and patient prognosis after open heart surgery. Circ J 2006;70(4):389–92.
36. Frasure-Smith N, Lesperance F, Talajic M. Depression following myocardial infarction. Impact on 6-month survival. JAMA 1993;270(15):1819–25.
37. House A, Knapp P, Bamford J, et al. Mortality at 12 and 24 months after stroke may be associated with depressive symptoms at 1 month. Stroke 2001;32(3):696–701.
38. Lloyd-Williams M, Shiels C, Taylor F, et al. Depression—an independent predictor of early death in patients with advanced cancer. J Affect Disord 2009;113(1–2):127–32.
39. Pinquart M, Duberstein PR. Depression and cancer mortality: a meta-analysis. Psychol Med 2010;40(11):1797–810.
40. Rudd MD. The assessment and management of suicidality. Sarasota (FL): Professional Resource Press; 2006.
41. Waraich P, Goldner EM, Somers JM, et al. Prevalence and incidence studies of mood disorders: a systematic review of the literature. Can J Psychiatry 2004;49(2):124–38.
42. Mitchell AJ, Chan M, Bhatti H, et al. Prevalence of depression, anxiety, and adjustment disorder in oncological, haematological, and palliative-care settings: a meta-analysis of 94 interview-based studies. Lancet Oncol 2011;12(2):160–74.
43. Kozlov E, Phongtankuel V, Prigerson H, et al. Prevalence, severity, and correlates of symptoms of anxiety and depression at the very end of life. J Pain Symptom Manage 2019;58(1):80–5.
44. Payne A, Barry S, Creedon B, et al. Sensitivity and specificity of a two-question screening tool for depression in a specialist palliative care unit. Palliat Med 2007;21(3):193–8.
45. Mitchell AJ. Are one or two simple questions sufficient to detect depression in cancer and palliative care? A Bayesian meta-analysis. Br J Cancer 2008;98(12):1934–43.
46. Jefford M, Mileshkin L, Richards K, et al. Rapid screening for depression—validation of the Brief Case-Find for Depression (BCD) in medical oncology and palliative care patients. Br J Cancer 2004;91(5):900–6.
47. Kroenke K, Spitzer RL, Williams JB. The PHQ-9: validity of a brief depression severity measure. J Gen Intern Med 2001;16(9):606–13.
48. Zigmond AS, Snaith RP. The hospital anxiety and depression scale. Acta Psychiatr Scand 1983;67(6):361–70.
49. Block SD. Assessing and managing depression in the terminally ill patient. ACP-ASIM end-of-life care consensus panel. American College of Physicians—American Society of Internal Medicine. Ann Intern Med 2000;132(3):209–18.

50. Widera EW, Block SD. Managing grief and depression at the end of life. Am Fam Physician 2012;86(3):259–64.
51. Lyness JM. Unipolar depression in adults: assessment and diagnosis. Waltham, MA: UpToDate Inc; 2016. UpToDate Web site. Available at: https://www-uptodate-com.ucsf.idm.oclc.org. Accessed July 21, 2019.
52. Robinson S, Kissane DW, Brooker J, et al. A systematic review of the demoralization syndrome in individuals with progressive disease and cancer: a decade of research. J Pain Symptom Manage 2015;49(3):595–610.
53. Hudson PL, Schofield P, Kelly B, et al. Responding to desire to die statements from patients with advanced disease: recommendations for health professionals. Palliat Med 2006;20(7):703–10.
54. Onderdonk C, Thornberry K. Psychological aspects of care. In: Sumser B, Leimena ML, Altilio T, editors. Palliative care: a guide for health social workers. New York: Oxford University Press; 2019. p. 71–96.
55. Chochinov HM. Dying, dignity, and new horizons in palliative end-of-life care. CA Cancer J Clin 2006;56(2):84–103 [quiz: 104–5].
56. Simon G. Unipolar major depression in adults: choosing initial treatment. UpToDate; 2019. Available at: www.uptodate.com. Accessed July 22, 2019.
57. Hart SL, Hoyt MA, Diefenbach M, et al. Meta-analysis of efficacy of interventions for elevated depressive symptoms in adults diagnosed with cancer. J Natl Cancer Inst 2012;104(13):990–1004.
58. Okuyama T, Akechi T, Mackenzie L, et al. Psychotherapy for depression among advanced, incurable cancer patients: a systematic review and meta-analysis. Cancer Treat Rev 2017;56:16–27.
59. Kissane DW, Grabsch B, Clarke DM, et al. Supportive-expressive group therapy for women with metastatic breast cancer: survival and psychosocial outcome from a randomized controlled trial. Psychooncology 2007;16(4):277–86.
60. Chochinov HM, Kristjanson LJ, Breitbart W, et al. Effect of dignity therapy on distress and end-of-life experience in terminally ill patients: a randomised controlled trial. Lancet Oncol 2011;12(8):753–62.
61. Breitbart W, Poppito S, Rosenfeld B, et al. Pilot randomized controlled trial of individual meaning-centered psychotherapy for patients with advanced cancer. J Clin Oncol 2012;30(12):1304–9.
62. Kendrick T, Dowrick C, McBride A, et al. Management of depression in UK general practice in relation to scores on depression severity questionnaires: analysis of medical record data. BMJ 2009;338:b750.
63. Lloyd-Williams M, Friedman T, Rudd N. A survey of antidepressant prescribing in the terminally ill. Palliat Med 1999;13(3):243–8.
64. Rayner L, Price A, Evans A, et al. Antidepressants for depression in physically ill people. Cochrane Database Syst Rev 2010;(3):CD007503.
65. Rayner L, Price A, Evans A, et al. Antidepressants for the treatment of depression in palliative care: systematic review and meta-analysis. Palliat Med 2011;25(1):36–51.
66. Ostuzzi G, Matcham F, Dauchy S, et al. Antidepressants for the treatment of depression in people with cancer. Cochrane Database Syst Rev 2018;(4):CD011006.
67. Fairman N, Hirst JM, Irwin SA. Depression and anxiety: assessment and management in hospitalized patients with serious illness. In: Pantilat S, Anderson W, Gonzales M, et al, editors. Hospital-based palliative medicine: a practical, evidence-based approach. Hoboken (NJ): John Wiley & Sons, Inc.; 2015. p. 71–91.

68. Theobald DE, Kirsh KL, Holtsclaw E, et al. An open-label, crossover trial of mirtazapine (15 and 30 mg) in cancer patients with pain and other distressing symptoms. J Pain Symptom Manage 2002;23(5):442–7.

69. Candy M, Jones L, Williams R, et al. Psychostimulants for depression. Cochrane Database Syst Rev 2008;(2):CD006722.

70. Goldman N, Frankenthaler M, Klepacz L. The efficacy of ketamine in the palliative care setting: a comprehensive review of the literature. J Palliat Med 2019;22(9): 1154–61.

71. Administration UFD. FDA news release: FDA approves new nasal spray medication for treatment-resistant depression; available only at a certified doctor's office or clinic. 2019. Available at: https://www.fda.gov/news-events/press-announce ments/fda-approves-new-nasal-spray-medication-treatment-resistant-depression-available-only-certified. Accessed July 20, 2019.

72. Substance Abuse and Mental Health Services Administration. 2017 National survey on drug use and health: detailed tables. Rockland (MD): Center for Behavioral Health Statistics and Quality; 2018.

73. Juurlink DN, Herrmann N, Szalai JP, et al. Medical illness and the risk of suicide in the elderly. Arch Intern Med 2004;164(11):1179–84.

74. Mezuk B, Rock A, Lohman MC, et al. Suicide risk in long-term care facilities: a systematic review. Int J Geriatr Psychiatry 2014;29(12):1198–211.

75. Harwood DM, Hawton K, Hope T, et al. Life problems and physical illness as risk factors for suicide in older people: a descriptive and case-control study. Psychol Med 2006;36(9):1265–74.

76. MacLean J, Kinley DJ, Jacobi F, et al. The relationship between physical conditions and suicidal behavior among those with mood disorders. J Affect Disord 2011;130(1–2):245–50.

77. Kanzler KE, Bryan CJ, McGeary DD, et al. Suicidal ideation and perceived burdensomeness in patients with chronic pain. Pain Pract 2012;12(8):602–9.

78. Rafanelli C, Guidi J, Gostoli S, et al. Subtyping demoralization in the medically ill by cluster analysis. Eur J Psychiatry 2013;27(1):7–17.

79. Rudd MD, Berman AL, Joiner TE, et al. Warning signs for suicide: theory, research, and clinical applications. Suicide Life Threat Behav 2006;36(3):255–62.

80. Substance Abuse and Mental Health Services Administration. SAFE-T: suicide assessment five-step evaluation and triage. In: .Rockland (MD) Substance Abuse and Mental Health Services Administration

Management of Urgent Medical Conditions at the End of Life

Benjamin M. Skoch, DO, MBA*, Christian T. Sinclair, MD[1]

KEYWORDS

- Emergency • End of life • Hospice • Cancer • Seizure • Hypercalcemia • Bleeding

KEY POINTS

- Medical emergencies often alter the prognosis of patients and, therefore, require exploration of the goals of care with the patient and family.
- A thorough assessment and wide differential diagnosis will help clinicians to identify situations where specific interventions may be helpful.
- Education and forming an emergency plan may help to increase the confidence and help patients and families handle difficult situations at home.

INTRODUCTION

Patients cared for by palliative care teams carry diagnoses which significantly impact quality and quantity of life. Palliative care teams are often tasked with identifying when a patient might be dying from complications of their serious illness, identifying goals of care based on this information, and helping to provide goal-concordant care for patients and their loved ones. This article cannot cover all potential emergencies at the end of life, but **Box 1** provides a partial list to highlight the importance of preparation for the most likely emergencies a patient and family may encounter. This article focuses on a few challenging emergencies with unique treatment options for patients at the end of life. Although many affected by hypercalcemia, status epilepticus (SE), hemorrhage, superior vena cava syndrome (SVCS), and spinal cord compression (SCC) carry a primary oncologic diagnosis, these can also be complications of various other diagnoses.

Increasing the difficulty of these situations is the lack of common vocabulary surrounding the end of life and prognostication. Hui and colleagues[1] extensively reviewed the literature in this area, noting that "end of life," "terminally ill," and "actively dying" are sometimes used interchangeably. Additionally, end of life was described as time

Division of Palliative Medicine, University of Kansas Medical Center, Kansas City, KS, USA
[1] Present address: 2330 Shawnee Mission Parkway, Mission, KS 66205.
* Corresponding author. 4000 Cambridge Street, MS 1020, Kansas City, KS 66160.
E-mail address: bskoch@kumc.edu
Twitter: @skochb (B.M.S.); @ctsinclair (C.T.S.)

Med Clin N Am 104 (2020) 525–538
https://doi.org/10.1016/j.mcna.2019.12.006
0025-7125/20/© 2020 Elsevier Inc. All rights reserved.

medical.theclinics.com

Box 1
Partial list of potential medical emergencies at the end of life

Hematologic and oncologic
  Hyperviscosity syndrome
  Neutropenia with fever
  Disseminated intravascular coagulation
  Tumor lysis syndrome
  Hypercoagulable state
  Pathologic bone fractures

Neurologic
  Increased intracranial pressure
  Seizures
  SCC

Gastrointestinal
  Esophageal varices
  Gastrointestinal bleeding
  Small bowel obstruction

Pulmonary
  Airway obstruction
  Symptomatic tachypnea
  Pleural effusion

Metabolic
  Syndrome of inappropriate antidiuretic hormone secretion
  Adrenal insufficiency
  Hypercalcemia
  Hyperglycemia/hypoglycemia
  Severe electrolyte abnormalities (sodium, potassium)

Circulatory
  Pericardial effusion
  Cardiac tamponade
  SVCS
  Stroke
  Symptomatic tachycardia, bradycardia
  Massive hemorrhage
  Hypertensive emergency
  Myocardial infarction
  Sudden cardiac arrest in patient with full code status

Psychiatric
  Suicide attempt
  Delirium
  Combative behavior

Environmental
  Abuse or neglect of patient
  Sudden lack of access to dependent medications (risk of drug withdrawal)
  Disconnection from critical infusions
  Power failure for ventilatory or high O_2 dependent patients
  Power failure for mechanical circulatory assist devices
  Loss of caregiver for fully dependent patient
  Traumatic fall or injury
  Severe burns
  Severe allergic reaction or anaphylaxis

periods as short as days by one source, whereas another offered a duration of years. The National Cancer Institute offers the following regarding end-of-life care for the oncology population: "Care given to people who are near the end of life and have stopped treatment to cure or control their disease . . . includ(ing) physical, emotional, social, and spiritual support for patients and their families."[2] Unless otherwise stated, for the conditions discussed, we presume the patients we describe have a disease that is no longer amenable to life-prolonging therapies, have goals consistent with a comfort focus, and are most likely in the days to week(s) range of time.

Treatment of urgent medical conditions at the end of life often necessitates a confirmation of goals with the patient and/or surrogate decision maker. This article presents options for treatment, but each clinical situation may have variables (eg, location, access to care, and goals) that may impact decision making. For more details on goals of care, please see Nelia Jain and Rachelle E. Bernacki's article, "Goals of Care Conversations in Serious Illness: A Practical Guide," in this issue.

HYPERCALCEMIA OF MALIGNANCY
Evaluation

Hypercalcemia of malignancy (HCM) is a complication commonly encountered by patients with advanced cancer. The number of patients with cancer who experience issues with hypercalcemia nears 30%. Hypercalcemia caused by an underlying malignancy is most often humorally mediated, with parathyroid hormone related peptide causing up to 80% of cases. Although this can occur with any malignancy, most commonly it is related to breast cancer, multiple myeloma, lymphoma, and lung cancer. Less commonly, osteolysis from bony metastases can cause hypercalcemia (about 20% of the time). Calcitriol-secreting lymphomas and ectopic production of parathyroid hormone are each responsible for less than 1% of malignant hypercalcemia.[3] Oft-cited as the syndrome that can cause stones, bones, abdominal moans, and psychiatric groans, HCM can present in myriad ways, with a direct association between the rate of development of elevated calcium levels and symptom severity.[4] Symptoms in these patients can be nonspecific, especially for patients at the end of life, making diagnosis particularly challenging in this population. Generally, in patients who experience mild (10.5–11.9 mg/dL) to moderate (12.0–13.9 mg/dL) hypercalcemia, symptoms include constipation, nausea and vomiting, anorexia, polyuria, and thirst. Severe HCM (>14.0 mg/dL) causes more distressing symptoms, including confusion, coma, neurologic symptoms, and sometimes lethal cardiac arrhythmias (**Box 2**). Since this population may also have low albumin from malnutrition, it is important to adjust the calcium level, because patients with hypoalbuminemia can have elevated serum total calcium, but normal ionized calcium, which is more physiologically relevant. Some patients with severe HCM can develop posterior reversible leukoencephalopathy syndrome, characterized by headaches, seizures, and subcortical edema noted on imaging studies.[5]

Prognostication

It is well-known that patients with HCM generally have poor overall prognoses. It would be reasonable to use a new diagnosis of HCM as a trigger to involve palliative care if not previously used. A median survival of 30 days regardless of treatments used has been suggested.[6] A more recent study specific to gynecologic malignancies suggests that certain risk factors (brain metastasis, >1 site of metastasis, ionized calcium ≥5.9 mg/dL, and serum corrected calcium ≥12.4 mg/dL) portend a shorter prognosis.[7] Initial treatment of HCM may improve some symptoms (polyuria, central

---

Box 2
Hypercalcemia

Signs and symptoms
  Polydipsia
  Polyuria
  Anorexia
  Nausea
  Thirst
  Constipation
  Weakness
  Confusion
  Coma

Common causes
  Breast cancer
  Multiple myeloma
  Lymphoma
  Lung cancer
  Bone metastases
  Total parenteral nutrition
  Adrenal insufficiency
  Thiazide diuretics
  Hyperthyroidism
  Immobility

---

nervous system symptoms, constipation, nausea and vomiting), whereas others (ie, pain) may persist. If a person experiences confusion or delirium that is reversed with treatment of HCM and there is a lack of clarity regarding future directions of care, priority should be given to addressing goals of care focusing on preferences for symptom management, desire for rehospitalization, and possibly even place of death should symptoms recur. Certain populations of patients with cancer, including breast cancer and some hematologic malignancies, may have further anticancer treatment options available to them if HCM resolves, making collaboration with the primary oncology team essential.

Management

Treatment options are often based on the severity of symptoms and the degree of hypercalcemia. With mildly symptomatic hypercalcemia (usually serum corrected calcium <12 mg/dL), reducing offending agents and close monitoring may suffice. For more symptomatic patients or those with serum corrected calcium of greater than 12 mg/dL, core treatments include intravenous (IV) hydration, calcitonin, and bisphosphonates; steroids, hemodialysis, and possibly denosumab may also have roles. A recent study suggests that even patients not receiving antineoplastic therapies should receive a trial of calcium-lowering therapies if consistent with their goals of care, because this treatment may still have a significant impact on lifespan and symptoms.[8] Patients less likely to have a response were those who were previously treated for HCM and of older age. Interspecialty differences (namely, between palliative medicine and oncology) likely exist in physicians' attitudes, beliefs, and reasons for not using these modalities for terminally ill patients with cancer.[9] For patients with advanced untreatable cancer, that is, at the end of life, it may be very reasonable to manage symptomatically without the use of traditional options. Instances where a patient has a very elevated calcium and has become comatose may focus more on reassurance to family members that the patient is restful, along with continuous monitoring.

A trial of IV fluids such as normal saline may be beneficial, but the goal of 200 to 300 mL/h of normal saline will overload patients with renal failure, heart failure, or those that are actively dying. Subcutaneous calcitonin (4 IU/kg every 12 hours) can rapidly lower calcium levels within 6 hours, but after 48 hours, patients develop tachyphylaxis and the efficacy is greatly reduced. Note that nasal calcitonin is not effective in HCM. For patients without renal insufficiency, IV bisphosphonates (pamidronate and zoledronic acid) can reduce hypercalcemia in about 2 to 4 days, and last for a few weeks. Decisions can then be addressed if zoledronic acid should continue on a monthly basis. Denosumab can be considered for patients who are refractory to bisphosphonates or with significant renal impairment.

Comfort medications should be selected based on a patient's constellation of symptoms. Patients with nausea and vomiting in addition to restlessness may benefit from regular low doses of antipsychotics such as haloperidol, benzodiazepines such as lorazepam, or some combination of the 2 agents. Dexamethasone may also be helpful with nausea for select patients. Signs and symptoms of pain should be treated with available opioid medications, bearing in mind these patients likely have some degree of renal failure, so avoidance of morphine may be beneficial. For patients who continue to take oral medications, special attention should be paid to deprescribing medications that may worsen hypercalcemia, including thiazide diuretics, antacids, lithium, calcium containing supplements, vitamin D, and even total parenteral nutrition, which may contain calcium.

STATUS EPILEPTICUS
Evaluation

Status Epilepticus (SE) is broadly defined as a continuous seizure lasting longer than 5 minutes without full neurologic recovery between seizures. The International League Against Epilepsy has proposed a revised definition that includes 2 operational dimensions to consider for treatment and prognostic purposes. The first time point (t1) is the time at which a seizure should be considered an "abnormally prolonged seizure," and is usually regarded as 5 minutes for tonic–clonic seizures. The second time point (t2) indicates the point at which negative long-term consequences can occur, including alteration of neuronal networks, neuronal injury, and neuronal death depending on the seizure type, usually regarded as 30 minutes for tonic–clonic seizures.[10] Theoretically, any type of seizure could evolve into SE. Although easily recognizable when the seizure is characterized by generalized tonic–clonic shaking, more subtle forms can be quite difficult to identify including nonconvulsive SE (NCSE). This distinction can be particularly challenging to make in the hospice or home setting for patients at the end of life where continuous monitoring is not possible. The incidence of SE in the general population is low, occurring in 41 cases per 100,000 people per year. This number is likely higher in the hospice population, although definitive data are lacking. SE is commonly associated with primary brain tumors and cerebral brain metastases but can also have several other etiologies including: intracranial hemorrhage, ischemic stroke, metabolic derangements as a result of organ failure (liver, kidney, lung), neurodevelopmental and neurodegenerative diseases, medication and/or drug withdrawal.

Classification

Further delineation of convulsive SE can help to define which treatment options may be most effective. Premonitory, established, refractory, and super-refractory SE are terms that can be used based on the length of a seizure. Premonitory SE maintains for 5 to 10 minutes. Established SE generally lasts from 10 to 30 minutes. Refractory SE are those seizures that continue despite treatment, lasting between 30 and 60 minutes. Super-refractory SE are those seizures lasting longer than 24 hours despite maximum medical therapy.[11]

NCSE is challenging to diagnose in the end-of-life population, particularly outside of a hospital setting. The only sign that may be clinically present in these patients is altered mentation. Management of these patients overlaps somewhat with convulsive SE, while other aspects may vary as discussed elsewhere in this article.

Prognostication

SE carries a mortality rate of up to 33% for the general population and can be a terminal event for those at the end of life and/or on hospice. The 1-year mortality for treated refractory SE in the elderly population can be as high as 80%. The most influential factor on outcome after SE is the underlying cause or disease. Other determinants of poor outcome after SE include old age, frailty, poor functional status, metastatic cancer, presence of severe comorbidities, and high severity of acute illness.[12] Fewer than one-third of people who experience SE will return to their previous level of functioning, again likely affecting the dying population much more significantly. Multiple tools have been identified to assist clinicians in prognostication after SE. Three tools—the Status Epilepticus Severity Score, the Epidemiology-Based Mortality Score in Status Epilepticus, and the Modified Status Epilepticus Severity Score—can each help predict mortality before hospital discharge. The Encephalitis Nonconvulsive Status Epilepticus Diazepam Resistance Imaging Tracheal Intubation score can help to predict outcome 3 months after hospital discharge.[12] Knowledge of risk factors, natural history, and general prognostic indicators for SE can help to guide advanced care planning discussions between patients, families, and clinicians.

Management

General principles

Although convulsive seizures are startling to observers, most often these events will be self-limiting. Decisions to treat seizures at the end of life should be congruent with patient wishes if known. It is reasonable to monitor patients and provide supportive measures (stabilize, monitor vitals, and, if possible, assess oxygen saturation and blood sugar) during seizures for patients known to have relatively short, recurrent seizures, and even for patients experiencing their first seizure near the end of life. Administration of antiepileptic drugs (AED), especially benzodiazepine medications, can alter mentation for hours or even days in critically ill people, limiting their ability to subsequently participate in goals of care conversations.[11] See **Table 1** for important pharmacologic properties of common AEDs. For patients with a long history of seizures, asking what they value if their seizure frequency increases is important, that is, if sleepiness owing to recurrent seizure medications would be acceptable to help control seizure frequency. Similarly, it can be helpful to identify patient wishes for people at risk of more seizures who lack evidence of recurrent episodes. The evidence is weak for routine prophylactic use of AEDs for people at risk for seizures, though some situations may warrant exploration such as postcraniotomy and malignant melanoma. Newer therapies for adults with refractory seizures are coming, such as the cannabidiol preparation for Dravet and Lennox-Gestaut epilepsy syndromes in the pediatric population, although research is ongoing.

Table 1
Pharmacologic properties of common AEDs

Medication	Half-Life	Available Routes	Dose Adjustments
Cannabidiol	56–61 h	PO	Hepatic
Carbamazepine	25–65 h (initial) 8–22 h (chronic)	PO	Renal
Diazepam	Highly variable but ≥18–24 h	PO, IV, IM, SC, PR	None
Fosphenytoin	8 min (children) 15–30 min (adults)	IV, IM	None
Gabapentin	5 h (children) 5–7 h (adults) 4 h (adult on HD)	PO	Renal
Lamotrigine	Highly variable, but often >24 h	PO, rectal	Hepatic
Levetiracetam	5–8 h	PO, IV, SC, rectal	Renal
Lorazepam	18–73 h (neonatal) 12–18 h	PO, IV, IM, SC, buccal	Renal, Hepatic
Midazolam	6–12 h (neonatal) 2–7 h (children, adults)	PO, IV, nasal, buccal	
Phenobarbital	110 h (children) 79 h (adults)	PO, IV, IM, SC, rectal	Renal
Phenytoin	Variable – usually near 24 h	PO	Obesity
Pregabalin	3–6 h	PO	Renal
Topiramate	Highly variable	PO, rectal	Renal
Valproate	Highly variable	PO, rectal	Hepatic

Not all routes are approved by the US Food and Drug Administration and may be based on limited published data.
Abbreviations: IM, intramuscular; PO, oral; PR, rectal; SC, subcutaneous.

Nonconvulsive status epilepticus

Patients with known NCSE, and likely even those with suspected NCSE given underlying diagnoses and clinical findings, may benefit from a trial of AEDs. The primary benefit of treatment in this population would be to restore communication function. It may be reasonable to withdraw AEDs and life support for patients with NCSE if they seem to be comfortable, are very near the end of life, and this is consistent with patient preferences.[13]

Convulsive status epilepticus

For seizures lasting at least 5 minutes, timely assessment and treatment is critically important. First-line therapy for these seizures is administration of a benzodiazepine because it quickly enters cerebral tissues after administration. Medication, dose, and route are often determined by the patient setting. For patients in the hospital setting with appropriate IV access, a longer acting benzodiazepine such as lorazepam is a reasonable first choice. For patients in a home setting, alternate routes likely need to be considered. Rectal diazepam is often recommended as an initial treatment in this setting, and if the rectal form is not available the IV form can be administered rectally via a syringe. Other options for home use include midazolam via buccal, intranasal, or intramuscular routes, depending on availability.[14] Practically speaking, lorazepam (about 3 weeks) and midazolam (about 8 weeks) for injection can be kept at the bedside at room temperature without risk of degradation or decreased effectiveness.[11]

Seizures that persist despite initial therapy likely need additional AEDs. Although there is good evidence that benzodiazepines are a good first-line option for SE, evidence is lacking to suggest an order of second-line and third-line AEDs that is superior to another.[15] It is important that institutions regularly treating people for SE have access to appropriate algorithms for treatment, with staff trained in how to deliver these treatments. The earlier SE is treated, the more likely it is to achieve seizure cessation. It is imperative to involve family members, loved ones, and patients (as able) in advanced care planning discussions amid the diagnosis of SE. It would be ideal to determine if the patient has a desired location when death occurs, because this knowledge would help to guide discussions of transport to and from home, hospital, and inpatient hospice settings.

HEMORRHAGE
Evaluation

Massive hemorrhage in trauma or postoperative scenarios or in patients with cancer, although relatively uncommon, can be particularly distressing to patients and even more so to their loved ones. Most often occurring in head and neck cancers, hemorrhage can also occur in people who suffer from hematologic malignancies, gastrointestinal tumors, and virtually any tumor that can cause a fungating mass. Significant bleeding may occur in up to 14% of patients with advanced cancer; terminal hemorrhage, or major bleeding from an artery that quickly results in death, has an incidence of 3% to 12%.[16] Other terms often used interchangeably with terminal hemorrhage are catastrophic hemorrhage and major hemorrhage. Definitive diagnosis, regardless of the terminology used, can only be made after a person dies from such an event. Significant bleeds that resolve after packing and pressure which do not result in death are often referred to as sentinel or herald bleeds, and may be a sign of impending larger bleeds. Commonly affected vessels that cause major bleeding at the end of life are the carotid artery, femoral artery, and intrapulmonary arteries.

Prognostication

There are no specific calculators or algorithms to help inform prognosis for patients with cancer at risk for bleeding at the end of life. Some disease-specific research has been published in recent years, with GI stromal tumors as an example.[17] Carotid blowout syndrome, a feared complication of head and neck cancers, has been reported to have a mortality rate of around 50%.[18] Additional research in this area would be invaluable to help guide conversations around end-of-life care for this population. Knowledge of risk factors that increase a person's chance of bleeding from their cancer can help in goals-of-care discussions with at-risk patients and their families. See **Box 3** for risk factors for massive hemorrhage.

Management

Specifically for patients at the end of life, management reviewed here focuses on patients who have exhausted invasive interventions including surgery, radiotherapy, and stenting. Conversations around this topic should proceed delicately, balancing the need to inform patients of the potential threat of bleeding while recognizing that such events may ultimately never occur. Following advanced illness conversation templates can help to determine how much information patients want to know about their situation, how to respond in the face of ambivalence, and how to educate family and caregivers in a way that ensures difficult information has been received and understood. Particular attention should be given to educating patients that major

| Box 3 |
Risk factors for massive hemorrhage
Type of cancer
Size of mass
Visible arterial pulsation
Proximity to major vessels
Presence of fistula
Prior surgery
Prior radiation
Age greater than 50 years
Greater than 10% weight loss
Myelodysplasia
Diabetes
Disseminated intravascular coagulopathy
Atherosclerosis

bleeding is not a painful occurrence, death usually happens quickly in these scenarios, and that any medications used will not expedite the dying process. Discontinuing anticoagulants and continuing antihypertensives (even in normotensive or hypotensive readings) may help to decrease the risk of a massive hemorrhage.

Harris and Noble[16] outlined 3 steps for the management of bleeding at the end of life. First, care should be taken to outline those at risk. Patients identified using the risk factors mentioned elsewhere in this article should be discussed among the interdisciplinary team, including oncologists, surgeons, nursing staff, chaplains, and any caregivers or hospice team that may be involved to ensure a unified approach to patient care. Considering a patient's performance status, perceived quality of life, and likely prognosis helps to guide recommendations moving forward. Second, general supportive measures should be in place should a patient develop bleeding. Someone should always be with patients who have a high likelihood of bleeding, and assurance should be given to patients who develop bleeding that someone is present. Regardless of the setting, patients should rest on a bed with dark linens, and dark towels should be available to apply pressure in the event of external bleeding. This measure will help to camouflage any major bleeding, making the event less distressing for those providing care. Suction should be available to help contain large volumes of blood. To decrease the visual impact of frank blood, consider covering the suction canisters. Specifically, for patients with centrally located lung cancers who develop massive hemoptysis, care should be taken to roll the patient into a lateral position with the affected side down to help control bleeding. Oxygen should be available if the patient is expected to have dyspnea. Last, the availability and use of emergency or crisis medication is suggested. Most often this is in the form of a sedative, although the drug and dose vary by source. Midazolam is often cited as the first-line medication in a dose of 5 to 10 mg given 1 time IV or intramuscularly, with additional doses available every 10 minutes as needed after the first. The usefulness of these medications is debated, especially for those patients who ultimately succumb to bleeding within a few minutes, because the onset of action is likely 10 minutes or more. Some sources reference the use of opioids in addition to sedatives for bleeding patients. These are likely useful for those patients that live longer than minutes who develop significant signs of discomfort or breathlessness. This sequence of events has been cited as the ABCs of terminal hemorrhage, referring to Assurance, Be there, Comfort and Calm.[19]

It is recognized that witnessing someone exsanguinate is extremely traumatic. Providing support to family, loved ones, and even trained caregivers after an episode of terminal hemorrhage is critical. Exploring and acknowledging emotions directly after and referral to grief and bereavement counselors after the event are important steps for ongoing healing. Disposal of soiled linens in colored trash bags can help to limit negative emotions as they relate to the sight of blood. It is also important to recognize that hypervigilance around the possibility of massive hemorrhage can produce significant trauma, and reassurance that hemorrhage is often less likely when blood pressure decreases during the normal dying process.

SUPERIOR VENA CAVA SYNDROME

Obstruction of flow through the superior vena cava from any source can lead to SVCS. Originally described in the 18th century as a complication of syphilitic aortitis, malignancy has become the most common cause of SVCS, causing approximately 85% of all cases. Lung cancers and lymphomas (especially in pediatrics) seem to be the most common causes, although any cancer that could metastasize to the pericaval area could cause SVCS. An increasing number of SVCS cases are thrombosis related, owing to the number of IV devices uses for patient care (central venous catheters, dialysis catheters, port catheters, etc.). Infectious, anatomic, hematologic, endocrinologic, and other iatrogenic sources have also been described.[20]

Patients with SVCS commonly experience facial plethora largely related to mechanical venous congestion of the SVC. As edema worsens, patients may also experience shortness of breath, cough, chest and/or shoulder pain, and possibly hoarseness from laryngeal edema. SVCS is often a slowly developing complication as tumors grow, sometimes taking weeks or months to be better appreciated. As a result of this gradual onset, bodies are physiologically better able to compensate as a result of the development of collateral circulation. When SVCS develops rapidly over the span of days, perhaps more common when due to thrombotic events, truly emergent situations can arise as collateral vessels have not had time to form, causing rapid onset of dyspnea and possibly airway emergencies. This is especially true if this is the initial presentation of a person with malignancy of unknown origin.

Prognosis

There is a paucity of data surrounding prognosis as it relates to SVCS. It has been suggested that less than 10% of patients will survive longer than 2.5 years after treatment of SVCS owing to the advanced nature of their disease.[21] Another indicated that patients who presented with combined malignant airway and superior vena cava obstruction had a worse prognosis, often with survival in terms of weeks to months.[22] For our purposes, the patient population discussed here are those at the end of life, where chemotherapy is felt to be ineffective for a given malignancy. Likely this means the patients we discuss are within days to weeks of death.

Management

Patients who rapidly develop symptoms attributable to SVCS without a known underlying etiology likely require advanced life support, particularly with aggressive or unclear goals of care. Often in this population, intubation and hemodynamic stabilization are required during ongoing workup and goals of care conversations.

Although steroids can be helpful in patients with SVCS, caution should be used in patients with rapid symptom development because this treatment could interfere with obtaining a viable tissue sample. Collaboration with intensivists and oncologists is important.

Care setting may determine which interventions are possible for a patient who is dying with SVCS. Patients in a hospital setting with advanced interventional radiology capabilities may benefit from evaluation for stenting of the SVC, even within weeks of death, which may relieve symptoms of plethora and breathlessness in as few as 24 hours. Some clinicians suggest stenting of the SVC can be used as a first-line treatment for patients with SVCS regardless of etiology, as well as for recurrent SVCS refractory to other treatments.

For patients without interventional capabilities, especially in a hospice setting, symptom control becomes paramount. Positional maneuvers may include elevation of the patient's head and avoiding needle sticks in areas of congestion. Dexamethasone 16 mg IV daily in divided doses can be initiated when SVCS is suspected. Symptom control will likely involve treating dyspnea and pain with opioids and benzodiazepines as appropriate. Particular attention should be given to patients who develops symptoms rapidly while on a comfort plan of care, because small doses of either medication may not alleviate the distress associated with this situation. It may be reasonable in this specific population to consider palliative sedation with a continuous benzodiazepine infusion such as midazolam, particularly if patients develop stridor from airway edema.

SPINAL CORD COMPRESSION
Evaluation

SCC occurs in approximately 5% of patients with cancer, increasing to about 10% of those with known spinal metastases. Originating cancers in adults include lung cancer, breast cancer, prostate cancer, lymphoma, and myeloma, whereas in pediatrics diseases like sarcoma, neuroblastoma, germ cell, and Hodgkin's lymphoma are more common. It is important to consider SCC early in the differential diagnosis of back pain in a patient with cancer, because the signs of lower extremity weakness and bowel and bladder dysfunction are often found later in the course of SCC and may limit the ability to maintain or restore function. Pain is often worse when supine, with percussion tenderness, and worse with cough or Valsalva. Possible band-like distribution with radicular components may also be seen. None of these findings are extremely specific or sensitive. Sites of compression are typically thoracic accounting for more than 70% of all cases. If the lesion is below L1, then typically examination shows no fasciculations and increased reflexes and tone (upper motor neuron). For lesions above L1, the examination may show fasciculations, and decreased reflexes and tone (lower motor neuron). Eighty-five percent of these lesions originate in the vertebral body, so MRI is the best imaging mechanism, and one must consider a scan of the entire spine, because of the variable locations and 35% of patients have multilevel metastases. Functional status, availability of treatment options, stability of the spine, and extraspinal disease status are additional factors to consider.

If the patient does have radiographic evidence of SCC, then many cases should be considered for hospitalization to facilitate urgent multidisciplinary evaluation by oncology, radiation oncology, palliative care, and surgery. Interventional radiologists and physiatrists may also provide unique insight if available. The immediate goal is to determine the urgency of the case, which will inform the prognosis, treatment options, and ultimately the goals of care.

Prognosis

If a patient is nonambulatory after diagnosis and definitive treatment of SCC, the median survival is 1 month. For patients who already have a prognosis in the weeks or less range, careful consideration and goal-focused conversations should be completed before transferring patients to a higher acuity setting. Providing comfort-focused care in a home setting via hospice may be a reasonable option for patients who already had a poor prognosis at the time of diagnosis of SCC.

In more functional patients, with better prognoses, the emergence of SCC often decreases a prognosis to the few to several months range, with more favorable prognoses for the minority of patients who successfully retain or regain function. The rate of change in the symptoms and signs may also be a prognostic factor, with improved functional outcomes seen when patients have slower development of motor deficits before intervention.[23]

If the patient is ambulatory and able to receive therapies for decompression, most people may avoid paralysis. If a patient has developed weakness, decompression may lead to improved function. If the patient already has paralysis from SCC, then the prognosis for walking again is bleak.

Management

The goal of SCC interventions is to decompress the spinal cord to halt further neurologic damage and potentially regain neurologic function. Decompression is achieved through external beam radiation therapy, surgical intervention, or a combination of both. Systemic therapies are unlikely to accomplish decompression without external beam radiation therapy and/or surgery.[24]

A single fraction of 8 Gy may be helpful for those with a shorter prognosis in the weeks to months range. If the prognosis is longer, then more complex radiation therapy regimens may be more appropriate and may involve surgery and/or radiation. For more detail, the American College of Radiology produces evidence-based guidelines on SCC, with a 3-year review cycle.[25] Stereotactic body radiation therapy may be an option at some hospitals, but has limited published evidence and requires more planning. If the patient has prior radiation exposure to the same spinal area, consideration for maximal doses and possible complications should be reviewed with the radiation oncologist.

Dexamethasone may help to decrease spinal cord edema and provide analgesia. Moderate dose strategies (10 mg loading dose, followed by 4 mg 4 times per day, with a 2-week taper) have similar outcomes to high-dose strategies, but with fewer adverse events.[26] There is no evidence for bisphosphonates to improve outcomes in SCC.

Beyond the immediate threat of SCC, the palliative care clinician should make sure to attend to bowel and bladder management, skin breakdown from immobility, and support in coping with this prognosis altering complication.

SUMMARY

A primary challenge facing palliative care teams is determining which patients are indeed in an end-of-life scenario. End of life refers to patients who have a disease that is no longer responsive to life-prolonging therapies, goals of care consistent with a comfort-based approach knowing they are dying from their illness and are likely within days to weeks of death. Some patients with HCM can be treated with known interventions, whereas for others who are near the end of their lives it may be reasonable to consider exclusively symptom control and reassurance. SE can develop from any prolonged seizure, and early recognition is critical for optimal treatment. Benzodiazepines are first-line treatment, and clear plans should be made for patients who do not respond to initial therapies. Terminal hemorrhage most often occurs in patients suffering from head and neck cancers, although it remains a rare occurrence. Care should be taken to balance the patient's and family's need to know about this dreaded complication with the fact that most people do not exsanguinate. SVCS can result from metastases from any malignancy to the pericaval area causing compression and reduced flow. When possible, stenting can provide symptomatic relief for patients, and in those who cannot be stented a combination of steroids and symptom medications can often comfort patients. SCC can be debilitating, particularly if not recognized early. Radiation therapy and/or surgery can often help patients to maintain function with early recognition and treatment, and radiation and steroids can provide symptomatic relief even in patients are have lost function. Regardless of the diagnosis, collaboration with specialists to determine a prognosis for each patient can help patients to identify their own goals of care for the remainder of their lives.

CONFLICT OF INTEREST DISCLOSURE

The authors have no financial conflicts of interest for this article.

REFERENCES

1. Hui D, Nooruddin Z, Didwaniya N, et al. Concepts and definitions for "actively dying," "end of life," "terminally ill," "terminal care," and "transition of care": a systematic review. J Pain Symptom Manage 2014;47(1):77–89.
2. National Cancer Institute. NCI dictionary of cancer terms. Available at: https://www.cancer.gov/publications/dictionaries/cancer-terms/def/end-of-life-care. Accessed August 11, 2019.
3. Stewart AF. Hypercalcemia associated with cancer. N Engl J Med 2005;352: 373–9.
4. Glare P, Griffo Y, Alickaj A, et al. Palliative care emergencies in hospitalized patients. In: Pantilat S, Anderson W, Gonzales M, et al, editors. Hospital-based palliative medicine: a practical, evidence-based approach. 1st edition. Hoboken (NJ): John Wiley & Sons; 2015. p. 171–94.
5. Mirrakhimov AE. Hypercalcemia of malignancy: an update on pathogenesis and management. N Am J Med Sci 2015;7(11):483–93.
6. Ralston SH, Gallacher SJ, Patel U, et al. Cancer-associated hypercalcemia: morbidity and mortality: clinical experience in 126 treated patients. Ann Int Med 1990;112(7):499–504.
7. Cripe JC, Buchanan TR Jr, Wan L, et al. Inpatient management of hypercalcemia portends a poor prognosis among gynecologic oncology patients: a trigger to initiate hospice care? Gynecol Oncol Rep 2019;28:1–5.
8. Mallik S, Mallik G, Macabulos ST, et al. Malignancy associated hypercalcemia-responsiveness to IV bisphosphonates and prognosis in a palliative population. Support Cancer Care 2016;24:1771–7.
9. Mori I, Shimada A, Maeda I, et al. Interspecialty differences in physicians' attitudes, beliefs, and reasons for withdrawing or withholding hypercalcemia treatment in terminally ill patients. J Palliat Med 2016;19(9):979–82.
10. Trinka E, Cock H, Hesdorffer D, et al. A definition and classification of status epilepticus – report of the ILAE task force on classification of status epilepticus. Epilepsia 2015;56:1515–23.

11. Grönheit W, Popkirov S, Wehner T, et al. Practical management of epileptic seizures and status epilepticus in adult palliative care patients. Front Neurol 2018; 9:595.
12. Kalviainen R, Reinikainen M. Management of prolonged epileptic seizures and status epilepticus in palliative care patients. Epilepsy Behav 2019;101:106288.
13. Marks S, Williams A, Peltier W, et al. Treat the patient, not the test when a hospitalized patient in status epilepticus transitions to comfort-focused goals of care. J Palliat Med 2018;21(8):1195–8.
14. Droney J, Hall E. Status epilepticus in a hospice inpatient setting. J Pain Symptom Manage 2008;36(1):97–105.
15. Glauser T, Shinnar S, Gloss D, et al. Evidence-based guideline: treatment of convulsive status epilepticus in children and adults: report of the guideline committee of the American Epilepsy Society. Epilepsy Curr 2016;16(1):48–61.
16. Harris DG, Noble SI. Management of terminal hemorrhage in patients with advanced cancer: a systematic literature review. J Pain Symptom Manage 2009;38(6):913–27.
17. Wan W, Xiong Z, Zeng X, et al. The prognostic value of gastrointestinal bleeding in gastrointestinal stromal tumor: a propensity score matching analysis. Cancer Med 2019;8(9):4149–58.
18. Gahleitner C, Hofauer B, Stock K, et al. Outcome of carotid and subclavian blowout syndrome in patients with pharynx- and larynx carcinoma passing a standardized multidisciplinary treatment. Acta Otolaryngol 2018;138(5):507–12.
19. Ubogagu E, Harris DG. Guideline for the management of terminal haemorrhage in palliative care patients with advanced cancer discharged home for end-of-life care. BMJ Support Palliat Care 2012;2:294–300.
20. Cohen R, Mena D, Carbajal-Mendoza R, et al. Superior vena cava syndrome: a medical emergency? Int J Angiol 2008;17(1):43–6.
21. Higdon M, Higdon J. Treatment of oncologic emergencies. Am Fam Physician 2006;74(11):1873–80.
22. Ren J, Cao C, Fu Y, et al. Double stent insertion for combined malignant airway and superior vena cava obstruction. Medicine (Baltimore) 2019;98(21):e15777.
23. Rades D, Heidenreich F, Karstens JH. Final results of a prospective study of the prognostic value of the time to develop motor deficits before irradiation in metastatic spinal cord compression. Int J Radiat Oncol Biol Phys 2002;53:975–9.
24. Yu JI, Park HC, Ahn YC, et al. Spine metastasis practice patterns among Korean, Chinese, and Japanese radiation oncologists: a multinational online survey study. J Radiat Res 2017;58(1):155–63.
25. Expert Panel on Radiation Oncology-Bone Metastases, Lo SS, Ryu S, Chang EL, et al. ACR appropriateness criteria® metastatic epidural spinal cord compression and recurrent spinal metastasis. J Palliat Med 2015;18(7):573–84.
26. Kumar A, Weber MH, Gokaslan Z, et al. Metastatic spinal cord compression and steroid treatment: a systematic review. Clin Spine Surg 2017;30(4):156–63.

Options of Last Resort
Palliative Sedation, Physician Aid in Dying, and Voluntary Cessation of Eating and Drinking

David A. Gruenewald, MD[a,b,]*, Gregg Vandekieft, MD, MA[c,d,e]

KEYWORDS

- Palliative sedation • Continuous deep sedation • VSED
- Voluntarily stopping eating and drinking • Physician-assisted dying
- Hastened death • Bioethics

KEY POINTS

- Requests for hastened death offer an opportunity to explore reasons underlying the request. Treatments of last resort may provide relief when severe suffering near the end of life persists despite vigorous efforts to mitigate the causes.
- In proportionate palliative sedation (PPS), sedating medication is titrated as needed to control symptoms. PPS for intractable physical symptoms in imminently dying patients is broadly endorsed by health care professional societies.
- Although voluntarily stopping eating and drinking is patient-initiated, extensive caregiver support is required and assistance from health care professionals to assess decisional capacity, plan care, and manage complications is highly recommended.
- Ethical and legal controversies regarding last-resort palliative treatments are best navigated through shared decision-making, with consultation from palliative care, ethics, and mental health specialists.
- Safeguards include determination of refractory suffering, assessment for decisional capacity and mental illness, discussion of alternatives, informed consent, second opinions, institutional policies and procedures, and reporting and review.

[a] Palliative Care and Hospice Service, Geriatrics and Extended Care Service, Veterans Affairs Puget Sound Healthcare System, (S-182-GEC), 1660 South Columbian Way, Seattle, WA 98108, USA; [b] Division of Gerontology and Geriatric Medicine, Department of Medicine, University of Washington School of Medicine, Seattle, WA 98195, USA; [c] Palliative Care Program, Providence St. Joseph Health Southwest Washington Region, Providence St. Peter Hospital, 413 Lilly Road Northeast, Olympia, WA 98506, USA; [d] Palliative Practice Group, Institute for Human Caring at Providence St. Joseph Health, 879 W. 190th St., Suite 1000, Gardena, CA 90248, USA; [e] Department of Family Medicine, University of Washington School of Medicine, Seattle, WA 98195, USA
* Corresponding author. Palliative Care and Hospice Service, Geriatrics and Extended Care Service, Veterans Affairs Puget Sound Healthcare System, (S-182-GEC), 1660 South Columbian Way, Seattle, WA 98108.
E-mail addresses: David.gruenewald@va.gov; dgruen@uw.edu
Twitter: @vandekieftg (G.V.)

Med Clin N Am 104 (2020) 539–560
https://doi.org/10.1016/j.mcna.2020.01.002
0025-7125/20/Published by Elsevier Inc.

medical.theclinics.com

INTRODUCTION

Excellent interdisciplinary palliative care for physical symptoms, and psychosocial, spiritual, and existential concerns, is usually, but not always, able to relieve patient suffering near the end of life. Patients with unrelieved suffering may request provider assistance to hasten death or attempt to hasten their death without provider involvement. Interventions to hasten death should be considered only as a last resort for intolerable suffering despite vigorous attempts to palliate its causes.[1]

In this paper, we discuss 3 potential options of last resort: palliative sedation (PS), voluntarily stopping eating and drinking (VSED), and physician-assisted death (PAD). All share the potential to mitigate suffering at the end of life, but they differ regarding the primary goal and intended outcome of the intervention (symptom relief, allowing natural death, or hastened death), the degree of active physician involvement, ethical and legal status, potential indications, and accessibility for patients not imminently dying.[2] In the following sections, the authors compare PS, VSED, and PAD with regard to these considerations, and suggest best practices. We conclude by outlining safeguards applicable to all 3 interventions to minimize risk of harms associated with their use.

Responding to Severe Suffering Including Requests for Hastened Death

When presented with severe suffering or a request for hastened death, the provider's first responsibility is to understand the underlying causes of suffering (**Box 1**).[3,4] After a concerted effort to identify and remediate potentially treatable causes of suffering, most requests for hastened death abate. For requests that persist despite these efforts, clinicians must clarify exactly what is being requested and explore mutually acceptable alternatives.[2]

These situations are ethically and emotionally challenging; clinicians should explore their own feelings and beliefs about the request and seek support from other health professionals. Second opinions from palliative care, ethics, and/or mental health professionals are highly recommended to ensure clarity in diagnosis and prognosis, optimization of palliative care, and consideration of treatments of last resort, including ethical aspects and pros/cons. After determining which treatment(s) are potentially appropriate, clinicians and patients should ascertain which options are ethically acceptable to the patient, family, and clinician, and their benefits, risks and burdens. Clinicians are not required to act against their principles, but they must not make moral judgments for their patients based on their personal beliefs.[5] It is usually possible to balance integrity and nonabandonment, even if common ground cannot be found on treatments of last resort.

PALLIATIVE SEDATION
Definition

PS has been defined as "the use of sedative medication to relieve intolerable suffering from refractory symptoms by a reduction in patient consciousness."[6] However, there is no consensus regarding indications, target depth of sedation, approach to titration, intermittent versus continuous sedation, or use in patients not imminently dying.[7]

Most guidelines and many commentators distinguish forms of PS based on goals of sedation and whether titration is performed.[7,8] In a classification by Quill and colleagues,[8] the term "ordinary sedation" describes the use of sedatives to relieve common symptoms, such as anxiety without reducing level of consciousness. In proportionate palliative sedation (PPS), sedatives are titrated to relief of suffering in imminently dying patients with refractory physical suffering, and only the minimum

---

Box 1
Recommended initial approach to requests for hastened death

- Ask patient what led them to make this request for hastened death

- Clarify the nature of the request: is the patient merely having thoughts about hastened death, exploring the possibility of pursuing hastened death in the future, or asking for immediate assistance to hasten death?

- Respond with empathy: ask open-ended questions, and make facilitatory comments to encourage the patient to tell their story

- Obtain palliative care and/or hospice consultation as appropriate

- Perform comprehensive assessment; involvement of interdisciplinary care team strongly preferred
  - Physical and psychological symptoms
  - Medical and mental health history and diagnoses
  - Response to previous treatments
  - Patient's understanding of their health condition
  - Patient's expectations for their care
  - Goals of care, advance directives, preferences for life-sustaining treatment
  - Decision-making capacity
  - Identify and document appropriate surrogate decision maker
  - Consider whether mental illness is present; perform suicide risk assessment for active desire to inflict self-harm or kill oneself; consult mental health professional or other qualified health care personnel to assist with suicide risk assessment and management as needed
  - Functional assessment
  - Prognosis, trajectory of illness
  - Social history including support system
  - Spiritual history

- Support the patient by offering your commitment to explore mutually acceptable care options

- Optimize palliative care: identify and make a vigorous attempt to mitigate potentially remediable causes of suffering

- Respond directly to request for hastened death only after completion of comprehensive assessment and intensification of palliative care

Data from Refs.[2–4]

---

sedation needed to relieve symptoms is used. Once symptoms are relieved, no further up-titration occurs. PPS sometimes involves sedation to unconsciousness to relieve symptoms; unconsciousness is considered an unintended but foreseen side effect when lower doses are ineffective in relieving symptoms.

Palliative sedation to unconsciousness (PSU) involves rapidly increasing sedation over minutes to hours to induce unconsciousness as the intended goal. Sedation then remains at that level until the patient dies. PSU may be appropriate for severe, intolerable physical symptoms despite optimal palliative care in imminently dying patients for whom continued consciousness is unacceptable (**Box 2**).[8] Some authors use the term continuous deep sedation (CDS) to describe the use of sedatives to achieve and maintain unconsciousness until death, but in contrast to PSU the process and intent of increasing sedation is generally not specified for CDS.

Ethical and Legal Considerations

PPS is broadly supported by health care professional organizations, including the American Medical Association, American Academy of Hospice and Palliative

---

Box 2
Potential indications for palliative sedation to unconsciousness

Palliative sedation to unconsciousness may be indicated initially if:
- Suffering is intense
- Suffering is definitely refractory
- Death anticipated within hours or a few days
- Anticipated time of death from disease is shorter than time of death from PSU-induced dehydration
- The patient's wish is explicit
- In setting of catastrophic end-of-life event, for example, massive hemorrhage or asphyxia

Adapted from Quill TE, Lo B, Brock DW, et al. Last-resort options for palliative sedation. Ann Intern Med 2009;151(6):421-4; and Cherny NI, Radbruch L, Board of the European Association for Palliative Care. European Association for Palliative Care (EAPC) recommended framework for the use of sedation in palliative care. Palliat Med 2009;23(7):581-93; with permission.

Medicine, National Hospice and Palliative Care Organization, and Hospice and Palliative Nurses Association as a last-resort option for intractable physical suffering at the end of life,[8] but sedation is ethically controversial if pursued with intent to hasten death. The doctrine of double effect (DDE) is often cited as an ethical basis of PS by those who oppose physician participation in hastened death.[9] In determining whether an action is ethical, the DDE distinguishes between what is intended and what is accepted as a foreseen but unintended consequence of the action. According to the DDE, intentionally causing death by PS is wrong but it is acceptable to administer high-dose sedation if the intent is to relieve suffering and not to hasten death.

PS has been distinguished from PAD and euthanasia based on intent (symptom relief versus hastened death), methods (sedatives for symptom relief versus lethal medication doses), and definition of successful outcomes (symptom relief versus death).[10–12] Some practitioners argue that the goal of PS is to relieve suffering and that the patient's death is foreseen but not intended.[8,13] However, with PSU/CDS the intent of the practitioner may not be easily discerned, potentially blurring the distinction between PS and euthanasia.[2] In PPS, practitioner intent may be inferred from actions, such as using the lowest sedative dose needed to control symptoms, and documenting signs and symptoms that justify dose increases.[10]

Some commentators focus the ethical justification for PS more on proportionality and autonomy than intent.[8,10] In PS, risks of hastening death and inducing unconsciousness are justified when other treatments and lower sedative doses are insufficient to control symptoms, and when life expectancy is short. Practitioners must ensure patient autonomy by discussing patients' values and care preferences, benefits and risks of PS, and treatment alternatives, and by documenting informed consent.

Several studies have examined whether PS is associated with hastened death. A Cochrane review comparing effect of sedation versus nonsedation on survival time near end of life found no difference in time from admission or referral to death.[14] A propensity score-weighted analysis of a multicenter prospective cohort study evaluated the effect of CDS on survival of patients with cancer in palliative care settings (n = 1827, 269 on CDS). Controlling for patient characteristics, disease status, and symptom burden at enrollment, median survival was 22 days from enrollment in CDS patients, versus 26 days in non-CDS patients (p = NS, median difference −1 day).[15] Although not definitive, these studies suggest that survival time is not significantly affected when PS is used in patients with prognosis of days to a few weeks.

PS is legal in the United States. In 1997, the US Supreme Court implicitly accepted "terminal sedation" as an alternative to PAD, but terminal sedation was not clearly defined. Justice O'Connor's concurring opinion supported the use of medication to relieve pain and suffering in terminally ill patients, even if it results in unconsciousness or hastened death. Since then, practitioners are cautioned that regardless of the patient's intent, the clinician's intent in using PS must be to relieve intractable suffering and not to hasten death, to minimize risk of breaching ethical and legal boundaries between PS and euthanasia.[8] The potential for unethical or inappropriate use of PS should be minimized by strictly adhering to ethical guidelines (**Box 3**) and a standardized checklist (**Box 4**).

Practice Standards

Despite efforts to standardize clinical practice of PS, marked variability persists. Striking variation is observed in use of PS across hospice and palliative care programs in various countries, ranging from 0% to 66% of deaths. Dosing and target sedation levels are highly variable; in some localities palliative care physicians administer sedatives continuously at the lowest possible doses for comfort,[16] whereas elsewhere PSU/CDS until death is commonly used.[17] Even PS guidelines exhibit marked variation in PS definition, indications, continuation of life-sustaining treatments, timing and prognosis, and medication selection.[18] Cultural differences are important determinants of practice variability, and many differences will likely remain.[18] These findings

---

Box 3
Ethical safeguards to determine the appropriateness of palliative sedation

- Doctrine of double effect: intention to relieve symptoms, not to hasten death

- Autonomy, goal appropriateness
  - Discern the patient's values and care preferences regarding symptom relief, longevity, maximization of alertness, interactivity, physical function, and other concerns
  - Discuss all medically appropriate and legal care alternatives including continuing other palliative interventions
  - Discuss expected benefits and harms of sedation
  - Obtain and document informed consent of patient or proxy decision maker

- Proportionality
  - Establish that death is expected within days to weeks
  - If PSU is planned, document that death is expected within hours to days, or that life-sustaining treatment is being withdrawn and death is expected
  - Establish need to relieve refractory suffering
  - Determine that other methods are unlikely to relieve suffering in anticipated remaining time frame
  - In PPS, proportionality also established by using the lowest dose of sedative that achieves goal of symptom relief
    - Increasing dose is permissible only if lower doses are ineffective
    - Criteria for increasing sedation should be specified (ie, visible signs of distress, such as restlessness, gasping, moaning, brow furrowing)
  - Temporary "respite" sedation (eg, 48 h) may be considered earlier in the dying process while awaiting relief from other interventions

Abbreviations: PPS, proportionate palliative sedation; PSU, palliative sedation to unconsciousness.

Data from Quill TE, Lo B, Brock DW, et al. Last-resort options for palliative sedation. Ann Intern Med 2009;151(6):421-4; and Lo B, Rubenfeld G. Palliative sedation in dying patients: "we turn to it when everything else hasn't worked". JAMA 2005;294(14):1810-6.

Box 4
Checklist: preparing for palliative sedation

- Establish that patient is terminally ill (days to a few weeks at most, unless respite sedation is planned)
  ○ If PSU is planned, establish that patient is imminently dying (hours to a few days)
- Review existing advance directive, documentation of care preferences, POLST or equivalent document
- Discuss and document current patient preferences for life-sustaining treatments, goals of care, treatment alternatives
- Determine that severe suffering is present that cannot be relieved by other means
  ○ Rule out treatable causes of distress, such as urinary retention or constipation
  ○ Ensure that all other reasonable means of controlling symptoms have been tried, and that other therapies are associated with unacceptable morbidity or are unlikely to offer relief within an acceptable timeframe
  ○ Rule out unrecognized depression or other mental health disorders
- Obtain informed consent for PS from patient or proxy, ensuring that PS decision is voluntary
- Seek a consensus decision with patient/surrogate, family, and participating team members
  ○ Discuss with nurse manager, charge nurse (or home care nurse for patients living at home)
  ○ Chaplain, social work, and/or psychologist for psychosocial, family and spiritual assessment and support as needed
  ○ Be explicit about goals, outcomes
  ○ Discuss common concerns and misunderstandings, including distinction from euthanasia, PAD
  ○ Participating team members must have input into sedation decision, opportunity to express concerns and right to opt out if concerns cannot be resolved
- Address nutrition/hydration issues and use of other life-sustaining treatments, such as antibiotics beforehand (these decisions are separate from decision to use PS)
- Ensure that DNR order is in effect
- Consider ethics consultation, especially if
  ○ PSU is planned
  ○ Provider inexperienced in palliative care and hospice
  ○ Patient is not imminently dying
  ○ Primarily existential distress
  ○ Lack of consensus regarding PS or care plan
- Discuss specific patient goals that need to be met before starting sedation, eg, visit from family member, rituals
- Assure peaceful, quiet setting
- Discontinue orders not contributing to comfort (eg, routine vital signs, fingerstick glucose)

Abbreviations: DNR, do not do not resuscitate; PAD, physician aid in dying; POLST, physician orders for life-sustaining treatment; PS, palliative sedation; PSU, palliative sedation to unconsciousness.

Data from Refs.[6,7,10,12]

highlight the need for institutional policies and procedures to standardize local practice.[8,18]

Establishing institutional policy and procedure involves culture change. Stakeholders in administration, providers, nursing, pharmacy, chaplaincy, and others may need PS education and training, including its ethical basis, distinctions between PS, PAD, and euthanasia; and differences between PS and monitored sedation for procedures. Nurses must become familiar with the use and monitoring of sedation in PS, sometimes with just-in-time training or a trained resource nurse. Medication administration policies may need modification to allow nurses to administer sedatives for PS. Pharmacy buy-in is essential, and certain sedatives may be unavailable in some settings because of institutional policy. Communication and coordination with pharmacists, nurses, and other staff covering all shifts and weekends is necessary to address ethical and moral distress concerns that may otherwise go unrecognized. A checklist of suggested best practices is shown in **Box 4**.

Medications

No controlled trials have compared medication efficacy in PS. Commonly used agents include benzodiazepines, barbiturates, propofol, and highly sedating neuroleptics. Opioids and haloperidol may cause significant sedation as a side effect but are not reliably effective for sedation, even at large doses, and are not indicated for PS. However, opioid infusions are commonly maintained at their previous rate: symptomatic treatments must continue alongside sedatives to avoid opioid withdrawal and treat unobserved pain or other symptoms. Opioid boluses are typically discontinued when adequate sedation is achieved.

Suggested initial bolus and infusion regimens are shown in **Table 1**.[12,19] There is no consensus on best monitoring and titration practices, including frequency of reassessment. The most important monitoring parameter is patient comfort, as demonstrated by absence of distress signs, including restlessness, moaning, brow furrowing, gasping, and patients' verbal report. Respiratory rate is monitored primarily to ensure there is no respiratory distress or tachypnea. During PPS, sedatives are titrated to visual evidence of comfort, at intervals typically ranging from hourly to daily depending on symptom severity.[8] When boluses are used, it is safe to re-bolus after the earlier bolus has reached peak effect. Infusion titration is based on medication pharmacokinetics; shorter acting drugs may be titrated more rapidly. If PSU/CDS is needed for severe symptoms, sedative down-titration may cause distress to recur and may be inadvisable. Respirations will gradually deteriorate as death approaches, and a decreasing respiratory rate by itself is not an indication to reduce sedation.[12,20]

VOLUNTARILY STOPPING EATING AND DRINKING

VSED is the deliberate, voluntary choice of a person with decisional capacity and unacceptable suffering due to advanced illness to stop ingesting food and drink with intent to hasten death. VSED is distinct from cessation of *artificial* nutrition and hydration, which involves withdrawal of invasive life-sustaining treatment to allow natural death, and from gradual involuntary reduction in eating and drinking accompanying terminal or advanced illnesses. In VSED, patients must overcome a strong physiologic drive to drink fluids, which may require considerable determination. Unlike other palliative interventions of last resort, VSED does not require clinician participation. Nevertheless, support from knowledgeable clinicians is highly recommended, for assessment of decision-making capacity, psychosocial support, care coordination, and active management of symptoms and complications.

VSED has become more widely recognized as a legitimate last-resort option to relieve suffering near end of life. VSED does not relieve acute symptoms in actively dying patients (for which PS may be a better option), but, unlike PS and PAD, VSED is available to people in any jurisdiction desiring hastened death, including seriously ill patients who are unlikely to die soon.[5,21] Even where legally available, PAD entails procedural hurdles and eligibility requirements, including terminal prognosis that

Table 1
Medications for palliative sedation

Medication	Titration	Usual Starting Dose	Usual Maintenance Dose	Comments
Midazolam	Onset: IV 30–60 s Peak: IV 3–6 min T½: IV 1–3 h	1–5 mg IV/SC bolus, repeat as needed, 0.5–1 mg/h IV/SC If rapid sedation needed, may administer 5–10 mg IV every 5 min up to maximum of 20 mg, eg, for profound agitation or catastrophic terminal event	1–20 mg/h	Most commonly used agent for palliative sedation. Brief duration of action because of rapid redistribution; continuous infusion generally required to maintain a sustained effect. Advantages: rapid onset. Can be administered IV or SC. Synergistic sedative effects when used with opioids and antipsychotics Disadvantages: does not always work for continuous deep sedation; ceiling on CNS depression with benzodiazepines
Lorazepam	Onset: IV 2–3 min Peak: IV 15–30 min T½: IV 12–14 h	2–5 mg bolus IV/SC, 0.5–1.0 mg/h IV/SC	1 mg/h up to usual maximum of 7–10 mg/h	Intermediate-acting, less amenable to rapid titration than midazolam because of its slower pharmacokinetics. Elimination not altered by renal or hepatic dysfunction Advantages: can be administered IV or SC. Compared with midazolam, less interindividual variability in sedation for infusions lasting >24–48 h Disadvantages: does not always work for continuous deep sedation; ceiling on CNS depression with benzodiazepines Propylene glycol (diluent) toxicity may occur at infusion rates >7–10 mg/h

Chlorpromazine	Onset: IV 15 min Peak: IV 2–4 h T½: 6 h	IV or IM 12.5 mg every 4–12 h, or 3–5 mg/h IV, or 25–100 mg every 4–12 h PR	Parenteral (IV or IM) 37.5–150 mg/d, PR 75–300 mg/d.	Advantages: antipsychotic effect for delirious patients. Can be given orally, parenterally, or rectally. Inexpensive. May be beneficial for dyspnea, nausea and vomiting, and pain Adverse effects: orthostatic hypotension, paradoxic agitation, extrapyramidal symptoms, anticholinergic effects. Reduce dose in hepatic failure
Phenobarbital	Onset: IV 5 min Peak: IV 30 min T½: IV 79 h	200 mg bolus IV/SC every 30 min until settled, then 10% of total loading dose every 12 h after that. Note: in midazolam failures, may need >1000 mg total load; may need to dose >200 mg at a time	Varies; typically 10% of loading dose every 12 h once adequate sedation achieved	Long-acting, long half-life. Anticonvulsant. No analgesic effect; continuing opioids is critical for pain patients Advantages: more potent than midazolam for sedation and may be used when midazolam fails to achieve adequate sedation. Useful for patients with severe agitation Disadvantages: cannot be mixed with other medications. Reversal of sedation is difficult. Accumulates with repeated dosing or continuous infusion. Long half-life makes it difficult to titrate upwards to address increased symptoms, or downwards if medication is causing preventable side effects

(continued on next page)

Table 1
(continued)

Medication	Titration	Usual Starting Dose	Usual Maintenance Dose	Comments
Propofol	Onset: 30 s Peak: 90 s	20–50 mg loading dose (may repeat) Initial recommended IV infusion rates vary from 1.2 to 8 µg/kg/min	15–70 µg/kg/min	Relatively expensive. Short acting, frequent dose adjustments may be required. Advantages: quick onset of sedation, ability to rapidly titrate, rapid washout Adverse effects: hypotension, respiratory depression, pain on infusion into small peripheral veins, infusion syndrome with risk of rhabdomyolysis, renal failure, cardiac arrhythmias, cardiac arrest with prolonged administration at higher doses Precautions: staff administering propofol should have training and experience with the drug. Use strict aseptic technique when administering propofol. Change infusion tubing every 12 h. Discard vial and any unused drug if not fully infused after 12 h Non-sedative benefits: antiemetic, antipruritic, and bronchodilation

Abbreviations: CNS, central nervous system; IM, intramuscular; IV, intravenous; PR, per rectum; SC, subcutaneous; T½, half-life.

Data from Cherny NI, Radbruch L, Board of the European Association for Palliative Care. European Association for Palliative Care (EAPC) recommended framework for the use of sedation in palliative care. Palliat Med 2009;23(7):581-593; and Bodnar J. A review of agents for palliative sedation/continuous deep sedation: pharmacology and practical applications. J Pain Palliat Care Pharmacother 2017;31(1):16-37.

many people with advanced illnesses cannot meet. Similarly, PS requires a prognosis of weeks or less and is available only to patients with severe symptoms.

Nevertheless, patients wishing to VSED may encounter barriers to clinician support, including moral or ethical objections, regulatory or legal concerns, and unwillingness of hospice agencies to enroll patients not yet terminally ill until several days after initiating VSED.[22] Residents of long-term care (LTC) facilities who want to VSED may find that VSED is not permitted at their facility. Administrators and clinical leaders may fear that cooperating with VSED requests could lead to abuse and neglect accusations, survey citations, or trigger mandatory reporting of suicidal intent. Understandably, resident safety and protecting vulnerable adults from harm are key priorities for LTC facilities. In responding to VSED requests, LTC facility administrators and clinical leaders can honor residents' right to self-determination while minimizing risk of harm by following sound processes of resident-centered care planning and delivery.[22]

Ethical and Legal Considerations

VSED remains ethically controversial. No consensus exists on how to distinguish morally and legally acceptable acts that hasten dying (eg, honoring requests to forego life-sustaining treatment, including artificial nutrition and hydration) from other acts that hasten death (eg, VSED, PAD).[23] Some commentators believe that VSED devalues the lives of people with disabilities and implicitly suggests that their lives are less valuable or even expendable,[23] and that, at least in some cases, patients who choose VSED are committing suicide. They believe that if a physician mentions VSED to patients as an acceptable option to address refractory end-of-life suffering, it is tantamount to collaboration in suicide and therefore morally wrong.[24]

Others believe that in some circumstances it is morally acceptable to permit people with decision-making capacity to hasten their death to avoid a greater harm of continuing to live with unmitigated suffering.[25] In this view, the ethical foundation supporting VSED rests on the voluntariness of the VSED decision, the persistence and determination required to VSED, and the reversibility of the decision while patients retain decisional capacity. These experts believe that physicians must provide necessary care and support during VSED, and that this neither implies endorsement of VSED nor that the patient's life is not worth living.[5,25]

One proposed way to reconcile ethical concerns about a patient's VSED decision is to determine whether it is a tragic choice born of impulsiveness or feelings of despair and abandonment (suggesting suicidal ideation), or whether it is a thoughtful and carefully considered decision to choose death when the alternative is unacceptably prolonged dying and intractable suffering.[5]

In a survey of hospice workers in Oregon, where PAD is legal, most participants perceived VSED as a natural process of "letting go of life," rather than a more active process of hastening death.[26] Most felt that VSED should be available to relieve end-of-life suffering, and would consider VSED themselves if they became terminally ill.[27] It is unknown whether hospice and other health care workers in locations where PAD is illegal hold similar views about the acceptability of VSED.

The legal status of VSED in the United States has only recently begun to be determined in US jurisdictions due to a paucity of court cases and legislative guidance. Several lower court cases ruled in favor of a patient's right to hasten death by VSED, but the matter has been not been adjudicated by a higher US court. In 2018 the Hawaii legislature recognized the legality of VSED, and the Supreme Court of British Columbia upheld a common law right of adults to refuse consent to oral nutrition and hydration. It has been noted that, based on shared common law principles and history, the decision in British Columbia has persuasive legal force in the United States.[21]

Absent explicit legal approval, the rationale for a right to VSED is based on the established right of patients to refuse life-sustaining treatments. Clinicians may not force feed patients or place a feeding tube without permission. In addition, legal scholars distinguish between active clinician involvement in processes that hasten death, for example, PAD or euthanasia, and passive acts of refusal that result in death, such as VSED.[21] Increasingly, professional health care organizations recognize the right of patients with decisional capacity near the end of life to choose VSED to hasten death, including the American Nurses Association, the International Association of Hospice and Palliative Care, and the American Academy of Hospice and Palliative Medicine.[28–30]

Still unresolved is the matter of "stopping eating and drinking (SED) by advance directive." Many people worry more about living mentally incapacitated for years with advanced dementia than about dying and death. Some people with early-stage dementia who retain decision-making capacity choose to die by VSED while still capable of doing so, but they may sacrifice years of high-quality life.[31] To address this dilemma, advance directives have been developed specifying circumstances under which a patient without decisional capacity would not want assistance with oral nutrition and hydration.[31–33] The feasibility and acceptability of these directives, and their legal status, remain to be determined.

Epidemiology and Patient Characteristics

The few studies examining how commonly VSED occurs are based on recollections of health professionals or informal caregivers.[34–36] In a survey of hospice nurses in Oregon, VSED was reported nearly twice as commonly as a cause of death than PAD.[34] In the Netherlands, population-based studies estimate that 0.4% to 2.1% of decedents chose VSED. A random national sample of 708 Dutch family physicians found that 46% had experience with VSED patients, 9% in the past year.[35–37] Most people choosing VSED are over 80 years of age, functionally dependent for daily care, and have a short life expectancy.[34,35] Common motivations for VSED include readiness to die, belief that continuing to live is pointless, poor quality of life, and desire to control the circumstances of death.[34]

Clinical Evaluation and Management

VSED requests are an opportunity for clinicians to explore and mitigate underlying causes of suffering (see **Box 1**). When a patient persistently intends to VSED after robust evaluation and attempts to mitigate suffering, clinicians must perform a comprehensive assessment and (if appropriate) prepare for VSED (**Box 5**).

During the initial phase of VSED, there may be opportunities for meaning making, reminiscence, reflection, and saying goodbye to loved ones. Patients may choose at any time to resume drinking and eating, but with continued abstinence, dehydration usually leads to death within 10 to 14 days.[11,34,35] Patients and caregivers must be told that ingesting even small amounts of fluids will significantly prolong the dying process. Survival time and intensity and duration of symptoms vary depending on nutritional and hydration status, underlying disease, and level of debility.

Patients who VSED usually experience a peaceful course characterized by progressive weakness and somnolence over days to weeks, eventually lapsing into coma before death.[38,39] However, some patients experience worsening suffering before death, difficult-to-manage thirst, and agitated delirium requiring intensive management.[25] In the Oregon hospice nurse survey, participants reported high overall quality of death by VSED in most cases. However, 8 out of 102 nurses felt their patients had bad deaths; these patients tended to be younger and in more pain

Box 5
Checklist of steps in evaluating patients requesting VSED and preparing for initiation of VSED

A. Patient evaluation
  - Before discussing details of VSED, perform initial assessment and management of requests for hastened death (see **Box 1**)
  - Assess decision-making capacity, rule out influence of mental illness, and rule out coercion to ensure voluntariness
  - Discuss all legally available treatment options appropriate to the patient's condition and goals, including potential benefits, risks, and burdens
  - Assess social supports available to the patient during VSED
  - Determine whether VSED is appropriate and consistent with goals and values. Factors suggesting appropriateness include:
    ○ Presence of terminal or severely debilitating illness
    ○ Presence of suffering refractory to excellent palliative care
    ○ Patient has decision-making capacity
    ○ Patient has determination and sufficient resolve to resist drinking despite thirst
    ○ Decision to VSED is voluntary and unaffected by mental health issues
    ○ Decision to VSED is consistent with longstanding values
    ○ Strong support from family or other informal caregivers for the duration of VSED process, or a willingness to VSED in an inpatient hospice or other health care facility that is able to support the practice
    ○ Surrogate decision maker is available and supportive of patient's decision to VSED
  - Obtain palliative care consultation; consider ethics, mental health, or other consultations when appropriateness of VSED is in doubt
  - Discuss whether you are personally willing to support the patient if VSED is chosen; if not, offer referral to another clinician

B. Preparing for initiation of VSED
  - Obtain and document informed consent to VSED
  - Ensure DNR/DNI order and formal designation of surrogate decision maker are in place
  - Update POLST form or equivalent document
  - Determine the setting where VSED will occur
  - Refer to hospice for interdisciplinary support if hospice not already involved
  - Provide education to patient, family/informal caregivers, and formal caregivers regarding VSED process and what to expect. Counsel that considerable support is needed from caregivers for duration of the process. Ensure patient understands that determination and perseverance is needed to carry out VSED in face of strong thirst, and that even small amounts of fluid intake will prolong the dying process
  - Discuss with patient, surrogate decision maker, caregivers, and care team how patient requests to resume eating and drinking are to be handled, particularly if delirium is present. Also discuss that some patients change their minds after starting VSED; the capacitated patient's decision to resume eating and drinking must be respected
  - Review care plan with all involved parties, discuss and attempt to resolve disagreements and concerns
  - Develop a plan to manage common symptoms during VSED and write appropriate orders
  - In anticipation of the loss of ability to take oral medications, identify alternative routes of administration for essential comfort medications, or alternative medications, that may be given subcutaneously, intramuscularly, transdermally, sublingually, buccally, intranasally, or rectally
  - Discuss whether palliative sedation, possibly with inpatient hospice admission, will be initiated in event of severe agitated delirium

Abbreviations: DNR/DNI, do not resuscitate/do not intubate; POLST, physician orders for life-sustaining treatment; VSED, voluntarily stopping eating and drinking.

Adapted from Gruenewald DA. Voluntarily stopping eating and drinking: a practical approach for long-term care facilities. J Palliat Med 2018;21(9):1214-20; and Wax JW, An AW, Kosier N, et al. Voluntary stopping eating and drinking. J Am Geriatr Soc 2018;66(3):441-5; with permission.

than patients with good deaths.[34] In the Dutch family physician survey, 80% felt the death went according to the patient's plans, and 42% had no symptoms in the last 3 days of life.[35]

Some patients abandon VSED after experiencing severe thirst, and some make more than one attempt. If the patient opts not to continue VSED, family and caregivers must support the patient's decision to resume eating and drinking. Patients may become delirious later in VSED and request fluids. It is a dilemma for family and caregivers to know how to respond, not wanting to worsen distress by withholding requested fluids but also wanting to honor the previous VSED request. Providers must discuss and document in advance how requests for fluids should be handled if the patient becomes delirious and incapable of decision-making. Strategies include reminding patients of their previous request together with aggressive oral care, distraction, and renewed attention to comfort. It may help caregivers to review written documentation of the patient's wishes. Patients must understand that caregivers cannot be required to enforce a "Ulysses contract" to withhold fluids no matter how strenuously the delirious patient requests them. Instead, patients have the option to VSED later if still desired.[22]

Symptom management suggestions are outlined in **Table 2**.[40,41] The most common symptoms during VSED are thirst and dry mouth. Anecdotally, it may be more comfortable to discontinue food intake 1 to 3 weeks before stopping fluids, depending on the patient's initial strength. Alternative routes of medication administration must be planned as patients lose the ability to swallow, and to minimize fluid intake.[40,41]

PHYSICIAN-ASSISTED DEATH

PAD is the practice of prescribing a competent, terminally ill patient a potentially lethal dose of medication, on the patient's request, that the patient intends to later ingest to hasten death. Disagreement persists regarding the terminology for this practice. We use the term PAD, and physician aid in dying is also widely used. Some prefer the term physician-assisted suicide (PAS) as a matter of linguistic precision since the individual *is* taking medication with intent to end their life. Critics argue that the term PAD equally applies to standard palliative care intended to ease the dying process without hastening death. Many PAD opponents consciously wish to link the practice with the negative connotations associated with suicide. Medical assistance in dying is an increasingly common term, particularly following passage of laws allowing PAD in California and Canada. The terminology distinction is further complicated in Canada and some European jurisdictions where both PAD as defined above and voluntary euthanasia administered by a physician or nurse practitioner are legal options.

Ethical and Legal Considerations

Ethical deliberations around PAD generally focus on the principle of autonomy to justify the practice, arguing that if a fully informed patient desires PAD and willing clinicians are available to support them through it, prohibitions infringe on their right of self-determination. Opponents note that autonomy has limits and is primarily a right to refuse unwanted treatments rather than demand therapies that are clinically futile or fall outside accepted clinical practice standards. Both proponents and opponents of legalized PAD invoke the principles of beneficence and nonmaleficence but diverge on how to interpret the duties to do good and avoid harm, respectively, when working with patients wishing to ease their death or avoid suffering via PAD.

Oregon became the first US jurisdiction to legalize PAD with the 1994 passage of the Oregon Death with Dignity Act. PAD did not take effect in Oregon until 1997 due to legal challenges, including an unsuccessful follow-up referendum to overturn the law. The first patient to use the law did so in 1998. Seven additional states and the District of Columbia have enacted similar laws (**Box 6**). Two PAD cases reached the US Supreme Court, which neither affirmed nor denied PAD as a constitutional right, instead deferring to "the laboratory of the states." The Supreme Court of Canada's

Table 2
Management of common symptoms during VSED

Thirst and Dry Mouth	Scrupulous attention to oral care; frequent use of moistened sponge sticks; atomized water spray; lip balm; artificial saliva spray, gel or solution; lubricating xylitol discs (XyliMelts); saliva stimulants, such as sugar-free candy or gum if able to suck or chew
Hunger	Well tolerated; no specific intervention generally needed
Dysuria	Opioids, bladder catheterization until anuric
Urinary incontinence	Bedside commode or bedpan may be helpful to facilitate urination. Incontinence briefs or either condom or indwelling catheter may be needed later
Pain	Analgesics previously in use for pain management should be continued but plans should be made for changing route of administration or substituting another medication as patient becomes unable to swallow Medication selection depends on underlying condition and severity and type of pain Options to consider when oral intake is no longer possible include: • Acetaminophen suppositories 650 mg PR every 4 h as needed for pain (or fever) • Diclofenac gel • Opioids: dosing adjusted based on previous use; laxatives should be initiated together with opioids (accumulation may occur as renal failure develops; consider dose reduction or less frequent administration as indicated): • Morphine concentrated elixir 20 mg/mL, 5 mg buccal every 4 h as needed, or morphine 2 mg SC every 4 h as needed (caution: if used regularly, glucuronidated metabolites may accumulate and cause neurotoxicity as renal failure develops) • Hydromorphone 0.5 mg SC every 4 h as needed • Oxycodone sustained release 10 mg PR every 12 h • Fentanyl transdermal patch (only in patients previously taking 60 mg oral morphine equivalents daily or more)
Nausea, vomiting	Identify and treat remediable underlying contributors (eg, constipation) Useful medications include: • Haloperidol solution 0.5–2 mg buccal every 4 h as needed (off-label) • Metoclopramide 10 mg SC every 6 h as needed (off-label; reduce dose by 50% in renal failure) Avoid dexamethasone, which may stimulate appetite
Fatigue and weakness	Provide progressive assistance with activities of daily living as needed
Constipation	Bisacodyl suppositories, phosphate enema, or digital removal of stool if impacted; avoid bulking agents, such as psyllium (may cause psyllium impaction, requires fluid intake) and polyethylene glycol (requires fluid intake)

(continued on next page)

Table 2 (*continued*)	
Delirium, confusion, restlessness, anxiety	In all cases, assess for uncontrolled symptoms (eg, pain, dyspnea, nausea), rule out urinary retention and constipation, consider medication adverse effects and withdrawal symptoms (eg, alcohol, nicotine, SSRI, opioids, benzodiazepines)
	For mild to moderate symptoms of confusion and anxiety: redirection, reorientation, natural light, reassurance, attention to comfort, put glasses and hearing aids on patient, use night light, avoid environmental over-stimulation. Continuous presence of a reassuring primary caregiver at the bedside is often very helpful
	For severe anxiety:
	• Lorazepam 1 mg SC (or 1 mg concentrated solution buccal) every 30 min until settled, then every 8 h (note: SC and buccal use not recommended by manufacturer but are reasonable alternatives in palliative care settings)
	For severe agitated delirium:
	• Haloperidol lactate 1 mg SC or IM every 30 min until settled, then every 8–12 h (note: SC use not recommended by manufacturer but commonly done in palliative care settings)
	If approved in advance by patient, use proportionate palliative sedation (often with inpatient hospice admission) if needed as a last resort (see **Table 1**)

Abbreviations: IM, intramuscular; PR, per rectum; SC, subcutaneous; VSED, voluntarily stopping eating and drinking.

Adapted from Wax JW, An AW, Kosier N, et al. Voluntary stopping eating and drinking. J Am Geriatr Soc 2018;66(3):441-445; and KNMG Royal Dutch Medical Association and V&VN Dutch Nurses' Association. Caring for people who consciously choose not to eat and drink so as to hasten the end of life. Available at: https://www.knmg.nl/web/file?uuid=1519ee45-2447-46a2-9cda-ec59d441 f8a8&owner=5c945405-d6ca-4deb-aa16-7af2088aa173&contentid=3658. Accessed Aug 10 2019; with permission.

Carter Decision ruled that laws prohibiting PAD were unconstitutional, after which Parliament created a legal framework regulating the practice.

US statutes allowing PAD, mostly modeled after Oregon's pioneering law, have similar requirements (**Box 7**). None allow euthanasia, and all have safeguards intended

---

Box 6
States with legalized physician-assisted death

Approved by voter referendum
• Oregon: 1994
• Washington: 2008
• Colorado: 2016

Approved by legislative action
• Vermont: 2013
• California: 2015
• Washington, DC: 2016
• Hawaii: 2018
• New Jersey: 2019
• Maine: 2019

Judicial decision
• Montana: 2009 (State Supreme Court ruled laws prohibiting PAD are unconstitutional, but no regulatory framework has been established)

Adapted from Nowels D, VandeKieft G, Ballentine JM. Curbside Consultation: Medical Aid in Dying. Am Fam Physician 2018;97(5):341-343; with permission.

Box 7
Common provisions of US statutes legalizing physician-assisted death

Patients
- Must be at least 18 years
- Must demonstrate residence in jurisdiction where request is made
- Must be capable of making and communicating their own health care decisions
- Must have a terminal diagnosis expected to cause death in 6 months or less

Physicians
- Must have license in the jurisdiction
- Must diagnose the patient with a terminal illness with a prognosis of 6 months or less
- A consulting physician must confirm the terminal diagnosis and prognosis, and that the patient has capacity to make the decision
- A referral to a mental health specialist must be made if either physician is unsure whether the patient has capacity to make this informed decision
- Must counsel the patient on various items, and inform the patient of alternatives, including palliative care, hospice, and others based on jurisdictional statutes

Patient request timelines
- Two oral requests at least 15 days apart
- Witnessed written request; timing and details vary among jurisdictions

Other
- All jurisdictions prohibit use of the law from impacting the patient's health or life insurance (ie, patients cannot lose coverage and benefits cannot be denied as a result of their decision)
- The terminal illness, not suicide, is listed as the cause of death on the death certificate
- No health care professional is obligated to participate

Adapted from Nowels D, VandeKieft G, Ballentine JM. Curbside Consultation: Medical Aid in Dying. Am Fam Physician 2018;97(5):341-343; with permission.

---

to assure that PAD is available only for patients with limited life expectancy, who have received excellent hospice and/or palliative care, and whose judgment is unimpaired by untreated mental illness, particularly depression.

Professional Considerations

Professional societies have deliberated whether to adopt policies or positions of support, opposition, or neutrality. The American Medical Association, American College of Physicians, and American Nurses Association all recently reaffirmed their opposition to laws allowing PAD. The American Academy of Hospice and Palliative Medicine maintains a neutral stance, and the American Academy of Family Physicians recently adopted a position of neutrality. The International Association for Hospice and Palliative Care believes that legalization of euthanasia or PAS should not be considered until universal access to palliative care services is assured.[42] Supporters of an organizational stance of neutrality argue that this approach is neither pro nor con, welcomes members along the full pro/con continuum, and is not passive since it encourages robust personal reflection and in-depth patient engagement to assure PAD is not pursued without first understanding the origins of the request and that it does not bypass comprehensive palliative care.[43] PAD opponents argue that "neutrality is not neutral," reasoning that adopting a neutral position is effectively "declaring a policy no longer morally unacceptable; the political effect is to give it a green light."[44] Opponents believe that a professional society's position on an issue so core to medicine's fiduciary responsibility to patients fundamentally affects how physicians view their obligations to patients and how the public views the profession. From this perspective, they argue, the profession's self-identity and image are compromised by any position other than formal opposition.

Practical Considerations

A survey of terminally ill Oregonians found that about 1 in 200 who considered PAD ultimately followed through with it, and about 1 in 25 who discussed PAD with a health care professional followed through.[45] Although these findings may not be generalizable, many patients who inquire about PAD will not follow through. Accordingly, all clinicians who may be asked about PAD need training to skillfully respond to these inquiries (see **Box 1**).

Oregon and Washington have robust data regarding PAD, publicly reported each year since their PAD laws took effect.[46,47] Typically, around 0.5% of all deaths in those states occur by PAD. Compared with the general population, those utilizing PAD are more likely to be Caucasian and have a higher level of education. Most are ≥65 years and 85% to 90% are enrolled in a hospice. These data identify common concerns that led patients to choose PAD (**Box 8**).

In 2012, a multidisciplinary panel established clinical practice guidelines for physicians participating in PAD.[48] Basic clinical competencies include knowledge and communication skills to sensitively respond to PAD inquiries, including exploration of concerns precipitating the request; the ability to assess decisional capacity and assess understanding of alternatives to PAD and symptomatic treatments along with hastened death; and knowledge and skills to respond to other issues that arise. Communication strategies regarding PAD have been previously outlined (see **Box 1**). Drugs used for PAD vary by location and rapid price increases have made some agents too expensive for most individuals, so new "cocktails" have evolved. This article does not discuss specific medications for PAD, but instead directs interested readers to PAD advocacy groups offering training or referrals to participating physicians.

Support groups for patients and families wishing to pursue PAD recommend initiating requests early enough to assure that the process, which frequently takes longer than the 2-week "waiting period" due to challenges identifying participating physicians and pharmacies, can be completed before patients lose the ability to self-administer the drug. They also advise waiting until shortly before the planned ingestion to pick up the prescription, to prevent family from having a large amount of unused lethal medication at home if patients become incapable of self-administration or elect to forego PAD. Oregon and Washington data indicate that about one-third of patients given a prescription for PAD never take the drug.

Box 8
Common end-of-life concerns for patients electing PAD

- Losing autonomy
- Less able to engage in activities making life enjoyable
- Loss of dignity
- Losing control of bodily functions
- Burden on family, friends/caregivers
- Inadequate pain control, or concern about it
- Financial implications of treatment

Box 9
Safeguards to minimize risk of harm for patients requesting palliative treatments of last resort

- Listen carefully to understand patient's suffering and reasons for the request
- Determine that the cause of suffering is accurately understood and not clouded by mental illness
- Ensure that the health care team, patient, and family have a clear understanding of the disease and prognosis
- Establish that suffering is refractory to excellent palliative care
- Assess decision-making capacity
- Consider your own values and legal limits, and search for treatment alternatives that are acceptable to both the patient and you
- Inform patients about all legally available treatment options
- Obtain an independent second opinion from a palliative care specialist, ethicist, and/or mental health consultant, especially if patient is not likely to die soon, there are concerns about capacity or mental illness, or there is lack of consensus
- Obtain informed consent
- Establish institutional policies and procedures for each palliative option of last resort, along with routine documentation, reporting, and review

Data from Quill TE, Lo B, Brock DW. Palliative options of last resort: a comparison of voluntarily stopping eating and drinking, terminal sedation, physician-assisted suicide, and voluntary active euthanasia. JAMA 1997;278(23):2099-104.

SUMMARY

Several practice recommendations apply for all last-resort options to relieve end-of-life suffering (see **Box 1**; **Box 9**). These include safeguards to ensure that when treatments of last resort are considered, patients are protected from clinical errors, abuse, and coercion (see **Box 9**).[2] The goal of practitioners considering these interventions should be to respond to a wide range of intractable patient suffering near end of life,[11] while attempting to balance nonabandonment and personal integrity. Individuals requesting PAD are vulnerable due to their underlying illness and the potential to trigger judgment or opprobrium if the physician is morally opposed to PAD, necessitating a high level of trust and/or courage to make the inquiry. This context creates opportunities for profound conversations and enhanced depth in the therapeutic relationship if the clinician has the courage, skills, and openness to explore the request with the patient, whether the physician supports and participates in PAD or not.

DISCLOSURE

The authors have nothing to disclose. This work was supported in part by the Department of Veterans Affairs. The views expressed herein are those of the authors and do not necessarily reflect the views of Providence Health and Services, the Department of Veterans Affairs, or the US Government.

REFERENCES

1. Quill TE, Lee BC, Nunn S, et al. Palliative treatments of last resort: choosing the least harmful alternative. Ann Intern Med 2000;132:488–93.

2. Quill TE, Lo B, Brock DW. Palliative options of last resort: a comparison of voluntarily stopping eating and drinking, terminal sedation, physician-assisted suicide, and voluntary active euthanasia. JAMA 1997;278:2099–104.

3. Quill TE. Doctor, I want to die. Will you help me? JAMA 1993;270:870–3.

4. Block SD, Billings JA. Patient requests to hasten death: evaluation and management in terminal care. Arch Intern Med 1994;154:2039–47.

5. Schwarz J. Exploring the option of voluntarily stopping eating and drinking within the context of a suffering patient's request for a hastened death. J Palliat Med 2007;10:1288–97.

6. de Graeff A, Dean M. Palliative sedation therapy in the last weeks of life: a literature review and recommendations for standards. J Palliat Med 2007;10:67–85.

7. Schildmann E, Schildmann J. Palliative sedation therapy: a systematic literature review and critical appraisal of available guidance on indication and decision making. J Palliat Med 2014;17:601–11.

8. Quill TE, Lo B, Brock DW, et al. Last-resort options for palliative sedation. Ann Intern Med 2009;151:421–4.

9. Quill TE, Dresser R, Brock DW. The rule of double effect—a critique of its role in end-of-life decision making. N Engl J Med 1997;337:1768–71.

10. Lo B, Rubenfeld G. Palliative sedation in dying patients: "we turn to it when everything else hasn't worked". JAMA 2005;294:1810–6.

11. Quill TE, Byock IR. Responding to intractable terminal suffering: the role of terminal sedation and voluntary refusal of food and fluids. ACP-ASIM End-of-Life Care Consensus Panel. Ann Intern Med 2000;132:408–14.

12. Cherny NI, Radbruch L. European Association for Palliative Care (EAPC) recommended framework for the use of sedation in palliative care. Palliat Med 2009;23:581–93.

13. Truog RD, Berde CB, Mitchell C, et al. Barbiturates in the care of the terminally ill. N Engl J Med 1992;327:1678–82.

14. Beller EM, van Driel ML, McGregor L, et al. Palliative pharmacological sedation for terminally ill adults. Cochrane Database Syst Rev 2015;(1):CD010206.

15. Maeda I, Morita T, Yamaguchi T, et al. Effect of continuous deep sedation on survival in patients with advanced cancer (J-Proval): a propensity score-weighted analysis of a prospective cohort study. Lancet Oncol 2016;17:115–22.

16. Vivat B, Bemand-Qureshi L, Harrington J, et al. Palliative care specialists in hospice and hospital/community teams predominantly use low doses of sedative medication at the end of life for patient comfort rather than sedation. Palliat Med 2019;33:578–88.

17. Miccinesi G, Rietjens JAC, Deliens L, et al. Continuous deep sedation: physicians' experiences in six European countries. J Pain Symptom Manage 2006;31:122–9.

18. Gurschick L, Mayer DK, Hanson LC. Palliative sedation: an analysis of international guidelines and position statements. Am J Hosp Palliat Care 2015;32:660–71.

19. Bodnar J. A review of agents for palliative sedation/continuous deep sedation: pharmacology and practical applications. J Pain Palliat Care Pharmacother 2017;31:16–37.

20. Schildmann EK, Schildmann J, Kiesewetter I. Medication and monitoring in palliative sedation therapy: a systematic review and quality assessment of published guidelines. J Pain Symptom Manage 2015;49:734–46.

21. Pope TM. Voluntarily stopping eating and drinking is legal—and ethical—for terminally ill patients looking to hasten death. Huntington, NY: ASCO Post;

2018. Available at: http://www.ascopost.com/issues/june-25-2018/voluntarily-stopping-eating-and-drinking-is-legal-and-ethical/. Accessed August 8, 2019.

22. Gruenewald DA. Voluntarily stopping eating and drinking: a practical approach for long-term care facilities. J Palliat Med 2018;21:1214–20.

23. Pope TM, West A. Legal briefing: voluntarily stopping eating and drinking. J Clin Ethics 2014;25:68–80.

24. Jansen LA, Sulmasy DP. Sedation, alimentation, hydration, and equivocation: careful conversation about care at the end of life. Ann Intern Med 2002;136:845–9.

25. Quill TE, Ganzini L, Truog RD, et al. Voluntarily stopping eating and drinking among patients with serious advanced illness—clinical, ethical, and legal aspects. JAMA Intern Med 2018;178:123–7.

26. Harvath TA, Miller LL, Smith KA, et al. Dilemmas encountered by hospice workers when patients wish to hasten death. J Hosp Palliat Nurs 2006;8:200–9.

27. Harvath TA, Miller LL, Goy E, et al. Voluntary refusal of food and fluids: attitudes of Oregon hospice nurses and social workers. Int J Palliat Nurs 2004;10:236–41.

28. American Nurses Association Center for Ethics and Human Rights. Position statement: nutrition and hydration at the end of life. 2017. Available at: https://www.nursingworld.org/~4af0ed/globalassets/docs/ana/ethics/ps_nutrition-and-hydration-at-the-end-of-life_2017june7.pdf. Accessed August 4, 2019.

29. Radbruch L, De Lima L. International Association for Hospice and Palliative Care response regarding voluntary cessation of food and water. J Palliat Med 2017;20:578–9.

30. American Academy of Hospice and Palliative Medicine advisory brief: guidance on responding to requests for physician assisted dying. Available at: http://aahpm.org/positions/padbrief. Accessed August 4, 2019.

31. Menzel PT, Chandler-Cramer MC. Advance directives, dementia, and withholding food and water by mouth. Hastings Cent Rep 2014;44:23–37.

32. Volicer L, Stets K. Acceptability of an advance directive that limits food and liquids in advanced dementia. Am J Hosp Palliat Care 2014;33:55–63.

33. End of Life Washington. My instructions for oral feeding and drinking. Available at: https://endoflifewa.org/wp-content/uploads/2017/10/Instructions-for-oral-food-and-water-FINAL-10-2-17.pdf. Accessed August 4, 2019.

34. Ganzini L, Goy ER, Miller LL, et al. Nurses' experiences with hospice patients who refuse food and fluids to hasten death. N Engl J Med 2003;349:359–65.

35. Bolt EE, Hagens M, Willems D, et al. Primary care patients hastening death by voluntarily stopping eating and drinking. Ann Fam Med 2015;13:421–8.

36. Chabot BE, Goedhart A. A survey of self-directed dying attended by proxies in the Dutch population. Soc Sci Med 2009;68:1745–51.

37. Onwuteaka-Philipsen BD, Brinkman-Stoppelenburg A, Penning C, et al. Trends in end-of-life practices before and after the enactment of the euthanasia law in the Netherlands from 1990 to 2010. Lancet 2012;380:908–15.

38. Berry ZS. Responding to suffering: providing options and respecting choice. J Pain Symptom Manage 2009;38:797–800.

39. Byock I. Patient refusal of nutrition and hydration: walking the ever-finer line. Am J Hosp Palliat Care 1995;12(8):9–13.

40. Wax JW, An AW, Kosier N, et al. Voluntary stopping eating and drinking. J Am Geriatr Soc 2018;66:441–5.

41. KNMG Royal Dutch Medical Association and V&VN Dutch Nurses' Association. Caring for people who consciously choose not to eat and drink so as to hasten

the end of life. Available at: https://www.knmg.nl/web/file?uuid=1519ee45-2447-46a2-9cda-ec59d441f8a8&owner=5c945405-d6ca-4deb-aa16-7af2088aa173&contentid=3658. Accessed August 10, 2019.

42. DeLima L, Woodruff R, Pettus K, et al. International Association for Hospice and Palliative Care position statement: euthanasia and physician-assisted suicide. J Palliat Med 2017;20:8–14.

43. Quill T, Cassel C. Professional organizations' position statements on physician-assisted suicide: a case for studied neutrality. Ann Intern Med 2003;138(3):208–11.

44. Sulmasy DP, Finlay I, Fitzgerald F, et al. Physician-assisted suicide: why neutrality by organized medicine is neither neutral nor appropriate. J Gen Intern Med 2018;33(8):1394–9.

45. Tolle S, Tilden V, Drach L, et al. Characteristics and proportion of dying Oregonians who personally consider physician-assisted suicide. J Clin Ethics 2004;15(2):111–22.

46. Oregon Health Authority. Death with dignity act annual reports. Available at: https://www.oregon.gov/oha/PH/PROVIDERPARTNERRESOURCES/EVALUATIONRESEARCH/DEATHWITHDIGNITYACT/Pages/ar-index.aspx. Accessed August 11, 2019.

47. Washington State Department of Health. Death with dignity act annual reports. Available at: https://www.doh.wa.gov/YouandYourFamily/IllnessandDisease/DeathwithDignityAct/DeathwithDignityData. Accessed August 11, 2019.

48. Orentlicher D, Pope TM, Rich BA. Clinical criteria for physician aid in dying. J Palliat Med 2016;19(3):259–62.

Burnout and Self Care for Palliative Care Practitioners

David J. Horn, MD[a,b], Catherine Bree Johnston, MD, MPH[b,c],*

KEYWORDS

- Burnout • Palliative medicine • Self-care • Mindfulness • Exercise • Sleep
- Compassion • Empathy

KEY POINTS

- Burnout is common among physicians and other practitioners caring for patients with serious illness.
- Consequences of burnout include depression, substance use, suicide, leaving the profession, and poorer patient care.
- Risk factors for burnout include working on smaller teams, working longer hours, high workload, burdensome documentation, and regulatory issues.
- Mindfulness, exercise, sleep, and adequate time off can help buffer against burnout.
- Institutional and team factors can promote or protect against burnout.

INTRODUCTION

Caring for patients with serious illness involves frequent, intense interactions with patients and their families. Emotions run high as patients and families work through intense physical suffering, grief, existential distress, and all the other challenging experiences that may occur at the end life. It is the role of the physician to help guide people through this variable and complex psycho-socio-medico-spiritual context, which is a powerful and self-affirming exercise. However, the personal burden of this work is great. The emotional and physical toll can pile up over years and decades of practice. This accumulation of stress can gradually erode one's well-being and lead to feelings of depression, dissatisfaction, and depersonalization. This process is called burnout, and the purpose of this article is to define burnout and its associated terms; address the scope of the problem in medicine; discuss

[a] Department of Emergency Medicine, University of Arizona, Tucson, AZ, USA; [b] Division of Geriatrics, General Internal Medicine and Palliative Medicine, University of Arizona College of Medicine, PO Box 245036, 1501 North Campbell Avenue, Tucson, AZ 85724-5036, USA; [c] Department of Medicine, University of Arizona, Tucson, AZ, USA
* Corresponding author. Division of Geriatrics, General Internal Medicine and Palliative Medicine, University of Arizona College of Medicine, PO Box 245036, 1501 North Campbell Avenue, Tucson, AZ 85724-5036.
E-mail address: Bree.johnston@bannerhealth.com

Med Clin N Am 104 (2020) 561–572
https://doi.org/10.1016/j.mcna.2019.12.007
0025-7125/20/© 2020 Elsevier Inc. All rights reserved.

personal consequences of burnout; identify tools for burnout prevention and mitigation; and recognize team, institutional, and health system factors that can promote or protect against burnout.

RELEVANT DEFINITIONS

This section offers working definitions of the important terms used later in this article. This facilitates a larger discussion of these terms in the practice of physicians caring for patients with serious illness (which we shorten to provider for simplicity).

Burnout

A definition of burnout is central to further discussion in this article. The World Health Organization now includes the following definition of burnout in its International Classification of Diseases-11 document: "Burnout is a syndrome conceptualized as resulting from chronic workplace stress that has not been successfully managed. It is characterized by three dimensions: (1) feelings of energy depletion or exhaustion, (2) increased mental distance from one's job, or feelings of negativism or cynicism related to one's job, and (3) reduced professional efficacy. Burnout refers specifically to phenomena in the occupational context and should not be applied to describe experiences in other areas of life."[1]

The most commonly used tool for assessment of burnout is the Maslach Burnout Inventory.[2] The Maslach Burnout Inventory was first published in 1981, and it has now been revised multiple times. It assesses three domains of symptoms: (1) emotional exhaustion, (2) depersonalization, and (3) personal accomplishment.

Burnout is often accompanied by a loss of existential meaning in one's work.[3] Burnout has also been extensively discussed in the psychology literature as a specific syndrome with distinct phases. These phases include an insidious process by which well-intentioned individuals gradually succumb to a high-stress work environment that offers poor feedback and little reward. This sows discontent, leading to a pathologic coping response, which often manifests as cynicism. This response gradually evolves into the burnout syndrome and, if not intervened on, can result in severe personal and interpersonal dysfunction, such as substance abuse, depression, and suicide.[4]

Resilience

Resilience is the capacity of an individual to recover after exposure to stressful circumstances or events. The American Psychological Association believes that resilience is a learned behavior, which is strengthened through an individual's dedicated effort.[5] **Box 1** lists factors contributing to high resilience.

Mindfulness

Mindfulness is the act of existing in the present moment. It is a term originating from religious contemplative practice, and it draws from thousands of years of Buddhist scholarly work.[6] Buddhist teachings have now been adapted into a secular practice and applied to various personal and workplace contexts. Secular mindfulness teachings instruct individuals to release concerns for the past and future, instead isolating their attention on the present moment. This allows health care practitioners, specifically, to more fully engage with their patients during clinical encounters. Evidence for mindfulness in the prevention and treatment of burnout is discussed further later in this article.

> **Box 1**
> **American Psychological Association core factors contributing to high resilience**
>
> - Ability to develop realistic plans
> - A positive self-image
> - Well-developed capacity for problem solving
> - Strong communication skills
> - Maintenance of supporting relationships inside and outside one's family
> - Ability to manage strong emotions
> - Control of impulsive thoughts and desires
>
> *From* Maslach C, Schaufeli WB, Leiter MP. Job Burnout. Annu Rev Psychol 2001;52:397-422; with permission.

Sympathy

Within health care, sympathy is defined as an emotional reaction of a caregiver to the suffering of another individual. Sympathy acknowledges a patient's suffering without seeking to understand it or emotionally attune to the patient's suffering. In general, sympathetic statements involve pitying language that inherently identifies a patient's distressing circumstance as outside the realm of the caregiver's experience.

Empathy

Empathy is a response to another's suffering in which the caregiver acknowledges the suffering and experiences a visceral, affective response. Empathy is divided into cognitive empathy, which includes acknowledgment of suffering and an effort to objectively understand suffering, and affective empathy, which involves the evocation of a patient-centered emotional response within a caregiver. Empathy is a process by which caregivers can attune to the patient's experience of suffering, thus gaining enhanced understanding of the patient.

Compassion

Compassion occurs when caregivers are empathetic, while also demonstrating a sincere desire to reduce the patient's suffering. Compassion combines an understanding of suffering (either one's own or another's) with the intention for enhanced wellness.[7] Compassion arises from altruism, allowing insight that occurs during emotional engagement to be transformed into effective action. Given that loss of meaning is a hallmark consequence of burnout, one can see immediately that the ability to work compassionately is a central pillar of prevention and amelioration of burnout (discussed later in this article).

The terms sympathy, empathy, and compassion are often used interchangeably, and therefore incorrectly, in medicine. The relationship between these three concepts is depicted in **Fig. 1**. In fact, the isolation of these different modes of interactions allows providers deeper understanding of their relationships with patients. This is especially important for providers who care for the seriously ill, given the high intensity of the clinical encounters, which often have life and death consequences for patients. In the book *Standing at the Edge: Finding Freedom Where Fear and Courage Meet*, Joan Halifax[8] discusses five "edge states," related to an individual's personal demonstration of altruism, empathy, integrity, respect, and engagement.

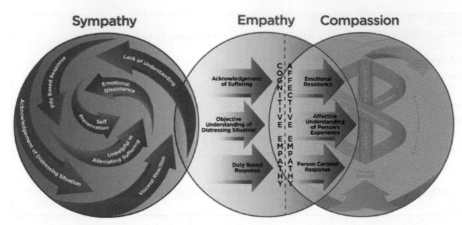

Fig. 1. The interplay among sympathy, empathy, and compassion. (*From* Sinclair S, Beamer K, Hack TF, et al. Sympathy, empathy, and compassion: A grounded theory study of palliative care patients' understandings, experiences, and preferences. Palliat Med 2017;31(5):441; with permission.)

These five qualities each facilitate meaningful and therapeutic connections with patients. However, each quality can also be taken too far, resulting in negative consequences. In the book, these are described as pathologic altruism, empathic distress, moral suffering, disrespect, and burnout, respectively. This is just one example of a mental construct that can be learned and applied to medical practice to better understand one's role in patient care. Overall, it is through the combination of reflective practice and the accurate, definitive use of language that inner life is delineated. With clear purpose and insight, one can increase resilience and become less susceptible to negative forces in the health care environment that might otherwise lead to burnout.[8]

MAGNITUDE OF THE PROBLEM IN THE HEALTH CARE SYSTEM

Physician, nurse, and other health care provider burnout is common, morbid, expensive, and increasingly recognized as a serious health care challenge. To highlight the magnitude of the problem, some experts now refer to the triple aim as the quadruple aim, adding the goal of improving the work-life of health care providers to the original aims of enhancing patient experience, improving population health, and reducing costs as the guideposts to optimize health system performance.[9] The prevalence of burnout varies between studies, in part because of differences in diagnosis and measurement, but rates near or exceeding 50% are reported in many studies.[10,11] A 2019 study estimated that approximately $4.6 billion in costs related to physician turnover and reduced clinical hours are attributable to burnout each year in the United States. At an organizational level, the annual economic cost associated with burnout related to turnover and reduced clinical hours is approximately $7600 per employed physician each year.[12]

Several risk factors for burnout have been identified, including poor control over workload, inefficient teamwork, insufficient documentation time, having a hectic-chaotic work atmosphere, lack of value-alignment with leadership, and excessive electronic medical record time at home. Younger, female physicians seem to be at particularly high risk.[10]

For providers, the most serious personal consequences of burnout include depression, suicidal ideation, family strain and divorce, substance abuse, motor vehicle crashes, and other dysfunctional behaviors.[10] According to a 2004 study, female physicians have a suicide rate 130% higher than the general population; for male physicians it is 40% higher.[13]

Burnout has an impact on patients and patient care.[14,15] Patients of practitioners who are experiencing burnout may feel a lack of compassion and human connection with their provider, which can lead to worse adherence and poor outcomes. Physicians who report higher levels of burnout have lower patient satisfaction scores, are more likely to be named in a malpractice suit, and perceive that they provide lower quality patient care and commit more medical errors.[16,17]

BURNOUT AMONG PROVIDERS CARING FOR PATIENTS WITH SERIOUS ILLNESS

Many factors contribute to burnout among providers who care for the seriously ill. Seriously ill patients are often frail; elderly; vulnerable; complex; and dealing with loss, grief, and intense emotions. Distress and conflict among seriously ill patients and their families is common, and providers sometimes become targets for the frustrations of families dealing with serious illness and a system that often does a poor job of supporting them. Many providers feel distressed when they cannot establish meaningful relationships with patients and their families or fully control symptoms of pain or existential despair. Providers often do not feel adequately trained to have conversations about prognosis, goals of care, grief, loss, or suffering or to manage refractory symptoms. Conflict may exist between different consulting teams with different ideas about prognosis or plans of care. Providers may feel the frustration of working in a system in which they care for patients who are uninsured, homeless, or lacking in resources and coverage for caregivers. Not all providers find meaning in the work of caring for patients with serious illness; some may see death as "failure" and think that there is "nothing they can do" if a patient cannot be cured. This lack of meaning may be a particular risk factor for burnout.

A 2016 study of burnout among hospice and palliative care clinicians in the United States reported an overall burnout rate of 62%, significantly higher than the average reported clinician burnout rates.[18] Nonphysician palliative care and hospice clinicians and home-based palliative care clinicians have particularly high burnout rates, which might be partly related to isolation. Other factors associated with burnout in hospice and palliative care include working in smaller organizations, working longer hours, being younger than 50 years, and working weekends. Other sources of burnout include increasing workload, tensions between nonspecialists and palliative care specialists, and regulatory issues.[18,19] Although not all providers who care for the seriously ill experience all the same set of stressors that hospice and palliative medicine practitioners do, there is likely to be some overlap.

PREVENTION AND MANAGEMENT OF BURNOUT

Burnout is a multifactorial process. It involves a complex interplay of individual characteristics with environmental effects. **Fig. 2**, based in part by a construct by Cotton and Hart,[20] demonstrates this schematically.

MINDFULNESS

In brief, mindfulness is the act of focusing on the present moment. This simple concept, when applied, can yield profound effects. Mindfulness can be practiced

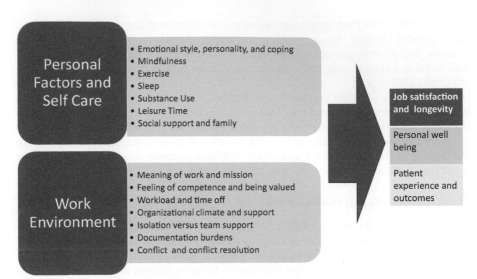

Fig. 2. Schematic demonstration of burnout as a multifactorial process. (*Adapted from* Cotton P, Hart PM. Occupational wellbeing and performance: A review of organizational health research. Australian Psychologist 2003;38(2):118–127; with permission.)

anywhere and at any time. It can be performed before, during, and after patient care. There is a growing body of evidence that suggests mindfulness practice can improve burnout in health care professionals. **Table 1** details a selection of individual studies and their relevant outcomes. A systematic review from 2016 that includes eight studies concludes that there is strong evidence that mindfulness reduces burnout in health care professionals and teachers.[21]

Many of these studies use a program called mindfulness-based stress reduction (MBSR). This program was developed by John Kabat-Zinn, who founded the MBSR clinic in 1979 at the University of Massachusetts Medical Center. MBSR is coordinated by trained facilitators. It occurs over 8 weeks, including weekly, 2-hour meetings and a single, 7-hour retreat. MBSR focuses on teaching a combination of yoga, meditation, and body awareness techniques. This approach has been subsequently modified by multiple groups to fit the parameters of different studies and populations. The Center for Mindfulness in Medicine, Health Care, and Society at UMass Medical School outlines this program in further detail, which can be explored on their Web site (https://www.umassmed.edu/cfm).

On an individual basis, there are many ways to begin learning and practicing mindfulness. There are innumerable books on the topic. Two introductions to the topic include *Wherever You Go, There You Are: Mindfulness Meditation in Everyday Life* by Jon Kabat-Zinn[22] and *The Miracle of Mindfulness: An Introduction to the Practice of Meditation* by Thich Nhat Hanh.[23] There are also multiple smart phone applications that offer guided meditation audio and video resources. Two notable applications include Insight Timer (www.insighttimer.com) and Headspace (www.headspace.com). These applications offer resources for first-time meditators and experienced mindfulness practitioners.

EXERCISE

There is a broad evidence base regarding the benefit of exercise in managing stress and maintaining good mental health. The Department of Health and Human Services

Table 1
Evidence for mindfulness in burnout reduction

Reference	Subjects	Intervention	Outcome
Happier Healers: randomized controlled trial of mobile mindfulness for stress management[2]	88 medical students	Randomized to control or cell phone–based mindfulness application	Improvement in well-being and reduction in perceived stress
A mindfulness course decreases burnout and improves well-being among healthcare providers[3]	93 health care providers from multiple disciplines	Continuing education course based on mindfulness-based stress reduction that met 2.5 h a week for 8 wk plus a 7-h retreat	Improvement in emotional exhaustion, depersonalization, and personal accomplishment per Maslach Burnout Inventory tool Improvement in mental well-being as measured by the SF12v2 tool
Mindfulness training for stress management: a randomized controlled study of medical and psychology students[4]	288 medical and psychology students	6 weekly sessions of 1.5 h each, a 6-h session in Week 7, and 30 min of daily home mindfulness practice based on a mindfulness-based stress reduction program	Significant improvements in mental distress, perceived stress, and subjective well-being
The effects of mindfulness-based stress reduction on nurse stress and burnout: a qualitative and quantitative study, part II[5]	27 individuals, including nurses, pastoral care, respiratory therapy, and social workers	8-wk-long intervention modeled after mindfulness-based stress reduction curricula	Improved in emotional exhaustion and personal achievement, as measured by the Maslach Burnout Inventory Improvement in emotional exhaustion at 3-mo follow-up

recommends that adults do at least 150 minutes of moderate-intensity exercise or 75 minutes of vigorous-intensity aerobic exercise per week. They recommend that this occur in episodes greater than 10 minutes and be spread throughout the week. They advise that some activity is far better than no activity.[24]

Studies have directly addressed the role of exercise in the management of burnout. Weight and colleagues[25] conducted an incentivized, team-based exercise program for residents and fellows. They found a statistically significant improvement in quality of life in the group that participated in the exercise program compared with residents and fellows who did not participate. Another study of medical students at the University of Pittsburgh School of Medicine found an association between lower exercise and lower professional efficacy.[26]

Psychiatric studies have also evaluated the role of exercise in generally improving mental health. A Cochrane systematic review published in 2013 included 39 trials with 2326 participants. They concluded that exercise was moderately more effective than controls in treating the symptoms of depression.[27] Another systematic review evaluated 12 randomized controlled trials examining the effect of exercise on anxiety. Although most studies included in the meta-analysis were methodologically limited, they suggest that exercise is more effective than placebo in reducing anxiety.[28] Overall, the link between physical activity and personal wellness is clear. Healthy exercise habits are a strong step toward resilience.

SLEEP

Maintaining high-quality sleep promotes resilience. In one study, individuals with high burnout had significantly greater sleep latency, greater daytime dysfunction, poorer sleep quality, and poorer sleep duration. Overall, this study found that high burnout predicted poor sleep.[29] No data examine the effect of sleep interventions to improve burnout; however, sleep and burnout seem to be intimately related, and the implementation of sleep hygiene techniques can only be beneficial in preventing burnout. Basic sleep hygiene tips are detailed in **Box 2**.

SUBSTANCE USE

Substance abuse is a significant public health problem with many deleterious mental and physical health effects. In one study, completed surveys from 7288 physicians regarding substance use found that 12.9% of male physicians and 21.4% of female physicians had use patterns consistent with the Diagnostic and Statistical Manual-IV definitions of alcohol abuse or dependence.[30] The use of other illicit substances was rare in this study, with 1.3% of physicians reporting opioid abuse and 2.7% reporting cannabis use. This study also found that individuals with alcohol abuse and dependence were much more likely to have burnout, depression, suicidal ideation, and lower quality of life. It is unclear whether substance use and abuse lead to distress or arise as a consequence of distress. However, it is clear that substance abuse suggests underlying pathology, and is likely to worsen or prolong distress. It is therefore recommended that clinicians with emerging or established substance abuse seek treatment of mental health problems, substance dependence, or both.[31]

Box 2
Tips for improved sleep hygiene

- Caffeine use close to bedtime disrupts sleep
- Nicotine use acutely and chronically disrupts sleep
- Alcohol may reduce sleep-onset latency, but it leads to sleep disturbance later in the night
- Regular exercise improves sleep
- Regular bedtime and waketime promotes improved sleep
- Bedroom noise reduction improves sleep by eliminating nighttime arousals
- Bedtime use of media devices (ie, smart phones, television) reduces sleep quality[12,13]

THE PURSUIT OF HAPPINESS

The sacrifice of personal life for work achievement occurs early in medical training. For trainees, incredible time and effort are necessarily devoted to the development of technical excellence. This often involves neglecting relationships and avocations. Once training ends, the subjugation of ineffable pursuits to medical practice has become habitual, and many physicians find themselves in a position of social isolation, where life has become a series of tasks designed to promote productivity. This type of behavior, sometimes described as a personal philosophy of "total work," is fertile ground for burnout and dissatisfaction.[30]

The solution to "total work" is the pursuit of activities that enhance meaning. What these include is highly individualized. Recreation may include spiritual pursuits, reading for pleasure, spending time with family, or any other venture that engages contemplation for its own ends. Moreover, work distractions during these ventures negate the experience. Setting clear boundaries between work and personal life is essential, which often includes eliminating work email, projects, or telephone calls during recreation. The importance of dedicated play cannot be overstated.

TEAM, INSTITUTIONAL, AND HEALTH CARE SYSTEM FACTORS CONTRIBUTING TO BURNOUT

Several team and institutional practices may be protective against burnout. The following discussion is based on interviews with dozens of palliative care practitioners and experts in the field in addition to published evidence.

According to one study, physicians who work in team-based settings where they feel better able to meet patient needs are less likely to report burnout. In that study, working with a social worker or pharmacist was protective against symptoms of burnout.[32] Other evidence supports that physician isolation contributes to burnout.[10] It is reasonable to assume that isolation is particularly difficult for physicians who care for patients with serious illness. There is a reason why palliative care and hospice are provided by teams; providers in isolation are lacking the important team "buffer" effect that hospice and palliative physicians rely on for support.

Approaches to the challenges of isolation are not always easy but may include creating virtual teams with other closely collaborating services, forming support groups (eg, several physicians who share similar practices coming together regularly to provide support). For providers who work in isolation or on small teams, it is particularly important to try to set clear limits about working nights, weekends, and taking clear time off with no work interruptions.

Highly emotional patient and family meetings can often be a source of stress, particularly if a practitioner experiences conflict personally or as a personal failing. Developing competence in conducting these difficult discussions empathically and competently can help providers feel less stress and find enhanced meaning. Such programs as VitalTalk (www.vitaltalk.org), the Serious Illness Communication Program through Ariadne Labs (https://www.ariadnelabs.org/areas-of-work/serious-illness-care/), is invaluable in improving communication and competence. The authors have found that family meetings conducted by two people (eg, physician and social worker or case manager) are often less stressful and can provide an opportunity to debrief, learn from one another, and reframe conflict so that it is less likely to be taken personally.

There is a growing sense within the medical community that the electronic health record (EHR) is driving professional dissatisfaction and burnout, some of which may be related to the burdensome documentation requirements to maximize reimbursement.[32,33] Many EHRs are cumbersome and add unnecessary time and complexity to the clinician's workload. In many instances, using time-based billing codes and using advance care planning codes can make documentation less burdensome for providers caring for patients with serious illness. All physicians need to advocate at the institutional and national level for EHRs that support quality patient care and making clinician's lives easier, not more difficult.

The hard work of caring for patients with serious illness and their families, including conducting lengthy meetings and goals of care discussions, tends to be incompletely captured by relative value units. Physicians who work in purely incentive- or performance-based income models report higher burnout rates than those in salaried positions,[34,35] and thus providers are likely to be particularly stressed in those settings. Moving away from fee-for-service and toward value-based organizations with salaried physicians is likely to make caring for patients with serious illness less burdensome.

Probably, the most important element to protect providers is finding deep meaning in caring for patients with serious illness[36] and feeling valued by colleagues and institutions for their role in the health care system. When physicians see the work of alleviating the suffering associated with serious illness and the dying process as important, meaningful, and valuable, they will feel the satisfaction that helps them remain resilient throughout a long career.

SUMMARY

Burnout is a growing problem in medicine and seems to be especially common in physicians who care for patients with serious illness. Solving this problem requires approaches at the individual, team, institutional, and policy levels. Providers who care for patients with serious illness need to find meaning in their work and practice self-care if they are to remain vibrant, present, and resilient through a full career.

DISCLOSURE

The authors have nothing to disclose.

REFERENCES

1. World Health Organization, W. ICD-11 for mortality and morbidity statistics 2018. Available at: https://icd.who.int/browse11/l-m/en. Accessed June 19, 2019.
2. Maslach C, Jackson C. The measurement of experienced burnout. J Organ Behav 1981;2:99–113.
3. Riethof N, Bob P. Burnout syndrome and logotherapy: logotherapy as useful conceptual framework for explanation and prevention of burnout. Front Psychiatry 2019;10:1–8.
4. Maslach C, Schaufeli WB, Leiter MP. Job burnout. Annu Rev Psychol 2001;52: 397–422.
5. American Psychological Association. The road to resilience. The road to resilience 2011. Available at: https://www.apa.org/helpcenter/road-resilience. Accessed July 26, 2019.
6. Rapgay L, Bystrisky A. Classical mindfulness: an introduction to its theory and practice for clinical application. Ann N Y Acad Sci 2009;1172:148–62.
7. Sinclair S, Beamer K, Hack TF, et al. Sympathy, empathy, and compassion: a grounded theory study of palliative care patients' understandings, experiences, and preferences. Palliat Med 2017;31:437–44.

8. Halifax J. Standing at the edge: finding freedom where fear and courage meet. New York: Flatiron Books; 2018.

9. Bodenheimer T, Sinsky C. From triple to quadruple aim: care of the patient requires care of the provider. Ann Fam Med 2014;12:573–6.

10. West CP, Dyrbye LN, Shanafelt TD. Physician burnout: contributors, consequences and solutions. J Intern Med 2018;283:516–29.

11. Shanafelt TD, Hasan O, Dyrbrye LN, et al. Changes in burnout and satisfaction with work-life balance in physicians and the general US working population between 2011 and 2014. Mayo Clin Proc 2015;90:1600–13.

12. Han S, Shanafelt TD, Sinsky CA, Awad KM, Dyrbye LN, Fiscus LC, Trockel M, Goh J. Estimating the attributable cost of physician burnout in the United States. Ann Intern Med 2019;170(11):784–90.

13. Schernhammer ES, Colditz GA. Suicide rates among physicians: a quantitative and gender assessment (meta-analysis). Am J Psychiatry 2004;161:2295–302.

14. Salyers MP, Bonfills KA, Luther L, et al. The relationship between professional burnout and quality and safety in healthcare: a meta-analysis. J Gen Intern Med 2017;32:475–82.

15. Dewa CS, Loong D, Bonato S, et al. The relationship between physician burnout and quality of healthcare in terms of safety and acceptability: a systematic review. BMJ Open 2017;7:e015141.

16. Rathert C, Williams ES, Linhart H. Evidence for the Quadruple aim: a systematic review of the literature on physician burnout and patient outcomes. Med Care 2018;56:976–84.

17. Shanafelt TD, West BP, Sloan JA. Career fit and burnout among academic faculty. Arch Intern Med 2009;169:990–5.

18. Kamal AH, Bull JH, Wolf SP, et al. Prevalence and predictors of burnout among hospice and palliative care clinicians in the US. J Pain Symptom Manage 2016; 51:690–6.

19. Kavalieratos D, Siconolfi DE, Steinhauser KE, Bull J, Arnold RM, Swetz KM, Kamal AH. "It is like heart failure. it is chronic … and it will kill you": a qualitative analysis of burnout among hospice and palliative care clinicians. J Pain Symptom Manage 2017;53:901–10, 18.

20. Cotton P, Hart PM. Occupational wellbeing and performance: a review of organizational health research. Aust Psychol 2003;38:118–27.

21. Luken M, Sammons A. Systematic review of mindfulness practice for reducing job burnout. Am J Occup Ther 2016;70:1–10.

22. Kabat-Zinn J. Wherever You Go ,There You Are: Mindfulness Meditation in Every-Day Life. 10th edition. New York: Hyperion; 1994. https://doi.org/10.1016/j.bbamcr.2005.12.011.

23. Hanh TN, Ho M, Vo-Dinh M. The Miracle of Mindfulness: An Introduction to the Practice of Meditation. 1st edition. Boston: Beacon Press; 1996.

24. Olson RD, Piercy KL, Troiano RP, et al, editors. Physical activity guidelines for Americans. 2nd edition. U.S Department of Health and Human Services; 2018. Available at: health.gov/paguidelines/second-edition/pdf/Physical_Activity_Guidelines_2nd_Edition.pdf. Accessed January 29, 2020.

25. Weight CJ, Sellon JL, Lessard-Anderson CR, et al. Physical activity, quality of life, and burnout among physician trainees: the effect of a team-based, incentivized exercise program. Mayo Clin Proc 2013;88:1435–42.

26. Wolf MR, Rosenstock JB. Inadequate sleep and exercise associated with burnout and depression among medical students. Acad Psychiatry 2017;41:174–9.

27. Cooney GM, Dwan K, Greig C, et al. Exercise for depression. Cochrane Database Syst Rev 2013;(9). CDOO4366.
28. Stonerock GL, Hoffman BM, Smith PJ, et al. Exercise as treatment for anxiety: systematic review and analysis. Ann Behav Med 2015;49:542–6.
29. Vela-Bueno A, Moreno-Jiménez B, Rodríguez-Muñoz A, et al. Insomnia and sleep quality among primary care physicians with low and high burnout levels. J Psychosom Res 2008;64:435–42.
30. Oreskovich MR, Shanafelt T, Dyrbye LN, et al. The prevalence of substance use disorders in American physicians. Am J Addict 2015;24:30–8.
31. Taggart A. If work dominated your every moment would life be worth living? 2017. Aeon website: Available at: https://aeon.co/ideas/if-work-dominated-your-every-moment-would-life-be-worth-living. Accessed August 13, 2019.
32. DeMarchis E, Knox M, Hessler D, et al. Physician burnout and higher clinic capacity to address patients' social needs. J Am Board Fam Med 2019;32:69–78.
33. Downing NL, Bates DW, Longhurst CA. Physician burnout in the electronic health record era: are we ignoring the real cause? Ann Intern Med 2018;169:50–1.
34. Tai-Seale M, Olson CW, Li J, et al. Electronic health record logs indicate that physicians split time evenly between seeing patients and desktop medicine. Health Aff (Millwood) 2017;36:655–62.
35. Shanafelt TD, Balch CM, Bechamps GJ, et al. Burnout and career satisfaction among American surgeons. Ann Surg 2009;250:463–71.
36. Shanafelt TD, Gradisher WJ, Kosty M, et al. Burnout and career satisfaction among US oncologists. J Clin Oncol 2014;32:678–86.

Printed and bound by CPI Group (UK) Ltd, Croydon, CR0 4YY

03/10/2024

01040480-0004